Prescribing Colonization

The Role of Medical Practices and Policies in Japan-Ruled Taiwan, 1895-1945

Prescribing Colonization

The Role of Medical Practices and Policies in Japan-Ruled Taiwan, 1895-1945

Michael Shiyung Liu

Asia Past & Present

Published by the Association for Asian Studies, Inc.

Asia Past & Present: New Research from AAS, Number 3

Asia Past & Present: New Research from AAS
A series edited by Martha Ann Selby, University of Texas at Austin

"Asia Past & Present: New Research from AAS," published by the Association for Asian Studies, Inc. (AAS), features scholarly work from all areas of Asian studies. In addition to scholarly monographs, translations, essay collections, and other forms of scholarly research are welcome for consideration. AAS particularly hopes to support work in emerging or under-represented fields.

Formed in 1941, the Association for Asian Studies (AAS)—the largest society of its kind, with more than 7,000 members worldwide—is a scholarly, non-political, non-profit professional association open to all persons interested in Asia.

For further information, please visit www.asian-studies.org.

Published by:
Association for Asian Studies, Inc.
1021 East Huron Street
Ann Arbor, Michigan 48104 USA
www.asian-studies.org

Printed in the United States of America on acid-free, archival quality paper.

Library of Congress Cataloging-in-Publication Data

Liu, Michael Shiyung, 1964–
Prescribing colonization : the role of medical practices and policies in Japan-ruled Taiwan, 1895–1945 / Michael Shiyung Liu.
p. cm. — (Asia past & present : new research from AAS ; no. 3)
Includes bibliographical references and index.
ISBN 978-0-924304-57-6 (pbk. : alk. paper) 1. Medicine—Taiwan—History—1895–1945. 2. Medicine—Japan—Colonies. 3. Taiwan—Politics and government—1895–1945. I. Title.
R644.T28L58 2009
362.1095124'90904—dc22
2009035475

Front Cover: (i) photo—Taiwanese carriers and a *keisatsu i* (police physician) in the white robe moving a body infected with plague. Courtesy of Chung Chin-shui; (ii) image of books—Igaku Chuo Zasshi, abstracts, journal of Japanese medicine and related fields, 1940's, Lane Medical Library, Stanford University, Palo Alto, California. Courtesy of Peter Kaminski.

Contents

Illustrations

Charts

Figures

Maps

Acknowledgments

Writing a history of colonial medicine is a risky undertaking. If it is written by a medical scientist, there may be too little history. Conversely, if it is written by an historian there is the danger that it may include too little sense of biotechnology. To prepare for the challenge, I have fortunately received professional help and went through training in economics, the history of medicine, and modern public health. Also the colonial aspect of medicine in Japanese-ruled Taiwan is a daunting subject. The dilemma between the brutality of imperialism and the mercy of modernization has haunted Taiwanese scholarship since the beginning of postwar era. Aware of both challenges, I decided early on that I would pursue my research by incorporating information from various disciplines.

I never imagined that I could write a book without help and guidance. The idea for this book began in 1996 at University of Pittsburgh in discussions about Japanese colonization first with Professor Evelyn Rawski of the History Department and later with Professor Thomas Rawski of Economics Department. Those discussions drew my attention to the nature of Japanese colonial medicine in Taiwan. The impetus to study Japanese colonization and medical services came not just from the topic's intrinsic interest but also from the Rawskis' detailed knowledge, critical judgment, and humorous compassion. A second impetus was a suggestion by Professor Iijima Wataru of Aoyama Gakuin University (Japan) and Dr. Robert Perrins of Acadia University (Canada) in 2003 that I should study medical modernization in Japan and its colonies, including Taiwan, a suggestion that has borne much fruit and continues even today to test my resourcefulness. Professor Kohei Wakimura of Osaka City University provided inspiration and knowledge along with bountiful moral support.

I am grateful to the National Science Council and Academia Sinica in Taiwan for financial assistance without which I could not have undertaken the travel necessary to visit scholars and search libraries and archives around the world. My task was made easier by the unfailing and courteous help of librarians and archivists in Taiwan, Japan, the United States, and the Wellcome Library in the United Kingdom. A significant portion of the early research for the book was conducted with the support of a Yoneyama Scholarship in 2003–04, through which I was extended the hospitality of Yokohama National University. Finally, grants from the Chiang Ching-kuo

Foundation (2005–07) and the Visiting Scholar Program of the Harvard-Yenching Institute (2006–07) allowed me to complete my archival research and finish preparing the manuscript.

A number of friends and colleagues have contributed substantially to this book. Professor Liu Ts'ui-jung has been a mentor to me, providing inspiration from the beginning; I express my sincere appreciation to her. Professors David Arnold and David Killingray have given generously of their knowledge of colonial medicine in British colonies, and I have profited immeasurably from it. Angela K.C. Leung has broadly inspired me and generiously offerred her support. From Dr. Stephan Morgan I have learned about anthropometric analysis and debates regarding Taiwan's colonial economy. I also owe a great deal to Fu Dawei, Charles Rosenberg, Li Shangren, Fan Yanqiu, Lei Xianglin, Wang Wenji, Wu Jialing, Bai Yubin, Chang Lung-chih (Zhang Longzhi), Peng Shuangjun, Zhang Kunjiang, Wu Yanqiu, Zhang Shuqing, Kuo Jinlin, Serizawa Ryoko, Joseph Wicentowski, and Judd Kinzley. I am grateful for their friendship and encouragement. For editing the text, Sara Jenkins' efforts are appreciated.

Finally, I remain in great debt to Grace (Yih-wen) Jwo, my wife, for her unbelievable support and understanding throughout this entire project. I would like to express my most sincere gratitude to her for caring for our children, Ariel (Szu-tung) and Brian (Chaowei), and for her constancy in cheering me up in times of difficulty.

Introduction

Taiwan's history with its powerful neighbors and foreign occupiers dates back to the seventh-century Sui dynasty in China. For many generations the Chinese rulers did not bring the island under direct control but left it under the dominion of aboriginals and open to refugees from China. Political outlaws from Japan also found shelter there, and Japanese pirates used it as a temporary base of operations. In the early part of the seventeenth century, the Dutch and the Spanish occupied Taiwan.[1] Later the Dutch expelled the Spaniards, but in 1661 they in turn were driven out by a Chinese general, Zheng Chenggong (or Coxinga), who refused allegiance to the New Manchu dynasty and established a native kingdom. After twenty-three years of independence Coxinga's kingdom surrendered to the Qing government, which ruled until 1895.[2] At that time, by the Treaty of Shimonoseki, Taiwan was ceded to Japan until the end of World War II.

Taiwan, an island of 15,000 square miles (one-third the area of Cuba), lies to the east of South China, opposite Fukien Province. A 1905 survey listed the population as 3,079,602—consisting of 2,915,894 Han natives, 104,334 aborigines, 53,365 Japanese, and 6,009 foreigners, including Chinese.[3] The main cities were on the west coast; towns and villages were scattered throughout the agricultural plains, where rice and sugarcane were grown, and the mountainous regions, where tea and camphor were produced. The economy was based on import-export businesses in the cities and agriproduction in the villages. Most people earned a living from agricultural work, and the standard of living was moderate until the first agricultural reform in 1918 when new breeds of rice and fertilizer were introduced.[4] Taiwan's society consisted of Han Chinese mainly from Fukien, Hakka from Canton, and aboriginals. While Han Chinese usually controlled the areas of plentiful arable soil, the Hakka lived in the infertile foothills and the aboriginals in the mountains.

Before 1895, some schools providing very basic education were supported for charitable reasons by the government and wealthy families. Home schools with private tutors provided elite education, but only for the offspring of affluent Taiwanese families. In 1896, the colonial government in Taiwan ordered the establishment of fourteen schools to teach Japanese. They were later upgraded to public schools. Before 1941, schools were segregated by ethnicity; *kôgakkô* (literally, "public schools") were established for Taiwanese children, while *shôgakkô* ("primary schools," the same term used in Japan) were restricted to the children of Japanese nationals. Schools for aborigines were established in aboriginal areas. By 1944, there were 944 primary schools in Taiwan with total enrollment rates of 71.3 percent for Taiwanese children, 86.4 percent for aboriginal children, and 99.6 percent for Japanese children. As a result, primary school enrollment rates in Taiwan were among the highest in Asia, second only to Japan itself.[5]

The judiciary of Taiwan under the Japanese was like that of the German colonial system and unlike the British system in that it was not absolutely independent of the administration. The governor-general had full power to establish and abolish courts and could suspend judges from active service while laws were administered under the supervision of the governor of civil administration. In the colonial administration, financial problems were of the highest importance and often difficult to solve. In 1896, for example, 6,840,000 yen were spent by the colonial government, chiefly for public works, sanitary and educational improvements, and the promotion of commerce and industry. In 1897, the figure was 5,959,000 yen.[6]

During the early years of the colonial period, the Japanese government in Taiwan encountered many obstacles, and its plans were not carried out as effectively as expected.[7] Plague and famine not only discouraged improvement and investment but often destroyed the good that had been accomplished. Under the Chinese regime, sanitation in Taiwan was altogether neglected, and the island was generally regarded as unsafe for civilized people. Even Taihoku, the capital, was in a chronic state of filth, swarming with flies and mosquitoes. Malaria, black fever, and smallpox were common among the natives. In the first year of Japanese occupation, the death rate of the Japanese was so high that it discouraged immigration.[8]

Taiwan was Japan's first overseas colony, and the Japanese intended to turn the island into a showpiece "model colony."[9] As a result, much effort was made to improve the island's economy, industry, and public facilities. The success in overcoming early obstacles increased Japan's confidence in being a great colonial empire. In October 1935, the governor-general of Taiwan held an "Exposition to Commemorate the Fortieth Anniversary of the Beginning of Administration in Taiwan," which served as a showcase for the achievements of Taiwan's modernization process under Japanese rule.[10] Throughout the 1930s, the themes of modernization and civilization through Japanese colonization were extensively promoted, and medical reform was an important element in those themes. Government propaganda usually implied that medical reform in Taiwan was guided by advanced Japanese medicine, which would enable it to catch up with the progress in Europe. That argument not only legitimized

Japanese colonial medicine, but also accidentally left a clue—picked up by Western scholarship in the 1980s—to reinterpreting popular concepts of colonial medicine.

Health Conditions in Taiwan before the Japanese Occupation

It is worth noting that during the early occupation the term *shinryôdo* (new territory) was preferred by Japanese intellectuals to describe Taiwan rather than the official term *shokuminchi* (colony) used in documents. On one hand, the implication of the term *shinryôdo* was that Taiwan had been claimed by the Japanese empire, but its administrative status was still unknown. *Shokuminchi*, on the other hand, meant a land under colonization, and colonization was merely a process that would integrate this new territory into the imperial map. A similar attitude can be found in many books about Japanese colonization. Although "*colonization*" is used to describe colonial policies, these policies are seen as necessary steps in the "civilizing" and "enlightening" of the colonial population.

To rule the new territory, Japanese colonizers in Taiwan had to deal with an unfamiliar environment with their limited experience of medical modernization. Acclimatization of the colonizers to the unhealthy Taiwanese environment would thus have first priority. As shown in official records and local gazettes before 1895, the island was notorious for its fatal epidemics and lethal miasmas—a good excuse for the Japanese to bring "civilization" and "science" to this savage land. Other negative images of Taiwan before 1895 in various Chinese records provided a conceptual base or political excuse for the development of Japanese colonial medicine there. Almost no systematic data related to health conditions in Taiwan are available prior to the twentieth century—only scrappy information collected from local gazettes and military records. However, based on current standards some of the data are reliable, and the colonial government later used them to reflect the achievements of Japanese colonial medicine.

Major Diseases and Health Problems

The terms most frequently used in many gazettes in Qing Taiwan to refer to environmentally based illnesses are *zhang* (miasma), *zhangqi* (pestilential vapors), and *zhangli* (miasmatic epidemics). The authors of these gazettes recorded large-scale *zhang*-related epidemics as *yi* and *dayi*. Some scholars suggest that these terms in fact refer to malaria or malaria-related epidemics.[11] However, because we cannot scientifically identify these traditional terms I will use them to keep the meanings as broad as possible.

A study shows that *zhang* was the most prevalent and virulent medical problem in Qing Taiwan.[12] In 171 local gazettes, *zhang*-related illnesses contributed to maladjustment, especially in unsettled areas. According to the descriptions, the symptoms of *zhang*-related illnesses could be linked to various diseases, including malaria and typhoid. Table I.1 shows records of *yi* in Taiwan's local gazettes with most of the records listing the cause as *zhang*. It is reasonable to doubt the completeness of such records, and it is not clear what standard was used to identify a disease as *yi* rather than *dayi*. Despite the insufficiency of the data, gazette materials still support my hypothesis that Qing Taiwan's environment was very conducive to the spread of disease. A crude death rate calculated from government records is 23.48 percent.[13]

TABLE I.1. Epidemic Records in Taiwan's Local Gazettes

Year	Location	Event	Season
1681	Taiwan Fu	*Yi**	Unknown
	Taiwan Hsien	*Yi*	Unknown
	Fengshan Hsien	*Yi*	Unknown
1820	Tanshui Ting	*Yi*	Autumn
	Miaoli Hsien	*Yi*	Autumn
1856	Penghu Ting	*Dayi***	Unknown
1857	Penghu Ting	*Yi*	Unknown
1864	Chiayi Hsien	*Yi*	Unknown
1866	Tanshui Ting	*Dayi*	Summer
	Miaoli Hsien	*Dayi*	Summer
1868	Penghu Ting	*Dayi*	Autumn
1874	Miaoli Hsien	*Yi*	Autumn
1883	Miaoli Hsien	*Yi*	Summer
1884	Penghu Ting	*Dayi*	Summer
1885	Penghu Ting	*Dayi*	Summer
1889	Miaoli Hsien	*Dayi*	Winter
1890	Miaoli Hsien	*Yi*	Summer

Source: Liu Ts'ui-jung and Liu Shiyung, "Disease and Mortality in the History of Taiwan," 101.

Note: Because no quantitative measurement is involved, there is no way to differentiate between *yi* and *dayi*; that is, in some cases *dayi* could be smaller than *yi*.

*Yi = epidemic

**Dayi = large-scale epidemic or pandemic

According to reports from missionaries and reports on the sanitary and health conditions of Japanese colonists in the 1890s, Taiwan was an unhealthy and often deadly place. Edward House, an American journalist who visited Taiwan around 1870, mentioned that malaria was endemic and outbreaks of contagious disease, specifically plague and cholera, were common.[14] George MacKay, a Presbyterian missionary with medical training who went to Taiwan around 1870 and lived there for about twenty years, confirmed House's observation, noting that malarial fever, the most malignant disease, was most common in northern Taiwan.[15] Both Chinese gazettes and westerners' observations described the critical health conditions on the island before 1895.

Demographic Features before and after the Colonial Period

There are no documented statistics about the Taiwanese population before 1895. By using local gazettes and diaries, Chen Shaoxin estimated the growth rate in Taiwan before 1895 (see table I.2).

TABLE I.2. Annual Growth Rate of the Taiwanese Population before 1895

Period	Time	Duration	Annual Growth Rate (%)
I	1650–1680	30 years	2.4
II	1680–1810	130 years	1.8
III	1810–1890	80 years	0.3

Source: Chen Shaoxin, "Taiwan renkoushi de jige wenti," in *Taiwan de renkou bianqian yu shehui bianqian* (Population and Social Changes in Taiwan) (Taipei: Lianjin, 1979), 18.

Chen Shaoxin suggests that the natural growth of the Taiwanese population had only a slight impact on growth rates and that immigration from China was the main factor driving population growth before 1895.[16] However, the Qing government stopped its prohibition on emigration after the mid–eighteenth century, and the Taiwanese population steadily grew thereafter. Although the Japanese blocked Chinese immigration after their occupation, the growth of the Taiwanese population was significant due to the fairly even sex ratio before the 1900s.[17] During the colonial period, natural growth was the primary factor in population growth in a comparatively static Taiwanese population. Due to severe epidemics and social unrest, the Taiwanese population suffered a high mortality rate before the 1910s. According to many governmental reports, there was a steady and continuous decline in mortality after the 1920s because of improved medical care and economic welfare. The improvement in the health conditions of the Taiwanese population continued throughout the colonial period, and the life expectancy of a Taiwanese born in 1945 was almost twenty years longer than that of a Taiwanese born in 1920.

Improvement in mortality and life expectancy obviously has a positive impact on increasing population size. Immigration was no longer a factor in population growth after 1895, but declining mortality and increased fertility caused rapid population growth.[18] Table I.3 shows the change in the ethnic composition of colonial Taiwan's population. The ethnic mix in the colonial period was more stable than in the Qing.[19] The proportions of Taiwanese and aborigines slightly declined while the population of Chinese and Japanese increased a little. Based on correlation analysis, the decrease of the aboriginal population had some relation to the increase of the Japanese but had no statistical relationship to the Taiwanese and Chinese population shifts.[20] As the Taiwanese population was largely stationary, the ethnic proportion was similarly stable and rarely changed. Generally speaking, the increase in Chinese residents in Taiwan and the decrease in the aboriginal population were not statistically significant.

TABLE I.3. Demographic Change in Colonial Taiwan

Year	Number of Doctors	Notes
1874	28,262	82% trained in Chinese medicine
1880	38,322	No detailed records
1890	40,215	21.28% trained in Western medicine
		78.72% already in practice[a]

Source: Chen Shaoxin, "Taiwan renkoushi de jige wenti," 96–97.

The changes in the Taiwanese population represent the major demographic trends during the colonial period. However, table I.3 does not provide information on the impact of colonial medicine on Japanese-ruled Taiwan. We certainly need more information and analysis if we are to evaluate the improvement in living and health conditions for Taiwanese after the Japanese occupation. The following chapters address the main figures involved in the modification of the Japanese state medicine model in colonial Taiwan, the compromises and cooperation with indigenous society, and finally the evaluation of the impact of Japanese colonial medicine.

Popular Concepts of Colonial Medicine

During the early eighteenth century, Europeans sought largely to avoid disease rather than actively to prevent it, but in the nineteenth century there were attempts in the colonies to modify the environment in ways that would reduce sickness. This was the primary impetus behind sanitary reforms in European cities and was applied to the colonies as well. In both African and Asian colonies, until the late nineteenth century medicine operated pragmatically to meet the medical needs first of colonial officers and troops, immigrant settlers, and laborers responsible for economic development and later of colonized populations and then only when their ill health threatened the well-being of the colonies. Still there were some important differences that reflected colonial power relationships such as the research fever over British India.[21] This has led some historians to write about "colonial medicine" as if it were a distinct entity that gave priority to the needs of colonizers and vital sections of the indigenous population and served as the underpinning of a racialist ideology. Seen in its political and economic capacity, medicine is therefore often considered a "tool of empire."

The "tools of empire" concept was broadened to include colonization of the mind as well as the body in late 1980s Western scholarship. Medical knowledge and sanitary regulations are said to have imparted very different cultural ideas and to have been an important colonizing force in their own right. This idea has recently inspired scholars to take a cross-disciplinary approach in engaging the theoretical, historical, and discursive aspects of colonialism. Rather than focusing on a particular colonial period or legacy, Western scholars often discuss the overarching theoretical assumptions that underlay colonial history and discourse, as well as the material, literary, and cultural practices that emanated from them.[22] Beginning in the late 1980s, the study of medicine as a way to understand colonial societies rather than simply illuminating the colonizers' physical needs became more common.

For historians studying medicine in colonial settings, Daniel Headrick's and David Arnold's works have been inspirational. In *The Tools of Empire*, Headrick lists medicine among the several technologies that were crucial to the success of European expansion and dominion over large parts of the globe.[23] He argues that the major concern of colonial medicine was ensuring the health of Europeans in the tropics, especially colonial troops, the ultimate guarantors of imperial rule. In a case study of quinine prophylaxis, Headrick remarks that "scientific cinchona production was an imperial technology par excellence. Without it European colonialism would have been almost impossible in Africa, and much costlier elsewhere in the tropics."[24] To him, medicine is a technology that helped ensure the survival of Europeans in the colonies and thus helped guarantee the success of the colonial project as a whole.

Arnold, whose studies do not completely support Headrick's conclusions, points out that some of Headrick's evidence is rather selective and that he exaggerates the effectiveness of medical intervention.[25] In these researchers' attempts to understand Japanese colonial medicine, it may be that both confused means with motives. At least in colonial Taiwan, imperial expansion provided the stimulus for technological innovation rather than the other way around, as Headrick describes. The improvement of health conditions in the military had little effect on colonial society in Taiwan as civilian physicians with steady support from the colonial government only later launched the reforms that would improve medical care for the troops. Moreover, Arnold also cites the coercive and divisive nature of colonial medical interventions. For example, in his famous *Colonizing the Body: State Medicine and Epidemic Disease in Nineteenth-Century India*, he explores the vital role of the state in medical and public health activities.[26] Focusing on three major epidemic diseases—smallpox, cholera, and plague—he demonstrates that Western medicine, as practiced in India, was not simply transferred from West to East but was fashioned in response to local needs and conditions.[27] Significantly, the diffusion of Western medicine in the colonies after the nineteenth century was a painful process of compromise between the needs of the colonizer and indigenous health demands.

Colonial politics and social conflicts are not the only approaches to evaluating colonial medicine; demographic analysis should also be included. In *Death by Migration: Europe's Encounter with the Tropical World in the Nineteenth Century*,[28] Philip Curtin studies mortality among European soldiers in the tropics between about 1815 and 1914. This book is partly a statistical exposition of the changing death rates in European Algeria, the British West Indies, and southern India by cause of death from disease, with data set against comparable figures for citizens who remained in France or Great Britain. About two-thirds of the book is devoted to a discussion of what Europeans at the time thought about the possible causes of "relocation costs," which refers to the added colonial costs incurred by death from disease, and how that problem was addressed medically. The author infers that for European soldiers in the tropics at the beginning of the nineteenth century the death rate was at least twice that of soldiers who stayed home. Besides technology and political economy, Curtin also "looks at disease as a factor [that] influenced migration"[29] to the colonies. Coincidently, demographic data and epidemic statistics in colonial Taiwan play a key role in current Taiwanese scholarship on colonial medicine, supporting the adaptation of many Western arguments, including "tools of empire" and "scientific modernization."

Seeing Europe as the birthplace of modern medicine and imperialism could falsely mean that Japan—a latecomer to colonialism in the late nineteenth century—was merely copying European systems. In addition, there are many works of Western scholarship based on the idea of colonial medicine as a European experience. Among them, British India has received the most attention. However, using British colonial medicine to understand the Japanese experience would be risky. First, as mentioned above, the colonial administration in Taiwan was copied from the German model rather than the British, which, according to Ramon Myers and Mark Peattie, are different in nature. In fact, there are three major models of colonialism: the British, the German, and the French. The British model allowed the possibility of autonomous development of the imperium's various components while still bearing the common burden of trusteeship. The German model paid more attention to the creation of "scientific colonialism." This approach was based on the German passion for methodical research and investigation, both of which were seen as prerequisites for economically sound administration and maximum efficiency in the extraction of wealth from colonial territories. The French model drew on the republican principles of 1789. French colonies were parts of an indivisible republic whose global purpose was a *mission civilisatrice*—the propagation of French civilization.[30] The French model was never applied in colonial Taiwan.

In addition, between the late nineteenth and mid-twentieth centuries, Britain might have been the largest colonial empire but it was far from the only one in the world. Germany, France, Italy, and Spain were also colonial powers. Moreover, in the late nineteenth century German medicine shared with French scientists the highest reputation for promoting modern medicine and was greatly respected for its *Staatsmedizin* (state medicine). Possibly because Germany lost most of its colonies after World War I, Western scholars have neglected to study how German medicine was applied in colonization. Also, the terrifying experience of the Nazi concentration camps has focused discussions of German medicine on the policies of the Third Reich.[31]

The loss of colonies after World War I does not mean, however, that German medicine had no colonial counterpart. Although rare, articles and books related to German colonial medicine have been published (mainly in German), though they had no significant impact on the British-centered study of colonial medicine after the 1980s. For the majority of anglophone scholarship on colonial medicine, British India is the only case thoroughly studied and thus became the paradigm for all research on the subject. Defining the study of colonial medicine in terms of the British experience not only restricts such study but also disregards the potential role of German medicine in the application of modern scientific medicine in colonies. Familiarity with anglophone scholarship, however, is crucial to understanding modern medicine in Japan, including its colonial medicine. German *Staatsmedizin* set the standard for many states in building medical systems, and Japan in the 1870s adopted the German model of medical modernization.[32] When Japan occupied Taiwan in 1895, the newly learned *Staatsmedizin* had to be transferred to a colonial format. There was no sign of British influence in Taiwan before the 1930s; the transformation there was effected by the colonizers' creative shaping of Japanized *Staatsmedizin* to meet local medical needs. Colonial medicine in Taiwan not only was established as an achievement of modern medicine in Japan but also reflected what German colonial medicine might have been like if Germany had not lost its colonies in 1918. As Japan occupied more territories in East Asia in the 1930s and 1940s, the influence of colonial medicine in Taiwan became stronger. The extent of Japanese colonial medicine in East Asia in the 1930s was greater than that of British India in South Asia.

Changing Viewpoints on Colonial Medicine in Taiwan

In Taiwan in the 1990s, the study of colonial medicine was still in its infancy but booming. With the relaxation of martial law in 1987, the study of Taiwanese history broke free of political taboos and eventually became fashionable in academia.[33] Historians have frequently approached colonial medicine in Taiwan from the perspective of scientific modernization—a concept inspired by current Western scholarship—and, not coincidentally, emphasized by the Japanese colonial government. Not until the late 1990s did the idea of medicine as a "tool of empire" begin to impact the work of young researchers—which led to the circulation in Taiwan of important works by David Arnold and Warwick Anderson. The efforts of postwar historians—who adopted the "tools of empire" and modernization theories in pursuing the traditional concerns of social history by exploring the colonial discourses of the Japanese-ruled period—usually ended in contradiction: brutal colonization was necessary to bring modernization to Taiwan. Practices such as the use of quarantine as a rationale for burning down entire villages, arrests of suspected but unproven carriers of disease by the sanitary police force, and severe discrimination against the Taiwanese within medical circles are discussed in the following chapters. In the end, postwar scholarship in Taiwan may have involuntarily enhanced images of medical development that were intentionally fostered by the colonial government.

Studies of colonial medicine in Taiwan fall into two groups, which can be roughly classified by their dates of publication. One group views medicine as an aspect of scientific modernization, and the other views it as an imperial tool. Studies before the 1970s were written primarily by hygienists and medical doctors who had a great deal of confidence in modern medicine and simply accepted the importance of medical technology in precolonial Taiwan, which was considered unsanitary. In their eyes, the medical history of colonial Taiwan was a history of technological progress in which the colonizer delivered modernity.

In 1974, Ôda Toshirô published his memoir *Taiwan igaku gojûnen* (The Fifty-Year History of Taiwanese Medicine).[34] Ôda was a medical doctor from Tokyo University who studied in Germany in 1925. He was appointed principal of the Taipei Medical School in 1934, the first director of the Affiliated Hospital of the Medical School at Taipei Imperial University in 1938, and dean of the Taipei Imperial University Medical School in 1942. Although he was forced to resign as dean when the Japanese left in 1945, he, like Maruyama Yoshito, held his professorship until 1947.[35] This book provides a personal account of medical education and disease prevention before the 1940s along with rumors and gossip that circulated within the Japanese medical community. In this book and other publications, Ôda seems to prefer using rumors and gossip to demonstrate the magnanimity of Japanese colonizers toward the indigenous people.[36] For example, he greatly admires the medical aid that the Japanese Red Cross delivered to a Taiwanese aboriginal tribe.[37] His writing obviously reflects a colonizer's view of modern/scientific medicine in colonial Taiwan.

Du Congming's *Zhongxi yixueshilüe* (A Brief History of Chinese and Western Medicine) should also be classified in this group. Du was born in 1893 and was the first person in Taiwan to earn a doctorate in medicine. He founded the pharmacology laboratory at Taihoku Imperial University's Faculty of Medicine (the predecessor of National Taiwan University's College of Medicine before 1945), which specialized in the three research areas of traditional Chinese medicine: opium, venom, and pharmacological extractions of herbs.[38] His book gives a brief description of medical development in Taiwan from the sixteenth to the early twentieth century. Du's narrative is an impressive synthesis of accounts of colonial research projects and interpretations of institutional processes.[39] Progress in medical science was always the prism through which Du interpreted public health improvements during the colonial period. In analyzing medical development using technological indexes, Du's understanding of the spread of Western medicine is consistent with George Basalla's idea in the 1960s.[40] The three phases of medical modernization in Taiwan correspond to the precolonization, colonization, and postwar eras.[41] Interestingly, Du thought that colonization hindered the "scientific study" of Chinese medicine. He believed that in postcolonial Taiwan Chinese medicine should be studied by scientists as carefully as Western medicine had been over the past one hundred years.[42]

To medical professionals such as Du Congming, who were trained in colonial Taiwan, "scientific medicine" appeared to be a key result of Japanese colonization. For example, although Du describes traditional Chinese medicine as "the precious experience of our ancestors," his advice to medical professionals is that "being Chinese, especially researchers of modern medicine, we should study traditional Chinese medicine from a scientific perspective."[43] Du also criticizes traditional Chinese medicine as being "conservative" and lacking "scientific evidence."[44] He appears to admire modern medical education in colonial Taiwan, which was meant to "develop Taiwanese culture and contribute to the culture in mainland China."[45]

Generally speaking, medical historians in Taiwan were rare before the 1980s and tended to follow the "scientific modernization" interpretation of colonial medicine. From this perspective, scientific medicine and civilization were the primary legacies of Japanese colonization, and these scholars did not probe the social reactions or economic-political reasons behind it. In fact, it seems that a sense of Chinese nationalism was the only thing that could incite criticism of Japanese colonial medicine by Du Congming and his colleague Li Tengyue.[46]

The history of Japanese colonial medicine was pursued as a hobby in a privileged circle of medical professionals. After the 1980s, historical demographers used colonial statistics to gradually unleash the legend of public health improvements in colonial Taiwan. In addition, a second wave of writing about Taiwan's colonial medicine emerged in the 1990s. Young scholars eager to integrate knowledge from sociology and political science into their field were influenced by current Western studies in history and medical sociology. Their examinations of medicine and public health under colonial rule were published by the end of the twentieth century. Although these researchers were trained in a standard historical approach, they brought innovative perspectives to their examination of Japanese colonial medicine. They tried to explain medical development from social and political viewpoints, accepting without question the conclusions drawn by medical professionals and demographers.

The new wave of research on colonial medicine in Taiwan started with a group of graduate students mainly from national universities.[47] They undoubtedly accepted the concept of "scientific modernization" and then added to their explanations ideas related to the "tools of empire" theory. The 1989 master's thesis "Riben zhiminzhuyi xia Taiwan weisheng zhengcezhi yanjiu" (The Study of Public Health Policy in Taiwan under Japanese Colonialism), by Xie Zhenrong, was the first work of this type.[48] Xie's account of the development of *eisei shokumin* (hygienic colonization) undertaken by the Japanese colonial administration places the growth of Western medicine in twentieth-century Taiwan in a social and political context. The thesis explores the introduction of Japan's policy on hygiene and the process by which medical science came to be an essential tool in the colonization of Taiwanese society. In his revelations about the important stages of colonial medical development in Taiwan, Xie makes a significant contribution to our understanding of vital policies; however, his argument is sometimes so convoluted as to preclude a clear conclusion.[49]

To bypass the difficulty of medical terminology, some historians turned to studying the social role of doctors and the activities of the colonial government in Taiwan. Writing about the luxurious lifestyles and active socializing among Taiwanese doctors in the colonial period became an academic fashion in Taiwan. In describing it, the medical historian Guo Wenhua claims that "[this] writing style reflects some of the self-identity and expectations of doctors in Japanese Taiwan."[50] In addition, the sociologist Yao Rendo states that the anticolonization attitude of many Taiwanese doctors was an unexpected result of the economic-political privileges they shared with the colonial government.[51] The two themes—"tools of empire" and the "self-identity" of Taiwanese doctors—were individually elaborated on by the historian Fan Yanqiu and the sociologist Miriam Ming-cheng Lo—two influential scholars of Taiwanese colonial medicine in books published after 1995.

Fan Yanqiu completed her master's thesis,—"Rijuqianqi Taiwan zhi gonggongweisheng: Yi fangyi weizhongxin zhi yanjiu (1895–1920)" (Public Health Policy during the Early Period of Japanese Occupation: A Study Focusing on Epidemic Prevention)—in 1994. In it, Fan focuses on the anti-epidemic campaigns and identifies the vital role of the colonial government in sponsoring medical and public health activities. She argues that these activities were a critical aspect of the interaction and conflict between Japanese authorities and their Taiwanese subjects.[52] After completing her thesis, Fan published the article "Xinyixue zai Taiwan de shijian" (The Practice of New Medicine in Taiwan), 1898-1906 in 1998.[53] This was followed in 2005 by "Redai fengtuxunhua, riben diguoyixue yu zhimindi renzhuanglun" (Tropical Acclimatization, Japanese Imperial Medicine, and Racial Discourses in the Colony),[54] which clarifies her argument that "medicine was a tool of Japanese colonization" and "biological principles are a conceptual guide for colonial medicine."[55]

In her dissertation, "Ribendiguo fazhanxia zhimindi Taiwan de renzhuangweisheng" (Racial Hygiene in Colonial Taiwan under the Japanese Empire), 1895–1945, Fan elaborates on her argument that colonial medicine in Taiwan was not only an application of biological principles, but also a design for underscoring colonial rule.[56] In it, she asserts that the Japanese colonial government took *Renzhung weisheng* (racial hygiene) as a scientific discourse for legitimizing colonization.[57] It was also a tool for ensuring that indigenous doctors would cooperate with the administration and employ various strategies within "scientifically proven" boundaries.[58] Generally speaking, Fan elaborates on the old argument of "scientific modernity" in her assertion that colonial medicine was scientifically necessary for the colonizer and the colonized from a technological as well as a political standpoint.

Miriam Ming-cheng Lo published her dissertation, "From National Physicians to Medical Modernists: Taiwanese Doctors under Japanese Rule," in revised form as *Doctors within Borders: Profession, Ethnicity, and Modernity in Colonial Taiwan* in 2002. In illuminating the identity of Taiwanese doctors in the colonial period, Lo's book on the education of a generation of Taiwanese doctors under the colonial regime offers an excellent account of medicine in the second half of the colonial period. Identifying Japanese rule in Taiwan as a kind of "scientific colonialism," she carefully examines the changing roles of Taiwanese doctors. She successfully unearths the points of convergence between medicine and politics in colonial Taiwan by integrating individual interviews and archival materials with discussions of political and social theories.[59] She argues that medical modernization policy in colonial Taiwan was the cradle of the first professional elite group in Taiwanese history and also laid the foundation for this group's hybrid identity as Taiwanese who worshipped Japanese colonial rule.

Lo's clear narrative provides an essential time frame and argument for medical modernization as she successfully interweaves personal memories and archival materials with political and social theories. On the one hand, she sees the development of modern medicine in colonial Taiwan as linear, and she describes the transition from the original medical plan to the colonial reality as "the history of hybridization."[60] This hybridization, a process of mixing ethnic identity with an appreciation for modernization, caused a decade of conflict and compromise. On the other hand, she heavily relies on interviews with doctors who practiced after the 1930s. That strategy greatly magnifies the self-identity of Taiwanese doctors and their role in Japanese colonial medicine. When Lo writes that "Japanese colonialism emphasize[d] the similarities between the colonizers and the colonized without collapsing their hierarchical distinctions," the argument that Taiwanese doctors "became increasingly incorporated into the expanding imperial medical system" after the 1930s comes as no surprise to the reader. [61]

As we have seen in the work of Taiwanese scholars, if the desire of colonies for modern facilities—electricity, plumbing, cars, modern medicine, radios, and so forth—is appreciated, then scholars should accept the position staked out by nineteenth-century evolutionists, which holds that Western civilization is of a higher material order than Eastern. Therefore, like colonial medicine in Western colonies, Japanese colonization was an inevitable process in which Western modernity was grafted onto premodern Taiwan.[62] Indeed, the Japanese occupation of Taiwan after 1895 brought the first anti-smallpox vaccinations of the indigenous population and the creation of the first civilian hospitals on the island.[63] Further progress, such as determining a large-scale health care policy, would be held off until the economic advance of the 1930s. Thus, the Japanese public health care mission was justified politically as well as economically for "humanitarian" reasons.[64]

Ironically, "medicine" and "civilization" were two of the main themes the Japanese colonial government repeatedly used to persuade indigenous societies to accept colonization. Meanwhile, since the colonial government intentionally nurtured Taiwanese doctors as professional elites and social leaders of the indigenous society, searching for self-identity could unintentionally mirror a process that was being explicitly undertaken by the colonial government. By accepting government propaganda and statistics in colonial Taiwan, scholars can easily conclude that medical reforms improved the survival chances of the Japanese in Taiwan and that the Taiwanese gradually enjoyed the benefits of advanced modern medicine. However, Japanese colonial medicine was not a constant concept or a policy; instead, it shifted over time. Without dynamically reviewing the characteristics of colonial medicine in Taiwan, the research is merely superimposing different ideals—such as "scientific colonization," "scientific colonialism," or "colonial modernity"—onto a "tools of empire" theory base.

As mentioned previously, although studies of the social history of medicine in colonial Taiwan gained in popularity in the twenty-first century, research has never gone beyond the assumptions of modernization theory and the functions of state medicine. Most scholars have studied individual cases in colonial Taiwan, but a general picture of Japanese colonial medicine and its origins is still unclear and largely veiled by the colonial intention. By responding to the "tools of empire" argument, this book integrates the vast scholarship of existing studies in three languages (English, Chinese, and Japanese) and constructs an overarching framework for Japanese colonial medicine. It then analyzes the possible factors that shaped medical reform in Taiwan and reassesses Japanese colonialism in the medical field. Through a detailed examination of public health policies and medical practice in Japanese-ruled Taiwan, this book tests assumptions about the nature of colonial medicine that arise from examining this subject exclusively through the anglophone paradigm of British India. Finally, it explores the formation of "scientific evidence" in colonial propaganda and illuminates the weaknesses in the derivational legend of Japanese colonial medicine in contemporary scholarship. In addition, this book was written not only to satisfy curiosity about the colonial past but to portray colonial medicine in Japanese-ruled Taiwan as a missing stage in the evolution of German medicine and a case to be compared to that of British India. Generally speaking, my aim is not simply to provide an account of the development of modern medicine and public health in colonial Taiwan but also to explore the major elements of Japanese colonial medicine in Taiwan as a way of showing the transformation of modern Japanese state medicine as a necessary process in the modernization of the colony.

Considering that the 1895 occupation of Taiwan occurred less than fifty years after the revolutionary leap forward of modern bacteriology in mid-nineteenth-century Europe and that Japan's medical modernization (of the 1870s) was still in its infancy, it is crucial to place the case of colonial Taiwan in the historical frame of developing Western medicine. While contemporary studies often treated colonial medicine in Taiwan an isolated case, this book shows the process of establishing colonial medicine in Taiwan in a dynamic fashion, linking it to the appropriate stage of medical modernization in the Japanese empire and to the technological capability of modern Western medicine as well. In sum, this book shows the link between colonial medicine in Taiwan and the influence of Japanese *Staatsmedizin*, as well as Taiwan's heritage from Western medicine. [65]

There is no way to study colonial medicine without considering the colonizers' political motives and the demographic and socioeconomic effects on colonial society; thus, this book is a combination of narrative and quantitative studies. One goal of the discussion in the following chapters is to describe the formation and adaptation of Japanese colonial medicine in Taiwan. The second goal is to understand Taiwan's experience in the context of the international diffusion of medical knowledge as it was funneled through the Japanese imperial system. Finally, the third goal is to analyze possible factors that shaped the original blueprint of Japanese colonial medicine in order to reassess the colonial system. Obviously, all these goals can be linked to broader topics that concern current historians. Therefore, this book is an integrated study of Japanese medicine in colonial Taiwan and also provides a broader viewpoint for reexamining the process through which colonial medicine was developed on the island.

Studies of Japanese colonial medicine in Taiwan are largely unknown to an anglophone readership and scholars have treated this issue as a local experience limited to Taiwan. This book is the first attempt to link the discourse of Japanese colonialism to the wave of globalization in the first half of the twentieth century. It closely examines Japanese colonial medicine by tracing its roots in medical modernization in Japan as well as the process of making Japanese colonial medicine in Taiwan a legend. I extend the scope of the discussion to understanding the medical practice and policy of Japanese-ruled Taiwan from the perspectives of Japanese state building and the globalization of modern/Western medicine. This means that colonial medicine in Taiwan is seen not only as a local experience of medical modernization/Westernization but also as a branch process of the globalization of modern medicine in which Japanese colonialism played a key role. Thus, the study of Japanese colonial medicine in Taiwan may modify theories of how Western science was passed to non-European regions, as it portrays Japanese colonial medicine as a comparative counterpart rather than a copycat of British colonial medicine.

1

Japanized *Staatsmedizin*
The Prototype of Colonial Medicine in Taiwan

A t the end of the nineteenth century, the European powers—
Spain, Holland, England, Germany, and France—had reached
the peak of their colonial activity, with a large part of the world
colonized. In the course of that century, Western imperialism resulted not
only in the relocation of European populations to tropical colonies but also in
the transmission of diseases[1] and the diffusion of Western knowledge.[2] The
expansion of European colonization provided a paradigm for Japanese politics
as well as medicine.

In the last decade of the twentieth century in Taiwan, there was a surge
of interest in the colonial period. Previous studies of medical development
in colonial Taiwan contributed a great deal of background not only on medical
events and the development of related institutions but also on the social response
to Japanese colonial medicine. However, further discussion is needed to link
colonial medicine in Taiwan to the relationship between the westernization of
medicine in Japan and the globalization of modern Western medicine.

During Taiwan's colonial era (1895–1945), the Japanese government
introduced new medical ideas, methods, education, and equipment to amend
or improve Taiwan's hygienic environment. These efforts dramatically shaped
the Taiwanese population and society in various ways. Undoubtedly, medicine
and health care services in colonial Taiwan benefited from the application
of modern medical science and technology as well as the implementation of
improved administrative and educational systems. The transmission of modern
medical knowledge to colonial Taiwan took place through two related processes:
the creation of medical resources in Taiwan and the implementation of new
policy goals and organizational models for maximizing the development and
distribution of new medical techniques and service delivery concepts. Both
processes involved political negotiation, economic compromise, and social
conflict, and both were particularly difficult because Japan's own process of
medical westernization had begun only in 1870, less than thirty years before.

Medical westernization in Japan was inspired by German medicine and
included three essential components: mass immunization, the creation of
laboratories in the medical education system, and the establishment of new

medical institutions. The important role that Japanese westernized medicine played in Taiwan's colonial medical system will be examined in the chapters that follow.

Before proceeding, it will be useful to clarify the basic definitions of terms used throughout this book: *medical reform, state medicine, social medicine,* and *social hygiene.* The Japanese learned these concepts from Germany but eventually developed their own definitions and implementation strategies in Japan as well as Taiwan. The concept of *Staatsmedizin,* which arose in the nineteenth century, was based on the idea that the state should bear the primary responsibility for protecting the public health and had the right to regulate hygiene and sanitation in ways that improve the public good. However, due to political upheavals, *Staatsmedizin* was not fully implemented until the establishment of the German empire in 1871.[3] The German concept of *Staatsmedizin* had a great impact on medical westernization in Japan and later on colonial medicine in Taiwan.

German *Staatsmedizin,* the Model for Westernized Medicine in Japan

New forms of medical administration began to appear in Europe in the nineteenth century. While historical events in the early nineteenth century led England to place considerable emphasis on local government institutions, England pursued medical reform through a national public health program. In the United States, community groups, private philanthropists, and activist physicians initially oversaw the protection of public health with local, state, and federal authorities becoming involved relatively late. Medical reform in Germany, and later in Japan, was highly centralized, resulting in a reform movement that tended to occur from the top down.[4]

Modern medical reform, based largely on the European experience, was accelerated with the emergence of a united Germany in the latter part of the nineteenth century. Germans were already making strides in science and technology, and under Bismarck the government began to foster medical reform as a means of strengthening the state. Mass immunization drives were usually sanctioned by state authorities and executed by medical professionals. Coercive smallpox vaccinations begun in 1906 marked the first time that a population became the object of a large-scale medical intervention resulting from recent scientific discoveries. The German government also expected that a state-controlled medical education system would support its goals of implementing mass immunization, the creation of laboratories in the medical education system, and the establishment of new forms of medical administration.[5]

The revolution in bacteriology in the 1880s and the 1890s provided further impetus to the development of state medicine. Louis Pasteur successfully cultivated chicken cholera bacteria in France in 1880, and in 1882 the German bacteriologist Robert Koch isolated the tubercle bacillus, the first microorganism scientifically identified as the cause of a human disease. Identification of disease-causing organisms did not result immediately in improved clinical treatment.[6] First it was necessary to discover how the disease was transmitted and define the role of carriers. Then antitoxins and vaccines had to be developed, which opened a role for the state as sponsor of the new medicine. New technologies required a unified process for training doctors, paying for expensive laboratory equipment, and supporting graduates in medical practices. These developments were too expensive to be undertaken by a single institution, so the locus of medical innovation moved dramatically from hospital and university pathology laboratories, where the emphasis had been on disease symptoms and clinical treatment, to new bacteriological research institutes concerned with developing scientific medical techniques for preventing disease.[7] Seemingly, the state could do it all.

In Germany, there was a long tradition of state medicine, whereas in other parts of Europe it remained more an idea than a reality. Eighteenth-century German political theorists were the first to develop the concept of state "medical police," a key executive power of state medicine in Germany and later in Japan.[8] By the mid–nineteenth century, through the advocacy of Wilhelm Schallmayer and J. P. Frank, the concept of medical police referred specifically to the idea that state agencies should regulate and administer disease control activities, organize and supervise state medical personnel, and oversee sanitation and environmental conditions.[9] To Frank, and later Schallmayer, the medical police force, which had already existed during the Bismarck regime, was intended to preserve the security of the interior affairs of the state by receiving orders from a centralized medical administration. This system was also designed to protect the human labor force, as emphasized by the cameralism of that period.[10] A centralized system of medical administration with a powerful police force was instituted after the establishment of a united German empire. Most of the reform policies were systematically passed into law after the unification of Germany in 1871 and the passage of Bismarck's health insurance programs in 1883.[11] Between 1871 and 1890, Bismarck's regime successfully established a state medical system with a centralized medical administration, which included a central Ministry of Health and Academy of Medicine to coordinate medical administration and standardize and regulate the training and licensing of medical professionals.[12]

In addition to institutional innovations, German *Staatsmedizin* was influenced by the popular concepts of social medicine and social hygiene. That is, socialism and revolution had an important impact not only on late-nineteenth-century European politics but also on medicine. Before the unification of Germany, German socialists such as Rudolf Virchow and Salomon Neuman gradually became committed to the view that "the poor and the oppressed who carry their burden here below because they are to be richly rewarded in Heaven, should meet with happier conditions on earth and not depend solely on future bliss."[13] They argued that every citizen had a constitutional right to a healthy existence, and it followed that state medicine must become the enterprise for facilitating the protection of public health.[14] The public health program envisaged by the reformers and articulated in such documents as Neumann's draft for a Public Health Law reflected the aspirations of numerous politically conscious physicians.[15] Doctors' perceptions of themselves as German patriots and civil servants, their belief in the efficacy of medicine as a means of solving social problems, and their demands that physicians play an active role in raising the level of health in society left a deep imprint on Bismarck's regime after German unification.[16]

The nineteenth-century German medical reformers, led by Virchow, accepted this concept and argued that social factors rather than biological causes were to blame for the fact that it was the poor who were hit hardest by disease. Thus, the protection of public health could be best achieved through socioeconomic reforms.[17] Offering a broad vision of public health that went beyond the old reliance on sanitation, German social medicine was invented by medical progressives who were typically politically left wing. They believed that social medicine should incorporate statistics, social science, and prevention. Supporters of social medicine in Germany claimed that medicine is about treating sick people not diseases and that the government had to treat individuals as social beings as well as diseased bodies. Under this logic, a physician of social medicine, they insisted, had to practice "clinical sociology" on a patient-as-person basis.[18] In this way, medicine could cure human diseases as well as alleviate social ills.

Advocates of social medicine such as Virchow were also socialists, an ideology heavily suppressed in Bismarck's Germany. In 1873, the anxieties and discontent stoked by the first of several major economic depressions caused Germany to move to the right politically. Nationalism and social Darwinism began to dominate German medicine. Subsequent developments in the social aspects of health and disease in Germany further elevated the role of medicine at the expense of political and economic analysis.[19] Afraid of a possible relationship between socialist revolution and social medicine, the new German empire needed a way to satisfy the supporters of social medicine while suppressing "violent" socialism. Although the German government could accept some features of social medicine and integrate them into a new medical system, it had to eliminate the socialist effort to decentralize the government's totalitarian power. Bismarck finally adopted a strategy of emphasizing technology to reduce health problems in German society rather than applying scientific principals to social reform.

Revolutionary developments in bacteriology and microbiology stimulated the German government to begin a major assault on contagious disease. The new German Kaiserreich, established in 1871, invested some of the war indemnity funds it received from France into new state medical research institutes that were independent of German universities. These state institutes, established in Berlin for Koch in 1891 and for Paul Ehrlich in 1896, were specifically intended to extend central state control over the production of antidiphtheria serum and other newly discovered serums and vaccines.[20] Between 1882 and 1898, many microorganisms that caused the major contagious diseases afflicting humankind were identified and their vaccines and serum antitoxins developed in Germany: rabies (1882–85), cholera (1883–93), diphtheria (1883–90), tetanus (1884–91), typhoid (1884–98), and plague (1894–95).[21] Utilizing diagnostic laboratories and vaccines and quarantining the sick in homes or hospitals reduced the devastation caused by many killer diseases. It seemed hard to overlook the social impact of Koch's bacteriology and its remedy. Although Virchow and other radical medical reformers called doctors using Koch's remedy "poisoners and murders," their criticisms never successfully jeopardized the rapid growth of the Robert Koch Institute of Infectious Disease.[22] In 1891, Robert Koch was made the first director of the new Prussian Institute for Infectious Disease by the government to illuminate his contribution to hygiene studies. The Institute was renamed the Robert Koch Institute (RKI) in dedicatation to Koch in 1930 and the name is hence well-known among medical professionals as RKI. In the short term, laboratory medicine was very popular in Germany. The government and the public almost immediately donated large sums of money to the bacteriological laboratories.[23]

Bacteriological research and the resulting prevention programs in Germany necessarily supported state centralization. To reduce mortality and morbidity caused by disease, the state had to create new administrative mechanisms such as a household registration system to enforce the contribution of laboratory innovations such as mass vaccination and tracing of the results. Also the development of new medicines, discovery of new bacteria, and sanitation control became increasingly expensive. These activities usually required financial support from the state, and therefore the development of medicine was generally politically and financially linked to public support and state policies. Finally, the state controls led to the development, approval, and distribution of new medicines or vaccines for the registered population. Eventually, state-supported laboratories and medical bureaucrats fixed the definitions of health and the solutions to major health problems. A physician thus had to rely on laboratories and the bureaucracy to deal with certain illnesses. Medical reform began with technological innovation but eventually involved other medical and nonmedical sectors of the state.

As Andrew Cunningham and Perry Williams have pointed out, it was "frequently stated and assumed by advocates of the medical laboratory that the new techniques and instruments of the laboratory had had the human element totally removed, so that they were completely objective."[24] The Koch Institute can thus be seen to symbolize the important role of laboratory bacteriology and potentially to emphasize the objectivity of laboratory knowledge. Moreover, the rigidity of the central state position of the Koch Institute greatly depended on a unitary hierarchy, which was supported by a government that favored centralism.[25] However, Koch was forced to resign from his own institute in 1904 due to political centralism. Without Koch, the institute continued to play an important role as a national research center, but later it succumbed to the racialization of medical science that arose in twentieth-century Germany.[26]

Another of Bismarck's needs was met by the ideal of social hygiene, which was easily linked to the notorious *Rassenhygiene* (racial hygiene). Developed by the renowned social hygienist Alfred Grotjahn (1869–1931), the theory of *Sozialhygiene* appeared at the right time to fit into Bismarck's *Staatsmedizin* design. Grotjahn resented the usurpation of hygiene by bacteriology and chose to follow what by the 1890s was Virchow's nearly forgotten path of examining social factors that contribute to ill health.[27] Unlike social medicine, social hygiene emphasized the need for state control, and its proponents depended on the state to fulfill its goals. Social medicine's proponents, however, especially the socialists, believed that the cause of the problems was political not technical, and they sought to prevent medical problems by changing the political relations of power.[28] Social hygiene relies heavily on laboratory theories of disease and notions of prevention and includes an analysis of the social roots of morbidity and mortality. It does not exclude public hygiene but extends the application of social controls and social enforcement to the population as a whole within four categories of control: moral, social, dietary, and police. The first dealt with moral acts, passions, and intellectual, religious, and educational life. Social control refers to the regulation of issues such as marriage, labor, poverty, charity, and cooperative action. Health controls monitored patterns of nutrition, exercise, sleep, reproduction, and habitation while the police enforced health laws controlling food adulteration, construction of dwellings, and control of epidemics.[29]

The extensive field of research opened up by the new racial degeneration theory of human relations led German physicians to abandon the term *"social medicine"* and to substitute *"social hygiene."* First introduced by Alfred Ploetz (1860–1940) in 1895, in his *Grundlinien einer Rassenhygiene* (Guidelines for Racial Hygiene), the idea of racial hygiene quickly became associated with social hygiene in *Staatsmedizin* after the Weimar Republic in Germany had ended.[30] As an extension of Darwin's work on evolution, Ploetz proposed that intelligent and solitary people be used for reproduction in order to create a better and more just world and that a panel of doctors decide which newborn children would live or die (those selected for death would receive a small dose of morphine).[31] On June 22, 1905, Ploetz founded a society for racial hygiene in Berlin with 350 members (mostly professors), which existed until World War I.[32] The German term *Rassenhygiene* is broader than the word *"eugenics"* and includes all attempts to improve hereditary qualities as well as measures directed toward population growth.[33]

The aim of social hygiene as a total system was to maintain the well-being of the community through a critical examination of the manifestations of social life, tracing these currents to their sources and undertaking regulatory and ameliorative works. In 1915, a series of medical essays following Grotjahn's concept argued that social hygiene had become associated in Germany with national health insurance and was thus too narrow in scope. Taken descriptively, social hygiene should address a wide range of chronic and infectious diseases. Supporters of social hygiene viewed racial degeneration as the basis for the evaluation of disease and thus the central object of concern.[34] Near the end of 1919, the German government passed laws that identified the elimination of poverty as the key issue in social hygiene, stating that without it community well-being would remain unattainable. German physicians then introduced new categories of social behavior (i.e., moral, intellectual, religious, and educational values) into the realm of medical responsibility.[35] Social hygiene was necessarily linked to a normative science that aimed to spread hygienic culture. Thus, in the works of social hygiene proponents general pathology was substituted for socioeconomic analysis and biotechnical engineering replaced economic welfare.[36]

The concepts of state medicine and social hygiene were important in German medicine from imperial Germany to the Weimar Republic. Despite some differences between social medicine and social hygiene, both concepts included an ideological continuum that ranged from primarily economic to primarily biological analysis. Finally, social medicine and social hygiene became a system of sociobiological planning that could be achieved through biotechnical engineering and social control as advocated in the first half of the twentieth century.[37] For its supporters, like the supporters of laboratory medicine, social hygiene depended on scientifically informed, technocratically determined actions by the state. This technocratic vision differentiated the ideas of social hygiene from social medicine theories in which the vision of the state was political rather than technical, and it was this vision that encouraged German medical reformers to support state medicine.[38] Actually, social hygiene and racial hygiene have much in common and were not incompatible strategies for improving national health. Until recently, there was a tendency in literature addressing the history of social medicine to view social hygiene as an unambiguously progressive discipline in contrast to the racist and reactionary racial hygiene movement.[39]

During the early years of the twentieth century, German *Staatsmedizin* expanded rapidly. By the turn of the century, most German cities had established health departments with their own medical bureaucrats and professionals on their staff. The head of the department was usually a bureaucrat with medical training, and the other members of staff included bacteriologists, sanitary engineers, statisticians, educators, and health inspectors, many of whom had some professional training. Germany became a leader in the field of medical reform, and so when Japan adopted its modernization policy in the Meiji period, it chose Germany as its model. Japanese medical experts were deeply influenced by German medicine and were well acquainted with developments in Germany at least until the 1940s. Did Japanese experts fully or partially learn German medicine? How much did they learn from England? And, finally, how did members of the Japanese medical elite create colonial medicine from their German-Japanese model?

Medical Westernization in Meiji Japan

By the late nineteenth century, state sponsorship of medicine was a major feature of medical reform in both Germany and Meiji Japan, which adopted it in the 1870s.[40]

In Asia, missionaries sporadically introduced Western medicine to Qing China (1644–1912), but it did not fundamentally impact the health conditions there. The same was true in nineteenth-century Japan. Before the Meiji regime officially took up the German medical model, the Tokugawa government (1603–1867) occasionally employed Western practices that had been learned from Dutch or Prussian physicians, but it did not systematically adopt Western medicine.[41] The Meiji government almost duplicated Germany's three primary achievements—the establishment of state medicine, the study of bacteriology, and the implementation of social hygiene—and later transferred them to Taiwan. The major difference between the Japanese and German forms was not in the administrative structure but in the way it was implemented.

The arrival of Commodore Matthew Perry of the United States in Japan in 1853 marked the end of more than 480 years of *sakoku jidai* (seclusion). This event heightened Japanese awareness of Western technology. The shogunate government showed great ambivalence in dealing with the American challenge.[42] In fact, before the Meiji Restoration in 1867, the *bakufu* government was already familiar with Western medicine. In Tokugawa Japan, European learning equaled *Rangaku* ("Dutch learning"), for the Dutch were the only westerners allowed even limited access to Japan. Beginning in the late eighteenth century, a group of dedicated Japanese scholars wrestled with the difficulties of the Dutch language and laboriously made the first translations, compiled the first dictionaries, and published the first Western treatises on subjects such as geography, astronomy, medicine, and other sciences.[43] In this turbulent era, Japanese reactions to Western medicine varied widely. From their residence in Deshima, Nagasaki, many Dutch doctors introduced their knowledge of Western medicine to the Japanese. Some Japanese, however, had an absolute hatred of everything Western. John Bower portrays Chinese and Western medicine in Tokugawa Japan as "fundamentally divergent" and in conflict with each other.[44] The first half of the nineteenth century, however, saw an increase in private physicians' interest in Western medicine (especially German medical texts written in the Dutch language).[45] For example, Hiraga Gennai (1728–79) was a traditional physician who studied Dutch medical texts in translation. The physicians Takano Chôei (1804–50), Itô Genboku (1800–1871), and Kurokawa Ryôan (1817–90) organized the first Western medical group and advocated Western medicine to the shogun.

Several schools of Western medicine appeared in late Tokugawa society. For example, Hermann Katz (resident in Japan in 1661–62) influenced the establishment of the Arashiyama-Katsuragawa School. The other school in the late Tokugawa period was the Narutaki School in Narutaki outside of Nagasaki City. A surgeon, Philipp Franz von Siebold (1786–1866; resident in Japan in 1823–29), founded the Narutaki School with the sponsorship of Narabayashi Sôken. Siebold, a German physician, was hired by the Dutch government to treat the employees of the Dutch factory in Nagasaki.[46] Some Japanese physicians, including Minato Chôan (?–1838) and Mima Junzô (1795–1825), were trained in both Chinese and Western medicine.[47]

Despite the introduction of Western medicine into Tokugawa society, medical practice at the beginning of the Meiji period was still largely in the Chinese tradition. Surveys undertaken between 1874 and 1890 revealed the dominance of Chinese medicine in Meiji medical practice (table 1.1).[48]

TABLE 1.1. Growth of the Number of Doctors in Japan

Year	Number of Doctors	Notes
1874	28,262	82% trained in Chinese medicine
1880	38,322	No detailed records
1890	40,215	21.28% trained in Western medicine
		78.72% already in practice[a]

Source: Takenaka, *The Development of Social, Educational, and Medical Work,* 39.

[a]That these physicians were already in practice indicates that most were traditional doctors or healers.

Medicine in the Tokugawa period pioneered the abandonment of home treatments and the publication of medical texts. Doctors were not as close to the centers of political power and kept their place in the private sector, which left them relatively free of official restraints on the new ideas and procedures that were disseminated through these texts.[49]

The Meiji Restoration, as its name implies, was backward looking. It sought to reconnect the emperor's new government with the Japanese people so as to create a more patriotic population. While on the surface Meiji leaders embraced Western-style reforms, in reality they preserved many traditional social structures, one of the most important of which was the samurai.[50] Most doctors in the early Meiji period came from the samurai class, a small, educated minority within the total population. Most doctors of Western medicine in this period had fathers with connections to Tokugawa intellectuals—Confucian scholars, scholars of Dutch studies, or Sino-Japanese-style doctors.[51]

Samurai families had a high regard for Confucianism,[52] and the characteristically Confucian "intimacy between mentors and pupils" became a virtue in Japanese medical circles.[53] In the list of 1,505 Japanese holders of medical doctorates in 1925, 95.7 percent were from samurai families. Among them, 87.32 percent had married into another doctor's family. Kurô Iseki in 1925 claimed that the Japanese medical professionals had a problem with "self-centralism," excessive concern for self-interest and personal connections.[54] That is, the first concern of these physicians was themselves, their teachers and students second, and friends third.[55] Generally speaking, it is a safe guess that the Confucian discipline of filial piety was extended from within samurai families to medical professionals, and the teacher-pupil relationship functioned like a family tie.

The Meiji physicians quickly put into effect the new medical and public health policies they favored. Some of their quick success may have been due to the broad use of the Jennerian vaccination after 1849.[56] The success of the vaccination program helped legitimize Western medicine and gained support for medical westernization. Some traditional physicians who were also trained in Western medicine eventually became leaders in the medical reforms of the Meiji government.

In early Meiji Japan, Western medicine was seen as an integral part of Western power and culture, not as a politically neutral science or benign welfare program. Prior to 1867, Japan had proved to be a particularly infertile ground for Western medicine. The restored Meiji government in 1867 decided to adopt Western medicine as part of its broader modernization effort. Following the strong recommendation of the Rev. Guido Verbeck (1830–98), an American missionary of Dutch ancestry, the Meiji government accepted Sagara Tomoyasu's (1836–1906) proposal and chose Germany as the model for Japan's medical westernization.[57] Only after the Meiji government issued the Ise (Medical Regulations) in 1874 did the westernized system of medical service become the model for state medicine in Japan, a model that eventually inspired medical modernization in other East Asian countries.

Adopting Western medicine was no easy matter, however. An entire institutional infrastructure had to be built from scratch, and it was accepted that the training and deployment of personnel would probably take at least a generation. Also there was not just one version of Western medicine to emulate. From the viewpoint of the Japanese reformers, there were two primary models: British hospital-based, clinically oriented medicine, which had a partial foothold in the country;[58] and the German university-based system, which gave greater prominence to scientific training and laboratory work and at the time held the position of world leadership. In the end, the latter was chosen. As William Johnston points out, German medical thought became increasingly influential as the Meiji period progressed, and educators required all medical students to study the German language.[59]

In addition, during the late nineteenth century Germany was transformed from an agricultural to an industrial society. Unlike Britain and France, where a similar transformation began earlier and extended over a longer period of time, German industrialization, to use Ralf Dahrendorf's well-known aphorism, "occurred late, quickly, and thoroughly."[60] Germany's success as a latecomer inspired many Japanese reformers in the early Meiji period when the introduction of German medicine reached its peak. After the German victory over France in the French-Prussian War (1870–1871) the Japanese, especially those in charge of the military, became more and more interested in the Prussian rise to power. Yamagata Aritomo (1838–1929), the military reformer of Choshu *han*,[61] who was one of the victors in the civil war, had gone on a long military inspection trip to Europe. On returning home, in his reports to the emperor he advocated the implementation of the Prussian military system.[62] When he later became the Vice Minister of War, he made sure that two military students were among the first Japanese scholars to leave for Berlin. One of them, Satô Susumu (1845–1921), was later to become a general medical officer in the Japanese army.[63] Therefore, before the Meiji government formally announced the adoption of the German medical program, the army had already included German medicine in its own military reforms.

Medical reform in the army eventually brought about a decisive turn in Japan's medical westernization program. That began when Sagara Tomoyasu officially recommended German medicine to the Meiji government in 1869 and cited the experience of the army. The relationship between medical reformers and the Japanese military was very close. The first German scientists to be recruited as teachers by the German diplomatic representative in Japan were two Prussian army medical surgeons. They laid the foundations of Western medical training, which were closely linked to the German system, even including German and Latin as required foreign languages. Adopting the Prussian system of education obviously implied opening the doors of Japanese institutions to German medical reform. After 1871, the Japanese government invited German doctors to serve in the army, in universities, and even the imperial court. In fact, German doctors brought Western medicine to Japan almost exclusively, and the Faculty of Medicine at Tokyo University was also in the hands of German professors and their Japanese students.[64] German scholars introduced their disciplines and established their own departments at the newly founded Tokyo University and, like the German doctor Erwin Baelz (1849–1913), who remained in Japan for more than twenty-five years (1876–1902), taught whole generations of Japanese students.[65] With Japanese students enrolled at universities in Berlin, the subject of medicine, along with law, economics, military science, and politics, played a significant role in placing a specifically German imprint on the medical, as well as political and social, development of modern Japan.

The number of German experts in Japan peaked in 1887–88 when approximately seventy to eighty resided in the country. Soon the German language not only provided the technical terms of medicine but also served as the *lingua franca* of the Japanese medical profession.[66] Meanwhile, the Japanese Ministry of Education awarded most of its grants to students studying in major German medical schools such as Berlin University and the Academy of War, which were then ranked highest among all German universities. These schools had a formative influence on the education of the future medical elite of Japan. Berlin University was the school most frequented by Japanese students; between 1870 and 1905, a total of 448 Japanese students were enrolled there. Of those students the largest number, about 42 percent, studied medicine.[67] Contacts with German physicians in Japan meant that Japanese medical students, both at home and abroad during their studies in Germany, made remarkably rapid progress. By the end of the Meiji period, Japanese medicine was enjoying world renown for its successes in bacteriology. Kitasato Shibasaburo (1852–1931), for instance, who was a pupil of Koch in Berlin from 1884 to 1891, developed vaccines against rabies and diphtheria and discovered the bacillus that causes bubonic plague.[68]

Bacteriology was not the only thing that Japanese doctors learned from their German mentors. The German physicians, whose political and social outlook was shaped in Bismarck and Kaiser Wilhelm's Germany, saw themselves as an elite whose main task was to protect the monarchical order and the German race from subversive and foreign influences.[69] Japanese doctors adopted this same self-image. They were greatly affected by German scholars' ideology, and were eager to adopt policies of state medicine and social hygiene from their German teachers. Those ideas reached Japan through the advocacy of both German experts living there and Japanese students studying overseas. One of these Japanese students, Kuwata Kumazo, applied his German teachers' ideology to Japan after a prolonged study trip to Germany. He suggested that Japan should remind itself of its social responsibilities and resolve the growing medical problems of its population.[70]

Gotô Shinpei (1859–1932), a "founder of modern medicine in colonial Taiwan," spent three years in Berlin where he adopted the idea of combining state medicine and social hygiene.[71] Early medical elites in Japan, like Gotô, were soon affected by Virchow's theory of social medicine, Bismarck's ideas about social policy, and Herbert Spencer's concept of social Darwinism.[72] A key concept among the Meiji medical elite was expressed by Gotô as a *seibutsugakû genri* (biological principle), a term that denoted a medical "social Darwinism" or, more simply, the "survival of the fittest" in medical matters. The Meiji medical elite, and certainly Gotô, usually preferred the term

Biologische principien, in part because it was German but also because it was "scientific" and implied the application of biological knowledge in order to promote Japanese survival in the face of global competition.[73]

If Japanese medicine during the early Meiji era bore the marks of German influence, recent studies reveal that Japan did not adopt the German medical model without modification and in fact had its own interpretation and definition of state medicine and social hygiene.[74] Japanese state medicine had some difficulties in the early period, such as insufficient manpower, poor quality of medical education, and dual systems of medical practice, but it was successful in establishing a centralized system to implement German *Staatsmedizin* and was even more successful in using Bismarck's idea of social hygiene to train medical and hygienic practitioners. However, before the Japanese occupied Taiwan in 1895 most of these important changes occurred in urban areas and inside the government. The executive capability and influence of Japanese state medicine may not have extended to rural areas and did not necessarily become a part of common daily life until later.

Sanitary Policemen

The modernizing Meiji government appropriated German concepts of state medicine, social hygiene, and regulation by the police, and the police system played a crucial role in the Japanese state medical system. Meiji reformers such as Fukuzawa Yukichi (1853–1901) and Ishiguro Tadanori (1845–1941) were particularly quick to establish state medical institutions. The idea of a hierarchically organized and bureaucratically managed medical force appealed to late-nineteenth-century Japanese policymakers, and when the Meiji police system was organized in 1874 the police were placed in charge of supervising sanitation and public health affairs. In 1877, the Meiji government formally announced that it would adopt the Prussian state medicine system. In 1879, the central government ordered all prefectural governments to form their own sanitation departments, and in 1886 the Ministry of the Home Affairs put county police forces in charge of enforcing most health and hygiene regulations at the local level.[75] Sanitary policemen usually had the right to arrest persons for unhealthy behavior, such as spitting in the street, to check the hygienic conditions of a household, to examine food and drink in the market, and most important, to enforce "sanitary law."

However, the police system in state medicine combined both evolving Japanese and German features. The idea of policing the public for medical and hygienic reasons was not an innovation that Japan learned totally from Germany. The written record clearly shows that as early as the seventh century, and also in the tenth, Japan had thoroughly adopted the Chinese system for monitoring diseases. Provincial and capital officials were charged with immediately reporting pestilence.[76] The tradition of officials monitoring certain diseases continued up to the Tokugawa period, and local policemen were in charge of reporting venereal diseases and illnesses such as leprosy.[77] In fact, the reorganization of the police system in 1874 only adapted a traditional police system to fit the specific needs of the Meiji modernization. Later, in 1884, a German police officer named William Hoehn trained a special unit of Japanese policemen, which from then on was considered to be the guarantor of social order and public health in Tokyo. This change was really the start of a police system that would enforce the traditional and modern functions of state medicine. From 1884 to 1891, Hoehn ran a police school in Tokyo where all the top officers of the Japanese police were required to attend special courses on medicine and community hygiene. After closing the school, Hoehn embarked on a series of wide-ranging inspection tours to ensure that the Japanese police force had been organized in the Prussian way all over the country.[78] It is possible to say that the Japanese sanitary police system in the Meiji period was inspired by the German system, but it had its roots in Japanese tradition.

Dual Systems of Medical Services

When the Japanese introduced state medicine into their medical westernization program, the tendency was to place great value on the achievements of German medicine. However, Chinese medicine already had a long history in Japan and was supported by a large group of physicians. Facing strong resistance from traditional physicians and their patients, the new medical education could not immediately supply enough professionals to accomplish medical reform. To bypass these barriers, in the late 1870s Japanese authorities held licensing examinations for doctors practicing Chinese medicine. In the subsequent years, several similar examinations were held, and supporters of Sino-Japanese medicine were allowed to build Chinese medical schools according to the standards of Western medical education such as required training in medical schools and a fixed period of internship.[79] Although the number of officially practicing doctors of traditional medicine dropped over time, Chinese medicine still had its share of adherents in the Japanese medical care system. In short, because of manpower shortages and resistance from traditional physicians Japan did not completely "westernize" its medical system. In 1887, it finally settled on an approximation of the German state medical system when the Central Bureau of Sanitation accepted traditional medicine as a legitimate medical specialization.[80]

As they developed state medicine, the Japanese modified not only German medical technology and institutions but also German ideology and values. Like the cameralism in German state medicine, the nationalism in Japanese modern medicine was essential and even stronger. The traditional values of being a doctor—mercy, and talent—were not only the main criteria in treating a patient but the best way to serve the state. One way in which the medical elite in Japan were influenced by German ideas of state medicine and traditional values was that they advocated the social responsibility of doctors to serve the state in the interest of patients. Accepting the role of simultaneously serving the state and society, Japanese medical elites at one point tried to change the title of Western-trained doctors to *gokenshi* (health protection officials), which emphasized that the doctors' duties were authorized and legitimized by the emperor and the Japanese empire. Although *gokenshi* never successfully replaced the common title, *ishi*, in Japanese society, physicians in the Meiji period acted like missionaries of state medicine and needed an official capacity in which to work in the centralized structure of state medicine.[81]

Nationalization of Medical Facilities

The ideological differences between Japanese and German state medicine were also revealed in the process of *kokuyoka* (nationalization). In the beginning, however, *kokuyoka* meant the incorporation of private medical facilities into the structures of the state. Unlike the case in Germany, the Japanese government attempted to own all of the institutions needed to run the state medical system. For instance, after Kitasato returned from Germany, Nagayo Sensai and Fukuzawa Yukichi proposed the establishment of a research institute for him. In 1892, the Institute of Infectious Disease was established as a private entity because Kitasato refused to work in a university, especially Tokyo University, and the government could not afford to support it. In Germany, the state always supported research institutes, private and public. However, Japan did not choose to follow the German path in this respect. In 1893, Kitasato's supporters asked the state to take over the institute. Many medical bureaucrats, including Gotô Shinpei and the chancellor of Tokyo Imperial University, Aoyama Tanemichi, believed that nationalization was the only way to implement state medicine and that private institutes would weaken its development. Despite Kitasato's opposition, the Institute of Infectious Disease was finally centralized; in 1899, it was placed under the supervision of the Ministry of the Home Affairs, which transferred it to the Ministry of Education in 1914. Finally, in 1916, the institute was put under the jurisdiction of Tokyo Imperial University.[82]

Several other institutes were centralized or established by the state: the National Serum Academy (centralized from the Institute of Infectious Disease in 1896), the Institute of Microbiology at Osaka University (established by the state in 1932), and the Institute of Public Health (established by the state under the supervision of Tokyo Imperial University in 1938).[83] Through these institutes, the Japanese government controlled virtually every resource in the medical system. In Japan, the university, rather than research institutes as in Germany, became the major place to promote state medical policy. The Japanese put more trust in public than private institutions, perhaps because government service was more prestigious. In addition, the educational curriculum in universities guaranteed that medical ethics would serve all the needs of the state. It thus follows that despite Germany's influence over Japan's medical reform Japanese state medicine was more integrated and authoritarian than the German model.

One traditional influence on Japanese medical westernization came from the hierarchical structure of Japanese society. Many medical reformers in Meiji Japan believed that *hôken jidai* (feudalism) had been overcome and the newly unified national state was looking ahead to a bright, progress-filled future. These reformers still regarded patriotism not as a natural thing but as a specifically Japanese traditional virtue.[84] For example, the hierarchical structure in universities exactly mirrored Japanese society and reinforced the medical elite's conviction that they were the select group meant to spiritually and morally educate the common people.

By the early 1890s, Japanese medical education had been established as a three-tiered, pyramidal system. At the apex of the pyramid, the medical department at the Tokyo Imperial University (1877–1945) and other medical departments in the imperial university system were established to fulfill the goal of medical westernization. The medical graduates of the imperial university were called *igakushi*, holders of a bachelor's degree in medicine. University graduates in the Meiji era were very elite and were expected to study German and absorb advanced training from Germany.[85] The second tier consisted of *igaku-senmongakkô* (medical colleges), which were medical vocational schools attached to high schools.[86] As high schools were the preparatory schools for the imperial universities, the medical colleges were considered to be above secondary education but below the level of the imperial universities. The colleges were institutionalized in order to produce professionals rapidly, but their lack of training in German meant that they depended on the knowledge that filtered down from the university elite.

Both university and college graduates could practice medicine without passing further examinations. On the other hand, there was another path to becoming a doctor: passing a Ministry of Home Affairs examination open to those without any educational background in medicine.[87] Tsuneo Ozeki has studied the career patterns of graduates from Tokyo University, finding that most of the university graduates became practitioners in various public hospital and government facilities while doctors of the lower ranks practiced in private dispensaries.[88] A rapid rise in the number of medical graduates and increasing competition in the job market between 1900 and 1910 meant that even university graduates had to work in private dispensaries due to the competition for positions in public hospitals. The hierarchical structure in Japanese medicine remained. When the Great Japan Medical Association was established in 1916, it was led and controlled by the *kaigyôi* (private clinicians), but a considerable proportion of the leading doctors consisted of university graduates.[89]

The Japanization of German Medicine

Japan started its medical westernization program in 1870 by studying German *Staatsmedizin, Sozialmedizin,* and *Sozialhygiene.* In the following years, state medicine in Japan was deeply inspired by social hygiene theory, which had become more centralized and technocratic. Moreover, as a disciple of the German empire in the 1870s, the Meiji government seemed to admire the concept of social hygiene more than social medicine. That concept was introduced to Japan by many German-trained physicians in the early Meiji era and was called *shakai eisei* (translated from the German *Sozialhygiene*) to distinguish it from individual hygiene. The theory of social hygiene in Japanese medicine, unlike that in the United States, was formed mainly under the influence of social democracy and the social reform movement.[90] At the beginning of the Meiji Restoration, teaching and research in Japanese public health took place under the rubric of general hygiene, and courses in general hygiene taught between 1870 and 1890 took an environmental approach to public health. Leading hygienists such as Matsumoto Ryôjun and Nagayo Sensai emphasized the impact of air, climate, and water on health and made proposals for sanitary reform.[91] Advances in bacteriology led Japanese general hygiene in another direction. Some bacteriologists attempted to take over the teaching of public health using recent successes in the laboratory, but not all general hygienists were convinced that their field could be confined to the laboratory. They recommended that courses on community and social hygiene be introduced to broaden the curriculum.

Academics at Tokyo and Kyoto Universities were the first to develop the theory of social hygiene in Japan. For instance, Tsuboi Jirô (1862–1903) was a second-generation social hygienist and the first dean of the medical school at Kyoto Imperial University. His career revealed how the theory of social hygiene spread from Tokyo University to other major universities. Since Tsuboi's father was an active medical reformer in the early Meiji period, Tsuboi probably knew something about German medicine before he attended Tokyo University. After graduation, he taught social hygiene at the university's Department of Hygiene. In 1890, he went to Germany and studied under Max von Pettenköfer at Ludwig Maximilian University in Munich. The study of social hygiene was encouraged by Nagayo and Mori Ôgai. Both were important medical reformers and believed that Tsuboi's studies would promote the development of the Japanese race in terms of global competition.

Between 1895 and 1903, Tsuboi served as a sanitary adviser to the Board of Mineworkers, the Kyoto Sanitation Committee, and the Taiwanese colonial government.[92] Tsuboi's multiple roles of hygienist, educator, and sanitation adviser were common for first- and second-generation Japanese social hygienists.

According to Takizawa Toshiyuki's study on social hygiene in Japan, the theory of social hygiene there stated that the target group for such policies—laborers, poor people, and consumers of medical services—should be encouraged to incorporate more self-government and autonomy into their lives. Japanese social hygienists conducted research on such diverse subjects as demography, the problems of collective life, nutrition, addiction, sexual life, and labor, to name but a few. In their prescriptive work, they were encouraged by the state to believe that social hygiene was relevant to all aspects of modernization.[93] In the middle Meiji era, the term *shakai eisei* was coined by Gotô Shinpei in an article.[94] Later Fukuhara Yoshie and Kunisaki Teidô developed the foundation for Japanese social hygiene theory at Tokyo Imperial University between 1896 and 1916.[95] Hoshino Tetsuo, a social hygienist in the late 1930s, emphasized the important link between health and human culture. He strongly believed that a "healthy" human culture could be created through the promotion of human health and that only a healthy population could build a strong country—a concept that would later prevail in the Taishô (1912–25) and Shôwa (1926–89) periods.[96]

The continuous agitation and advisory work of social hygienists eventually yielded positive results. From the 1890s on, medical services that had previously been accessible only to the urban middle and upper classes were offered to more people, and regular visits to a professional doctor became increasingly common. From the beginning of the twentieth century, more and more cities extended and intensified their communal health services. The National Health Insurance Act was passed in 1938, and the number of hospitals consequently rose from 63 in 1875 to 4,732 in 1940.[97] As public health measures advanced,

Japanese social hygiene became a crucial component of social policy. Communal health services were offered to compensate for the risks to life inherent not only in the industrial mode of production but also in the social conditions connected with state development. At the same time, they were meant to facilitate the process of social integration by introducing the lower classes to official standards of health and cleanliness. In the long run, education and social control were seen as ways to close the cultural gap between the various social classes.[98] Good health, the ability to work, and decent morals all seemed to be aspects of social hygiene, and the state investment in physical fitness and efficiency paid off. These developments led in two directions. On the one hand, the emphasis on catching up with medical advances in the West called attention to the development of bacteriology and public health. On the other, the growing emphasis on social responsibility directed attention toward the value of preventive hygiene. Like some Germans, many Japanese physicians began to stress the importance of social conditions as a cause of disease.[99] This led to the development of Japanese social hygiene.

Japanese social hygiene bore some resemblance to both traditional Japanese community medicine and German *Sozialhygiene*. Social hygiene was not merely a medical idea. In Japan, medicine and medical ethics seem to have been influenced at an early stage by social Darwinism. Japanese such as Fukuzawa advocated social Darwinism in the mid-1870s. They viewed medical reform as one vast struggle for existence dominated by the "survival of the fittest." This motive stimulated a variety of medical reforms, ranging from a drive to improve public morals to the establishment of social hygiene as a means of survival.[100] Thus, social hygiene was established both as a discipline in medical schools and as a research field in specialized government institutes.[101]

Despite its association with social Darwinism, early Japanese medical reformers seemed hesitant about German *Rassenhygiene* (racial hygiene) until the 1920s. Although George Fredrickson thinks the fact that "the traditional belief of the Japanese that only people of their own stock can truly understand and appreciate their culture" reveals racist tendencies among the Japanese elite, the German concept of *Rassenhygiene* was not foremost in the establishment of Japanese state medicine before the 1940s.[102] It was not until after the Japanese Society for Racial Hygiene was established in late 1930 and began to publish its academic journal in 1931 that some German *Rassenhygiene* issues were introduced.[103] Before that, a eugenic argument about how to improve the Japanese race was a key aspect of Japanese racial hygiene, which seems to more closely resemble international *Eugenik* (eugenics) than *Rassenhygiene*.[104]

Evidence presented in the final chapter of this book indicates that before 1945 Japanese medical professionals never reached enough common ground to fully accept German *Rassenhygiene*.

Another Japanese modification of German medicine was the close relationship between the medical and pharmaceutical establishments, which greatly influenced postwar Japan as well as Taiwan.[105] Rejecting a separation between prescribing and dispensing, Japan gave the right to dispense to the doctor. The Japanese Ise (Medical Regulations) of 1874 were virtually identical to a German law issued in 1801.[106] Likewise, Japanese regulations for the pharmaceutical industry were drawn from a copy of the German *Revidierte Apothekerordnung* (Revised Pharmaceutical Regulations), which were issued the same year.[107] According to the original regulation 41, the pharmaceutical industry in Japan, with the exception of traditional herbal medicine (i.e., Chinese and Japanese medicine), had to strictly separate prescribing and dispensing.[108] In 1884, only ten years after the issuance of the Medical Regulations, this rule was modified due to "different social conditions and the historical heritage of herbal medicine in our country [Japan]."[109]

According to the new regulation, the government allowed private practitioners to operate dispensaries where the functions of prescribing and dispensing were combined under the supervision of dispensary clinicians.[110] The reason given for this change—the "different social conditions and historical heritage of herbal medicine"—strongly indicates that doctors of Western medicine were an elite power in the process of Japanese medical westernization and that compromises were made in accordance with the customary way in which Chinese medical therapies were dispensed. After obtaining the right to dispense, private pharmaceutical clinics soon outnumbered public hospitals and became the most common type of medical facility for the rest of the twentieth century.[111] Describing the structural characteristics of Japanese medicine in 1970s, Brian Abel-Smith notes, "the extreme development of open access is to be found in Japan where it is common for the doctor to have his own little 'hospital' at his place of practice."[112]

During the first half of the twentieth century, professional training for Japanese pharmacists was not an issue of foremost importance. In 1873, the Department of Manufacturing Pharmacy in the Faculty of Medicine of the University of Tokyo was established to train pharmacists to dispense imported Western drugs. Pharmaceutical laboratories, not regular pharmacies, were the main workplaces of these university graduates. Only twenty-nine schools of pharmacy (equal to the high school level) were built in the Meiji era; however, twenty of these schools closed after the revision of regulation 41 in 1884 and the rapid increase in pharmaceutical clinics.[113] Meanwhile, in the early Meiji period the government was the major importer, as well as distributor, of Western drugs.[114] During the Taishô era and the first half of the Shôwa, seventeen pharmaceutical colleges (on the same level as the medical colleges) were built while universities continued to train pharmaceutical professionals in laboratories.[115] The majority of graduates worked as regular pharmacists. Chart 1.1 shows the hierarchical relationship between medical practitioners and pharmacists along with the training of each group.

CHART 1.1. Careers of Japanese medical and pharmaceutical professionals, 1884–1945. Shaded areas indicate major activities. (Data from Koseisho, *Iseihyakunenshi,* 45–47; and Yamakawa, "A History of a Hundred Years of Pharmaceutical Education in Japan," 446–51.)

Training	Medicine	Pharmacy	Botanical Pharmacognosy
Professional/elite (university)	Governmental facilities and private dispensaries	Few in research institutes	Only in botanical research
Vocational (college)	Majority in private dispensaries	Majority in regular pharmacies	Few in pharmaceutical factories
Lay practitioners and others	Rare after the 1920s	Pharmacies and drugstores	Majority in botanical drugstores

The revision of regulation 41 in 1884 did not bode well for Japanese pharmacists. To survive, Japanese botanical pharmacists took advantage of a shortage of imported medicine during the Sino-Japanese (1894–95) and Russo-Japanese (1904–05) wars. In 1885, *kanbô* (herbal medicine) was revamped to produce Western-style over-the-counter (OTC) drugs. However, the importation of Western drugs in Meiji Japan proceeded without interruption. The market for herbal medicine was continuously shrinking due to the increasing popularity of Western medicine, both imported and domestically produced. The shortage of imported medications caused by World War I frequently interrupted the flow of Western medicines and eventually increased the domestic demand for herbal medicines as a substitute. The major change occurred just after the first world war when the first generation of pharmaceutical scientists returned from Germany to begin large-scale production of medicines using German methods. Until the 1940s, German pharmaceutical standards provided the guidelines for Japanese prescription medicines, OTC drugs, and even so-called "scientific Chinese medicines."[116]

The revision of the *Nihon Yakkyokuho* (Japanese Pharmacopoeia) in 1891 also promoted scientific Chinese medicine. The first edition of the *Pharmacopoeia,* published in 1886, was a translation of its German counterpart, *Deutsches Arzneibuch.*[117] The revision greatly expanded the Western category of pharmaceutical botanicals and included many materials from traditional Chinese medicine.[118] The second edition of the *Pharmacopoeia* gave new criteria for the classification of medicine into three categories: fundamental medicine; OTC drugs; and botanical medicine. In the 1891 edition, scientific Chinese medicine was classified as legal and was listed in the official *Pharmacopoeia.* The Western classification of prescription medicine and OTC drugs vanished in the *Pharmacopoeia* after 1891 and was replaced by a hybrid standard that combined scientific manufacturing and experiential effectiveness. Medicine that fit either criteria would be considered legal if dispensed by means of a doctor's prescription and a pharmacist's sale. While pharmacists in Japan had lost the sole right to dispense medicine to private practitioners, they may have been compensated by their ability to sell prescription medicines and botanicals as modern OTC drugs with no clear differentiation between them.

In general, the medical elite in Meiji Japan seemed concerned about their traditional duties while retaining their great faith in German medicine. They clustered around the imperial house, patriotism prevailed, and fraternalism gave rise to the goals of state medicine. These thoughts framed a German-style medical system in Japan. In short, advocates of medical westernization in Japan saw working for the glory of the new state and the health of society as their historical responsibilities, which were mixed up with the elite's traditional role in Japanese society and the expectation of a doctor's social responsibility in German *Staatsmedizin.*

Ambiguous Concepts in Japanese Colonial Medicine

Modifying elements of German medicine to meet health needs in Japan, and later in colonial Taiwan, was a tedious and vague process. Numerous terms have been used to describe modern medicine in Japan and its evolution: *public hygiene, social medicine, social hygiene, preventive medicine, state medicine, sanitary engineering,* and *public health.* According to official documents, the colonial government in Taiwan only enforced the *shakai eisei* (social hygiene) and *koshū eisei* (public hygiene) programs. In fact, the term *"public health"* (*gonggong weisheng* in Chinese, *kokyô eisei* in Japanese) did not appear until medical experts from the Rockefeller Foundation proposed their "American new medicine" in 1938.[119] The term was prevalent in postwar Taiwan but rarely used in the colonial period. However, medical historians usually addressed Japanese *shakai eisei* and *koshû eisei* using a modern concept of public health without considering the nuances of meaning in earlier usage.

The meanings of various confusing Japanese terms related to concepts of sanitation, hygiene, and public health could be, as Ruth Rogaski writes, "impossible to translate into English."[120] Indeed, from the mid–nineteenth to the mid–twentieth centuries, Japanese *eisei* could be translated into many different English words and terms. Instead of a single English translation, I use several terms in order to retain the original meaning(s). For example, the term *eisei,* picked up by Nagayo Sensai from an ancient Daoist text to translate the German *Gesundheitsflege,*[121] is best rendered in English in this context as "health care." Moreover, the wide variety in terminology indicates that more than one set of ideas and objects of inquiry were involved. A cursory glance at the medical westernization program in Japan in the past century highlights the need to reconsider the different meanings of those terms. The confusion surrounding the meaning of terms such as *social hygiene, public hygiene,* and the more modern *public health* was created when the Japanese mixed up German concepts—for example, from the German *Sozialhygiene*—with traditional ideas, which only served to muddy modern historical interpretations.

Fortunately, compound terms in Japanese are much easier to translate accurately than single words. For instance, the term *koshû eisei* is often used incorrectly by historians in a way that presents modern public health as *shakai eisei.* René Sand, the Belgian historian, offers a clear distinction between public hygiene and social hygiene.[122] Public hygiene means the construction of a sanitary urban environment; indeed, it is the science of urbanism itself and essentially includes sanitary engineering and city planning as its tools.[123] Public hygiene deeply relies on mechanical solutions to solve medical problems caused by the urban environment, while social hygiene incorporates the use of medical theories of disease and notions of prevention.[124] It was exactly this case that Iguchi Jowakai discussed in his examination of the relationship between urbanization and hygiene.[125] On the contrary, in the 1930s *shakai eisei* was commonly defined as the German concept that every medical problem is rooted in social problems and only social order and discipline can cure a society and prevent medical crises.[126] Generally speaking, in the Japanese context *shakai eisei* treats a community or country as a whole while *koshû eisei* focuses primarily on urban populations.

In Japanese, *shakai eisei* and *shakai igaku* (social medicine) have almost the same meaning.[127] The similarity of these two terms could be due to their relationship with the original German terms. German theorists of social medicine enthusiastically developed a theme that can be traced to social pathology, a theory that treated society as an organism and interpreted social problems in medical terms.[128] In their studies, they eventually replaced the term *medicine* with *hygiene* in the German context.[129] Edward Reich defined the application of social hygiene as "intended to maintain individual and social health and morality, to destroy the causes of disease and to ennoble man physically and morally."[130] To attain that goal, the state in Japan was given the right to police the population for medical reasons.[131]

In addition, the antisocialism policy adopted after the mid-1920s was catastrophic to social medicine in Japan. Japanese physicians who were seen as socialists or sympathizers of social medicine during the heyday of the left-wing movement in the 1920s were soon expelled or kept under surveillance.[132] Among those physicians, Komiya Yoshitaka (1900–1976), Soda Takemune (1902–1984), and other leftist activists organized the Research Committee for Social Medicine at Tokyo Imperial University. After Komiya and Soda were arrested for "disturbing social order" in 1930, Komiya moved to Shanghai as a scientist at the Institute of Natural Science.[133] Soda worked for the Central Institute of Research in Taiwan and obtained a professorship at Taihoku Imperial University in 1940.[134] In short, although public health arose in nineteenth-century Europe, the concept was rarely mentioned by medical professionals in prewar Japan. Meanwhile, *shakai igaku* was identified as a synonym of *shakai eisei* and brought policing power to Japan, focusing on people who were at high risk for or vulnerable to certain diseases.

It is important to clarify that, although contemporary Japanese and Taiwanese historians of medicine often translate *shakai igaku* or its derivate, *koshū eisei*, as "public health," only *shakai igaku* and *koshū eisei* appeared in prewar Japan. The concepts of *shakai igaku* and *koshū eisei* both arose in the nineteenth century as a way for the state to address the health problems of the society as whole. The differences between public health and social medicine have been identified by the English historian J. Alfred Ryle, who writes that public health is essentially an environmental philosophy regarding the origin and prevention of communicable disease; social medicine, by contrast, unifies preventive and remedial services and encompasses all diseases and the whole spectrum of hospital practice.[135] Although both concepts guided the government in applying statistics to prove the "social postmortem" and define the meaning of "normal" in the measurement of health, subsequent developments in social concepts of health and disease in Japan further elevated the role of medicine at the expense of political and economic analysis.[136] Under the great influence of German medicine, medical professionals in prewar Japan seemed to overlook public health, a concept that was more popular in Britain and France.

German *Rassenhygiene* (racial hygiene) was another ambiguous concept in Japan's medical westernization. As mentioned previously, racial hygiene was an aspect of German state medicine, but its influence on Japanese medicine was not significant. As early as 1900, Baelz had carried out research on racial hygiene, which for a long time Japan claimed was essential to the race.[137] However, when the Japanese Diet passed the National Eugenics Law in 1940, the terms for improvement of the Japanese race were *yûseigaku* (eugenics) and *minzogu eisei* (racial hygiene).[138] The confusion surrounding the definitions of *racial hygiene* and *eugenics* in Japanese scholarship lasted for nearly thirty years and caused the Japanese Society for Racial Hygiene, established in 1930, to have very selective criteria for its membership and research.[139] For our own clarification, Robert Proctor provides a clear way to distinguish *Rassenhygiene* and *Eugenik* in German: *Rassenhygiene* is a German-oriented idea for improving the Aryan race while *Eugenik* is based on an international and "neutral" concept of evolutionary biology.[140]

Two other factors caused the Japanese racial hygienists to accept the ideas of *Eugenik* while keeping the name *minzogu eisei*. As early as 1909, at the annual meeting of the German Society of Racial Hygiene, a debate arose over whether membership in the society should be limited to "whites" or should include "the yellow race."[141] When Ploetz referenced the debate over excluding nonwhite races in his formulation of so-called Nordic supremacy in mid-1910, advocates of racial hygiene in Japan felt humiliated by their skin color and the fact that they spoke a non-Aryan (Indo-European) language.[142] To Japanese racial hygienists, Germany's racially defined *Rassenhygiene* was less acceptable than English eugenics, developed by the naturalist Francis Galton in the 1890s, which was internationally acceptable and could be neutrally applied to a nonwhite race. In addition, the close relationship between overseas Japanese students in the early Meiji period and their Jewish teachers could be another factor that hindered the acceptance of *Rassenhygiene* in Japan. Although *Rassenhygiene* became the essence of Hitler's policy after the 1930s, Japanese medical theorists hesitated to follow in those footsteps.[143] Despite Fan Yanqiu's declaration that the colonial government in Taiwan practiced some aspects of racial hygiene,[144] there were actually several strategies that could be described as representing both social and racial hygiene.

Early Japanese medical reformers knew what and why they learned from Germany. It is also reasonable to suppose that the Japanese knew how and why they wanted to apply certain features of Japanese colonial medicine in Taiwan. By the time the Japanese occupied Taiwan, state medicine in that country was sufficiently institutionalized. The establishment of the Central Bureau of Sanitation, the sanitary police system, centralized medical education, and laboratories was part of the institutionalization process. The increasing formalization of standards for professional practice inevitably affected the composition of the body of officially recognized health care providers. It produced conflicts among university-educated physicians (mostly Western-influenced doctors), traditional doctors trained through apprenticeship, and empirical practitioners with no documentable training at all.

Although the Japanese were eager to demonstrate their success in implementing medical westernization programs, they did not choose Taiwan as their showroom for these programs. Rather, Japanese colonial medicine was developed by historical accident. Originally, Japan's strategy was to defeat Qing China in 1895 and subsequently occupy some major treaty ports; instead, international pressure forced Japan to abandon this original plan and take Taiwan as compensation. In the context of resources, acquiring Taiwan at this time placed a great burden on the Japanese medical elite. Without sufficient manpower and experience, medical professionals in Japan had to adapt state medicine to the needs of this new colony.

Colonial archives in Taiwan contain dossiers on major diseases, public health practitioners, and Japanese-run facilities and reports on epidemics and their eradication. In addition to such practical issues as disease identification and treatment, colonial physicians continually wondered about the relationship between Taiwan's tropical climate and physical degeneration. However, as Mark Harrison points out in his study of the construction of race and environment in medical texts in British India, a hardening of racial bias in theories of human difference in the early nineteenth century underlay the increasing pessimism about acclimatization in the colony.[145] Although microbial "tropical medicine" was immature in the 1890s, it provided new hope to colonial administrations, including those in Japanese Taiwan.[146] Moreover, because of the German impact on medical reform in Meiji Japan the original pattern of medical services in colonial Taiwan was influenced by the German system rather than the British experience in India. In British India, there was serious neglect of public health due to a policy of noninterference with Indian beliefs and customs.[147] A similar situation never arose in colonial Taiwan because of strong interference by the state in its imposition of German/Japanese medicine. Additionally, the conflict between military surgeons and civilian physicians in antimalaria programs in colonial Taiwan (described in chapter 2) shows how Japanese colonial medicine switched from the German to the British type. It is evident that historians can learn far more about modern medicine in colonial Taiwan than they ever thought possible.

Moreover, as described in the review of Western scholarship in the introduction to this volume, academic purpose, socioeconomic impact, and the nature and political significance of colonial medicine often helped drive the development of colonial medicine in general, and colonial Taiwan was no exception. In the following chapters, I examine familiar themes, such as medicine's role in the consolidation of colonial rule and its impact on the Taiwanese population, in a new and more critical context, thus exposing the gap between the rhetoric and the reality of colonial medical policy. In short, I place modern medicine in Taiwan in the context of the debates about state-society issues under Japanese colonialism. Japanese experts of the colonial government drew their blueprint for Taiwan's medical system without considering nonmedical factors in Taiwanese society. However, their original plan was eventually compromised for economic, political, and even cultural reasons. The importation of Japanese state medicine into Taiwan should be viewed as a collective process rather than the achievement of one or two individuals.

Nor should Japanese colonial medicine in Taiwan be viewed in a vacuum. In Taiwan, changing medical knowledge, technologies, and ways to handle related affairs were deeply influenced by medical developments in Japan and Europe. Compared to previous studies of medical development in colonial Taiwan, this book offers a broader focus. For Japanese colonization, the medical infrastructure in colonial Taiwan represents Japan's attempt to emulate European colonial empires and Japanese confidence in exporting their medical knowledge. For the history of medicine, this was the transition period from traditional to scientific medicine. From the beginning of their occupation of Taiwan, the Japanese knew that "tropical climates" could be fatal. Later they came to understand that it was disease, not climate, that killed. This change in etiology was related to the Japanese acceptance of germ theory. From a broader viewpoint, the development of colonial medicine in Taiwan also marked the introduction of modern scientific medicine. Finally, for historical demography the colonial period was crucial to our understanding of mortality and epidemiological transitions. These transitions are also the key to a more global understanding of demographic history.

2

Japanese Colonial Medicine in Taiwan
The Chaotic Beginning

Initially, Taiwan's primitive and dangerous conditions discouraged the ambitions of the Japanese colonizers. From the first year of the occupation (1895), rebellions and epidemics were the primary killers of the transplanted Japanese,[1] notably even a prince consort who died from the plague.[2] According army reports, only one-fifth of the initial wave of Japanese troops had survived by the end of September 1895.[3] Financial deficits also served as a stumbling block for Japanese colonial planners, at one point leading Diet members to attempt to put Taiwan up for international auction.[4] During the first year of occupation, nearly 29 million yen were drawn from Japan, chiefly to meet the cost of subjugating the insurgents. To suppress military resistance and fund public works, 6,940,000 yen were spent in 1896 and 5,959,000 in 1897. However, colonial rule still could not be carried out as effectively as expected. Within three years, three governors-general and four *minsei chokan* (deputy chiefs of civil affairs) resigned because of the ongoing turmoil. Pessimistic views regarding the outcome of Japan's first colonial venture were widespread.[5] In 1895–96, of the 25,000 Japanese soldiers stationed in Taiwan, 90 percent suffered from various illnesses and 2,104 died of their diseases. Although Japan sent medical experts to Taiwan to deal with epidemics and endemic diseases, the famous surgeon Mori Ôgai had to admit failure, stating that sanitary conditions in Taiwan were so bad that it was futile to apply modern medicine.[6]

Another obstacle to providing medical expertise for Taiwan was Japan itself. Medical westernization had begun in Japan only thirty years before its occupation of Taiwan, and Japanese resources for and experience with Western medical practices were still insufficient. Gotô Shinpei (1857–1929), a politician with a medical background, seized the opportunity to rebuild his professional reputation and political career by focusing his attention on this newest territory in imperial Japan. Gotô's plan for establishing a public health administration in colonial Taiwan emphasized two functions of the Japanese system: a sanitary police force and a public medical service. However, Gotô was unable to implement his idea because of personal factors—his family background (he was descended from low-ranking samurai), his mediocre medical education, and obstacles in his political career—as well as various difficulties such as armed resistance and financial deficits in early Japanese-ruled Taiwan. To realize his goals required the help of others who could compensate for his weaknesses.

In contrast to Gotô Shinpei, Takagi Tomoe (1858–1943) was a descendent of a high-ranking samurai clan and one of the famous "Kitasato pupils." After graduation from the Medical College of Tokyo in 1885, Takagi took a position at Fikui Hospital. From 1893 to 1897, he worked in the Kitasato Institute and from 1897 to 1899 at the Koch Institute in Germany. On his return to Japan, Takagi concentrated on epidemic prevention, and in 1902 Gotô Shinpei invited him to serve as a consultant on the anti-epidemic program in Taiwan. Later that year Takagi moved to Taiwan, and by 1904 he was formally in charge of the Department of Sanitary Police and the Central Sanitary Committee of Taiwan (CSCT). He traveled to Europe and the United States for advanced training, represented the colonial government abroad, and published the first book on sanitation in Taiwan. For his contribution to medicine, he was awarded a doctoral degree in 1913.[7] In 1919, he resigned from the government to head the Taiwan Electric Power Company. After Gotô Shinpei's death in 1929, Takagi retired from the power company and returned to Japan. He died in Tokyo at the age of eighty-six.[8] Takagi followed through on Gotô's ideas but compromised Taiwan's medical services by mixing the Western approach with that of local practitioners. Among his contributions in bringing important public health and medical practices to colonial Taiwan were the institutionalization of laboratory medicine, an emphasis on clinical training in medical education, and establishment of the Confucian/samurai concept of the teacher-pupil relationship as the norm within the medical profession.

Through Gotô and Takagi, the hybridized German-Japanese *Staatsmedizin* model was adapted to the needs of colonial Taiwan. The following discussion illuminates how these two colonial administrators utilized this model in developing a Japanese blueprint for medicine during the early colonial period.

Gotô Shinpei's Career as Doctor and Politician

Most Taiwanese historians studying Gotô's career view medicine as the least significant part of his legacy. Although his contemporaries and recent Japanese biographers portray him as an arrogant, ill-tempered politician whose achievements were negligible, his enthusiastic promotion of medical westernization resulted in a substantial improvement in health care in Taiwan.[9]

From Local Practitioner to Deputy Chief of the Central Bureau of Sanitation

Compared to his contemporaries in the early Meiji bureaucracy, Gotô Shinpei was a grand braggart but a mediocre doctor.[10] He practiced medicine for only five years, from 1881 to 1885, and spent almost fifteen years in administrative positions related to public health in Japan.

Gotô was born in 1857 into an old samurai family that turned to agriculture after the Meiji Restoration in 1868. After their loss in status, Gotô's family struggled to retain their heritage of Western learning, and their former glory could not ameliorate their poverty.[11] While Gotô worked at the age of thirteen in the prefectural government as a *kyôji* (low-ranking assistant), the local magistrate, Yasûba Ichihira, supported his education. Gotô completed his primary school education in *Fukushima shôgaku daiichi yogakô* (Western studies) and his *Sukagawa igakkô* (medical school studies) in Fukushima Prefecture. The two schools provided only the most basic education in Western learning and medical training.

By the early 1890s, as discussed in chapter 1, Japanese medical education was established as a three-tiered pyramidal system. *Igakushi* (medical graduates of the imperial university system), were at the apex of the pyramid, and *igaku-senmongakkô* (medical colleges) were primarily designed to train clinicians.[12] Some of the colleges had formerly been *igakkô* (medical schools) such as the school where Gotô studied.[13] The pre-WWII system of medical education in Japan had three layers. Medical training at medical schools (usually the level of vocational high schools) was poor and merely had two or three years of basic clinical knowledge. Medical colleges provided three years of vocational training to clinicians while universities provided four years of high-quality undergraduate training for elite students in both laboratory and clinical medicine. Since a medical school education did not provide sufficient training in German and was merely vocational training for clinicians, Gotô was no way a member of the medical elite. Although both university and college graduates could go into practice without taking further examinations, the license indicated nothing about the quality of a doctor's practice since some examinees with minimum knowledge passed the licensing examination.[14] Unable to rely on family heritage or educational background, Gotô could not become a member of Japan's medical elite through any of the traditional channels.

Gotô graduated from the Sukagawa medical school in 1876 and immediately afterwards served at the Aichiken prefectural hospital as a resident physician. According to the biography written by his son-in-law, Gotô's administrative career began in Aichiken Prefecture. While Gotô was still a resident, he was influenced by two colleagues who were knowledgeable about medical developments in Germany and became a *kensaku byôkanja* (petition addict), flooding local and central government offices with petitions and suggestions recommending Western medical practices and concepts. He believed that medicine could save not only individuals but the whole of society. In 1880, he gave a speech in Nagoya, quoting a familiar Chinese saying: "A regular physician can cure diseases, and a good physician can cure patients, but a brilliant physician could manage the state."[15] Such Chinese moral sayings were fashionable in Japanese medical circles in the Meiji period. Another, "A member of the elite should aspire to be a politician, otherwise a physician," was often quoted to stir ambition in medical students.[16]

In February 1877, *seinan sensô* (civil war) broke out between Saigô Takamori, leader of the Satsuma Rebellion, and the Meiji government. Gotô went to Osaka to help Ishiguro Tadanori at a temporary hospital set up at the front. Ishiguro was one of the founders of *gunjin igaku* (modern military medicine) in Japan and an important promoter of medical westernization in the Meiji government. During their tenure together, Gotô was impressed by Ishiguro's coercive quarantine and isolation measures and the efficiency of military medicine. In addition to Ishiguro Tadanori, in Osaka Gotô met Nagayo Sensai, Takagi Kawahirô, and other members of Japan's new medical elite and built connections with the sanitary administration and medical bureaucracy of the central government.[17] Gotô, still a low-ranking country doctor from the Aichiken hospital, began to pay close attention to the administration of public sanitation and to believe strongly that Western medicine was the path to a strong and healthy Japan.

After returning from Osaka, Gotô began to act more like an administrator than a doctor. He was promoted to deputy chief of the prefectural hospital and became the acting principal of its affiliated medical school, through the support of the prefectural magistrate Yasûba. While in Aichi Prefecture, Gotô built a reputation as a medical educator and a bureaucrat.[18] As early as 1878, he proposed the founding of a sanitary police system in a petition to Yasûba titled *Kanû Aichiken setsuritsu eiseikeiisatsu no kaiiryô* (On the Establishment of Sanitary Police in Aichi Prefecture).[19] Later he revised the proposal and submitted it, along with another proposal to modify the medical school system, to Nagayo Sensai, then the deputy chief of the Chûô eiseigyoku (Central Bureau of Sanitation, or CBS).[20] As Sawada Ken points out, the creation of a modern sanitation administration in Japan relied heavily on Nagayo Sensai's authority in the central government and Gotô Shinpei's implementation.[21] During this period, Gotô enjoyed a close relationship with Nagayo and gradually ingratiated himself with members of the medical elite who supported medical

Westernization. Because of his low-ranking samurai background and mediocre training in medicine, Gotô had to do even more to attract the lasting attention of this elite group. Despite his lack of fluency in German, he published two monographs promoting German *biologische Principien* (biological principles), the primary purpose of which was to serve as a stepping-stone to advance his career in medical administration.[22] The two monographs—*Kokka eisei genri* (The Principles of State Hygiene, 1889)[23] and *Eisei seidôron* (On the Sanitation Administration, 1890)—emphasized the importance and application of German *Staatsmedizin* in medical westernization.[24] In *Kokka eisei genri*, most of Gotô's statements were taken from Louis Pappenheim's *Handbuch der Sanitätspolizei* (Handbook of Sanitary Police), and he repeatedly emphasized the need to adhere to biological principles.[25]

For many Meiji intellectuals, those principles reflected the biological determinism of social Darwinism.[26] The impact of such biological principles on Japan was enormous. Scholars in Meiji Japan were excited by the prospect of founding a science of man based on biological principles, and they quickly began to apply Darwin's principles of natural selection to the ethics of human society.[27] The medical elite wanted to use biological knowledge as a tool to enhance the survival chances of the Japanese in the escalating competition with other societies, notably Western ones.[28] Gotô was heavily influenced by these concepts but did not consider applying them to the colony of Taiwan because practical matters such as the filthy environment and severe epidemics there were a much more urgent priority.

In 1890, Gotô received official permission to study medical administration in Germany. He spent time visiting several universities and government institutes both in Germany and in the United Kingdom. After his return to Japan in 1892 he submitted his *Doktorarbeit* (doctoral thesis)—completed at the Robert Koch Institute in Berlin and titled "Vergleichende Darstellung der Medizinalpolizei und Medizinalverwaltung in Japan und Anderen Staaten" (A Comparative Description of the Medical Police and Medical Administration of Japan and Other States)—to the Ministry of Education in Japan for a doctoral title. Gotô was not interested in laboratory techniques such as bacteriology but paid far more attention to broad questions affecting social medicine. In particular, he was heavily influenced by politician-physician Rudolf Virchow's theory of social medicine and his works on *Kulturkampf*. Virchow meant *Kulturkampf* to be a term of praise, signifying the liberation of public life from sectarian impositions, that is, anticlericalism.[29] In general, Gotô's studies in Germany (he also traveled to England) increased his understanding of state medicine and social welfare systems. We may also assume that his experiences abroad improved his political stature.

In 1892, at the age of thirty-six, Gotô returned to Japan and took a position as deputy chief of the CBS, which he used to aggressively promote a German-style state medicine system for Japan. However, the sanitary administration Gotô supported resembled, but did not duplicate, German *Staatsmedizin*. He was cognizant of the controversies surrounding the German system and willing to compromise. Two major differences were that his administration gave the medical board the power to monitor the sanitary police force and gave doctors the right to dispense medicine. Since the sanitary police were under the executive direction of the CBS, giving power to the medical board threatened the CBS's position as the top administrator of all medical affairs. In addition, giving doctors the right to dispense medicine harmed Gotô's reputation as a supporter of medical modernization because it compromised a very traditional pattern of practicing medicine in Japan. Since sanitary policing was a direct executive power of the CBS, giving that power to the medical board could devastate the CBS's position. There was some disagreement about the role of the CBS at the local level. For example, Ishiguro and Nagayo strongly criticized granting the sanitary police force excessive coercive power.[30] Therefore, the activities of the sanitary police were supervised by the medical board and became an executive force on it. Another compromise Gotô had to tolerate was the relationship between medicine and pharmacology. Regulation 41, which separated the prescribing and dispensing of medicines, in the 1874 Ise (Medical Regulations) was virtually identical to a German law issued in 1801.[31] However, Regulation 41 was revised in 1884, a mere ten years after the Medical Regulations were issued.[32] Because of the compromises made in the 1880s, when Gotô was in charge of the CBS, Japanese state medicine became a hybrid system with elements of both German *Staatsmedizin* and traditional Japanese medicine.

From the Center of the Japanese Empire to a Peripheral Position in Colonial Taiwan

In the 1890s, Japan's medical westernization remained controversial, and most members of the medical elite had little chance to consider the relationship between modern medicine and colonization on the eve of the Sino-Japanese War.[33] Instead, Gotô was still heavily committed to the arguments he had put forth supporting the 1884 revision of the Medical Regulations.[34] Ten years later, in 1894, a scandal known as the Sôma incident seriously damaged Gotô's rising career at the CBS. A member of the Sôma family, which had belonged to Meiji nobility, committed the last lord, Sôma Makotoreki, to an insane asylum, sparking an acrimonious rift among family members. To ease the friction, Gotô Shinpei was invited to examine the lord. The court did not accept Gotô's diagnosis that the lord was mentally unstable and sentenced him to five months in prison for perjury.[35] While in prison, he received emotional and monetary support from his former colleagues Ishiguro and Takagi Tomoe. After Gotô's release, Ishiguro recommended him to General Kodama Gentarô, who presented him with the task of establishing a quarantine station in Ninoshima for veterans of the Sino-Japanese War. In 1895, after the war, Gotô and Takagi were both placed in charge of the quarantine station in Osaka. Within two months, Gotô had established three fully equipped quarantine stations and examined 687 ships and more than 232,000 soldiers.[36] During his stay in Ninoshima, Gotô worked closely with Takagi. To prevent an outbreak of cholera, Gotô helped Takagi produce an anticholera serum, thus initiating the first mass immunization against this disease in modern medical history.[37] Although Gotô's efforts in Ninoshima helped him win back his former position at the CBS in August of 1895 and build strong connections with several of the elite in the medical community, he was never able to fully regain the support of Premier Itô Hirobumi and thus could not put what he had learned in Germany into practice in Japan.[38]

Despite Gotô's professional frustrations, his relationship with Takagi and General Kodama remained close. Kodama helped Gotô build his reputation in military medical administration. When Kodama was appointed governor of colonial Taiwan in 1897, Gotô was invited to serve as deputy chief of civil affairs.[39] Five years later, because of the ongoing conflict between the Kitasato Institute and Tokyo Imperial University, Gotô seized the opportunity to invite Takagi to resign from his position at Keio University to become an *eisei komon* (consultant on sanitary affairs) and assist in Taiwan's medical reforms. In short, both General Kodama's political support and Takagi's scholarship helped drive Gotô's reform plans in Taiwan.

Kitasato Shibasaburo and Colonial Medicine

The field of bacteriology and related knowledge about infectious diseases also significantly aided medical westernization in Japan. Infectious and parasitic disease studies began at Tokyo Imperial University (Todai) in 1885 with the support of German bioscientists such as the famous Dr. Erwin Baelz. Baelz taught at Todai from 1876 to 1902 and became the leading figure in introducing modern parasitology to Japan. With the support of Baelz and his German colleagues, the first generation of Japanese parasitologists appeared at Tokyo Imperial University after Iijima Isao (1865–1921) returned from Germany. Many Japanese students worked at his laboratory, including Gotô Seitaro (1876–1935), Miyajima Mikinosuke (1872–1944), Yoshida Sadao

(1873–1964), Koizumi Makoto (1882–1952), and Kobayashi Harujiro (1892–1964).[40] Todai's position as the central figure in modern parasitology in Japan was challenged by Kitasato Shibasaburo in 1892.

Institutes for the Study of Infectious Disease and Kitasato's Pupils

Trained by the faculty of parasitology at Todai, Kitasato Shibasaburo was the leading bioscientist in the establishment of Japanese infectious and parasitic disease studies. In 1883, upon his graduation, Kitasato joined the CBS and built a close relationship with Gotô Shinpei. Between 1885 and 1891, Kitasato studied in Germany under Robert Koch, who focused on bacteriology. In 1892, after Kitasato's return from Germany, the Meiji government announced plans to establish a central institute for infectious and parasitic diseases, which Kitasato was expected to head. However, a conflict arose between Kitasato and Todai. Kitasato hoped to establish an institute modeled after the Koch Institute in Germany, while Todai wanted to maintain the status quo. To bypass Todai, Kitasato created the Shiritsu densenbyo kenkyujyo (Private Institute of Infectious Disease) in 1892, which was supported by the Dainippon shiritsu eiseikai (Private Association of Hygiene in Japan).[41] At the new research institute, with the support of Gotô Shinpei, Kitasato and his pupils strove to control infectious and parasitic diseases.[42] Because of the *kokuyoka* (nationalization) policy and pressure from Todai, the Private Institute of Infectious Disease was put under the control of the Department of Public Health in the Ministry of Home Affairs. In 1899, it became the Kokuritsu densenbyo kenkyujyo (National Institute of Infectious Disease).[43]

While Kitasato Shibasaburo was in charge of the institute, he mentored a new generation of bacteriologists and parasitic medicine researchers. Referred to by recent scholars as *Kitasato no monsei* (Kitasato's pupils),[44] Takagi Tomoe, Kitajima Taichi (1870–1956), Asakawa Norihiko (1865–1907), Shiga Kiyoshi (1870–1957), and others greatly impacted the development of modern bacteriology and parasitology in Japan, becoming key researchers in the field and making crucial contributions to disease control.[45] Kitajima Taichi, who had a close connection with Kitasato later, became the dean of the Medical School of Keio University. Because of Kitajima, Kitasato's pupils were able to maintain their relationships and support networks despite the crisis merger with Tokyo Imperial University in 1914.[46]

The Conflict between the Kitasato Institute and Tokyo Imperial University

In 1914, when control over the National Institute of Infectious Disease was transferred to the Ministry of Education and placed under the Medical School of Tokyo Imperial University, political leaders in the cabinet did not consult with Kitasato Shibasaburo. It was rumored that the transfer resulted from a conspiracy generated by Aoyama Tanemichi to harm Kitasato's reputation.[47] Kitasato and his colleagues, who did not agree with this transfer, resigned from the National Institute of Infectious Disease and established their own organization, the Kitasato Institute. Because of the help they received from Kitajima Taichi, Kitasato and the scientists of his institute went on to establish the Medical School of Keio University in 1916, and, as mentioned above, Kitasato became its first dean.[48] After the transfer, Aoyama Tanemichi, a professor at the Medical School of Tokyo Imperial University, became the deputy chief of the Institute of Infectious Disease under Tokyo Imperial University. Aoyama's staff at the institute comprised a new generation of Japanese bacteriologists—Yokote Chiyonosuke, Hayashi Haruo, and Nagayo Mataro—who had their educational background in Todai.[49]

The conflict between the Kitasato Institute and the Institute of Infectious Disease of Tokyo Imperial University persisted, and this affected the structure of Japanese colonial medicine.[50] Many scientists from the Kitasato Institute went abroad to study, influenced by their close connection to Gotô Shinpei. The transfer of the former National Institute of Infectious Disease to the medical school of Todai could have been a disaster for Kitasato and his pupils, but with Gotô Shinpei's new appointment in Taiwan, the 1914 incident instead turned into an advantage for colonial Taiwan. During this time, Takagi invited former researchers on the Kitasato team to conduct important studies in Taiwan. Since Japan was still short on medical resources and manpower in the 1900s,[51] the 1914 friction in Japan drove out many of Kitasato's best pupils and brought unanticipated support for expanding colonial medicine in Taiwan. Japan's loss was Taiwan's gain.

Developing the Prototype of Japanese Colonial Medicine

Literature prior to the 1890s on Japan's motives for colonizing Taiwan is extensive but highly polemical, and it is likely that there will never be any agreement on the precise mixture of the commercial, financial, social, strategic, and powerful political forces that were involved. From a practical vantage point, Japan and the colonial government of Taiwan paid a heavy price in social apathy, riots, and financial deficits during the early stages of the occupation.[52] Given these circumstances, many Japanese thought of Taiwan as more of a burden than a gold mine.

Thus, when Gotô moved into the Office of Civil Affairs in Taiwan in 1897 he was confronted with mixed views as to the best direction colonial policy should take. For instance, a group of scholars at Todai claimed that any effort to reduce Taiwan's medical problems would end in failure because of the island's climate, which seemed to foster disease, and because of its residents' unsanitary habits.[53] Nevertheless, Gotô proceeded with plans for a major step forward in Japan's colonial medical policy. He set up a medical reform program to reduce the colony's social unrest, heavy expenditure for medical care, and high mortality rates.[54] In a speech delivered during a graduation ceremony at Taiwan Sôtokufu Medical School, Gotô insisted that medical reform would increase Taiwanese confidence in colonial rule and reduce the colony's financial dependence on Japan. He went on to announce two goals of the medical reform program: acclimating Japanese to the Taiwanese climate and convincing the Taiwanese to accept modernity.[55] Although he resigned in 1906 to accept a new position in Manchuria, Gotô's ideas and goals continued to influence medical reform in Taiwan. Moreover, his successors expanded his original plan and sought to implement an even more comprehensive health reform program.

Gotô Shinpei: The Agent of Japanese Colonial Medicine in Taiwan

Gotô's plan for medical services in colonial Taiwan in some ways can be viewed as an attempt to complete the project he started in Japan—instituting the Western medical model. He had promoted his concept of German *Staatsmedizin* in both *Kokka eisei genri* and *Eisei seidôron*, but the medical elite never gave him the opportunity to fully implement his blueprint. In Taiwan, however, he had the full authorization of Governor Kodama to apply his theories about medical administration. Unhindered by the political and medical roadblocks he faced in Japan, Gotô's first priority was to follow the steps of medical westernization taken in Japan and to partially institutionalize the medical system. During this period, the establishment of a sanitary police force and a medical care system would institutionalize "advanced" Japanese medicine in the "uncivilized" colony. Both systems would come to symbolize Gotô's *Staatsmedizin* plan in colonial Taiwan.

The application of German "biological principles" in colonial Taiwan was meant to increase the chance of survival for the Japanese colonizers by helping them better adapt to the climate and environment of the island.[56] Although Gotô's colleagues, namely, Takagi Tomoe and Horiuchi Takeo, expanded on Gotô's original plans, even into the 1930s the countryside was seen as a reservoir of dangerous disease inhabited by "uncivilized" Taiwanese. In fact, colonial medicine was restricted to a few Japanese settlements, most of which were located in urban areas.

The Sanitary Police

Japanese attitudes toward Taiwan and its inhabitants were varied and often contradictory. Yet there was one basic assumption: a belief that the unique Taiwanese environment and its maladies required an infusion of fundamental medical knowledge from "modern" Japan. This was especially obvious when Gotô (who was still at the CBS in Japan) invited Tsuboi Jirô, a professor of hygiene at Kyoto Imperial University, to conduct the first official investigation of Taiwan's hygienic conditions in 1898. Tsuboi Jirô had graduated from Tokyo Imperial University and continued his study of hygiene in Germany. On his return, his application of German *Socialmedizen* was rejected by Todai, but he soon became the first professor of hygiene at Kyoto Imperial University (1899).[57] In his final report, Tsuboi suggested that Taiwan's environment and human habitat presented a great opportunity to study many diseases: cholera, plague, malaria, and others. Belief in the distinctiveness of the island's tropical disease environment raised two fundamental questions for colonial administrators: was it possible for the Japanese to acclimatize their bodies to the new surroundings, and how could their medical practices could be adapted to suit the new environment?[58] The question of medical practices prompted Japanese administrators to consider the utility of the medical knowledge being imported to Taiwan. The "acclimatization question" was of great political significance because potentially it cast doubt on the long-term success of the Japanese presence there. The tendency to view Taiwan as part of the "sanitation problem" confronting Japan was evident even in the earliest days of the occupation. Gotô's plan increased the call for sanitary surveillance and regulation of the Taiwanese population.

An amendment to the Meiji 34 (1901), code no. 354, was the colonial government's response to these concerns. The act provided a system in which sanitary policing would be carried out by police officers, and regulations were laid down that set up sanitary measures, listed nuisances, regulated drainage, and outlawed unlicensed practices such as those used by traditional healers.[59] However, the original amendment was not pursued further because of local resistance and the incomplete administrative system.[60] Gotô later expected that funding for the sanitary police system would be raised by profits generated in Taiwan. Hygienic imperatives laid down in the law were vitally important to the process by which the Japanese would teach the Taiwanese about the hygienic discipline that Japan had itself only recently learned from the West. In general, for Gotô and his colleagues the sanitary police force was a good way to ensure the cleanliness of the immediate environment for Japanese residents without asking them to pay for it.[61]

Greater concessions had to be made to local elites in terms of representation if the Taiwanese population was to be asked to bear the burden of medical reform expenditures. In response, at the same time that Gotô strengthened the surveillance capabilities of the sanitary police (all funded by local taxes) by allowing them to collect fines, he also groomed the local medical elite, specifically medical students,[62] to become local leaders of the colony.[63] Despite Gotô's long-term strategy of creating a new elite that would help implement his medical reforms, in the short run the sanitary police played a larger role in colonial society.

To fund the program, Gotô levied a sanitation tax and issued bonds that subsidized the activities of the sanitary police. In general, based on the new regulations laid out in Meiji 35 (1902), the sanitary police in urban areas were mainly in charge of regulation and sanitary surveillance (the punishment for hygienic transgressions was a fine), but the act officially subsidized medical practices in rural areas.[64] It is also worth noting that the colonial police were to work in tandem with Taiwan's indigenous *ho-kô* (*baojia* in Chinese)[65] system to promote several of the colony's sanitary measures.[66] The *ho-kô* system was the most fundamental mechanism of social control in colonial Taiwan. The Japanese adopted traditional Chinese methods of neighborhood organization, putting local police in charge of surveillance. Usually five households were one *ho*, and ten households were two *ho* or one *kô*. The colonial government also used the *ho-kô* system to reorganize the Taiwanese social structure and mobilize residents to address hygienic issues.[67] Generally speaking, in addition to providing a solid social base for colonial rule the *ho-kô* system helped the Japanese regime carry out its sanitary goals.[68]

Gotô also called on the police to monitor Taiwanese doctors' practices and enforce cooperation with the surveillance reporting system. The urban population was the major target. Qin Xienyu has argued that the colonial medical police provided an omnipresent surveillance system used to control the Taiwanese population medically and even socially.[69] Her argument is particularly accurate in describing activities of the sanitary police in urban areas prior to the 1920s, when major cities were filled with Japanese inhabitants and the economy was stronger.

Quarantine Stations and Public Hospitals

The colonial government also built a variety of medical facilities in accordance with Gotô's design. If we see the system of sanitary police as a governmental tool to supervise medical and sanitary conditions, then medical facilities were used to promote good health.

While the sanitary police looked after problems within the colony, a new

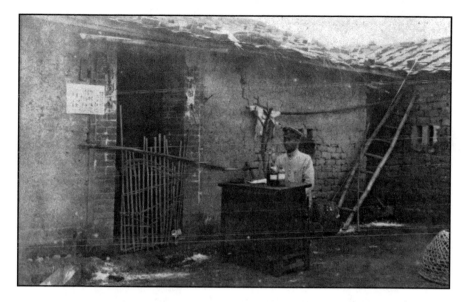

FIGURE 2.1. Enforcing quarantine on patients' families. Photo courtesy of Chung chin-shui.

quarantine system was established to prevent disease from entering the island. Influenced by Western germ theory, the colonial government enforced sanitary regulations at ports in order to prevent the spread of infectious diseases such as cholera, dysentery, and bubonic plague. In 1896, Utilizing his experience in setting up quarantine stations in Japan, Gotô issued the Enforcement of Notifiable Diseases Act. Temporary quarantine services in five major ports were quickly established.[70] Three years later, in 1899, permanent quarantine stations were established in Keelung and Tanshuei (Danshuei) harbors, two of the five major harbors in Taiwan, northern ports used for shipments to Japan. In 1918, the government attempted to enforce bylaws concerning health conditions in the colony's harbors. These conditions included epidemic relief, notification of infectious diseases, isolation of infectious cases, and immunization registration. According to the regulations, each port was required to have three to five health inspectors, an isolation hospital, and a quarantine station.[71] In order to coordinate the activities of the sanitary police force, the colonial government requested that it carry out surveillance and inspection beyond the harbor while the Bureau of Harbor Affairs officially dealt with incidents within it.[72] Only in the event of a crisis such as the plague epidemic of 1919 in China would the sanitary police enter the harbor area and offer free vaccinations for sailors.[73]

As quarantines blocked the intrusion of diseases into the island and the sanitary police monitored domestic conditions within it, medical facilities such as hospitals and dispensaries provided ways to cure or reduce the impact of illnesses within Taiwan. Gotô believed that firm state control was the only way to effectively offer basic medical protection for the population. In addition, for Gotô and his colleagues, medical facilities such as hospitals and quarantine centers were the hallmark of advanced Japanese medicine.[74] The main difficulty was finding qualified health workers and providing services at an affordable level. The former led to the construction of a medical school to ease the shortage of medical workers at the village and local community levels. On Gotô's advice, the governor-general took steps similar to those undertaken in early Meiji Japan; a particular focus was on the rearrangement of medical resources, especially the regional distribution of hospitals and dispensaries.

Western hospitals have existed in Taiwan since the seventeenth century.[75] During the first years of the Japanese occupation, the colonial government occasionally built military-style field hospitals or army dispensaries for the treatment of local citizens and erected police hospitals to accommodate the sick and destitute during epidemics.[76] It was not until 1898, however, that Gotô first suggested building a public hospital in every major city on the island. Following a proposal made by Takagi Tomoe, the Rinji Taiwan kyukan chôsa iienkai (Temporary Committee for Investigating Taiwanese Customs) convened in 1901 to investigate the possibility of establishing public hospitals in major Taiwanese cities with large Japanese populations.[77] From Gotô's proposal in 1897 to Takagi's plan in 1901, public hospitals steadily increased and accompanied the advancement of Japanese medicine in cities such as Taipei and Tainan.

Gotô's reforms did not yield immediate results, however. It was not until the second half of the occupation era (1920–45) that the number and distribution of medical institutions began to grow and serve a wider public purpose. An important factor in this development was the establishment of *kôi shinrôsho* (public dispensaries) rather than hospitals. Gotô initially did not expect this as the colonizers believed that public dispensaries were effective only in the alleviation of disease and did not assist in its study or cure.[78] The establishment of public hospitals clearly benefited the Japanese inhabitants because the funds appropriated and services allocated were almost exclusively for the Japanese.[79] Gotô always tended to favor hospitals as a way for Japanese medicine to "civilize" Taiwanese society and left dispensaries to the rural areas. In 1912, he returned from Manchuria and visited the public Taihoku hospital. After close inspection, he proudly proclaimed that this "modern" public hospital symbolized the success of Japanese rule.[80]

The spread of public dispensaries played another important role in establishing colonial medicine. The public dispensary system provided government-hired medical assistants (*kôi,* "public doctors") to treat the rural population without encroaching on public hospital services in the cities. The *kôi* who worked at the public dispensaries had to follow the directives set forth by the government and coordinate their activities with local police departments.[81] The establishment of public dispensaries for public doctors in 1896 and 1897 was another attempt to provide westernized Japanese medicine to the Taiwanese people, particularly those living in the countryside. In 1896, after taking the position of hygienic consultant for Taiwan Sôtokufu, Gotô proposed that the public doctors serve as "missionaries" for Japanese medicine and key supporters of colonialism in its promotion of social hygiene as well as in its curative work. In one speech, Gotô compared the cooperation between the public doctor and the sanitary police to the cartwheels of Japanese colonization in Taiwan. That is, while the police force focused on executive power, the public doctor should shoulder the responsibility of teaching modern medicine to the Taiwanese.[82] Like hospitals in the cities, public dispensaries became local centers of hygienic education and mass vaccination, further reflecting Japan's medical superiority to "uncivilized" Taiwan.[83] The number of these dispensaries increased considerably in the early decades of the twentieth century. In 1900, there were only 68 public dispensaries in Taiwan, but by 1940 there were more than 291.[84]

The Japanese *kôi* system in Taiwan was rooted in the German *Feldsher* (field doctor), a concept that originated in the fifteenth century. The term *Feldsher* was used in the medieval era for barber-surgeons and later for army field surgeons for the German and Swiss *Landsknecht* (teams of pikemen) until real military medical services were established in Prussia in the early eighteenth century. The term was then exported with Prussian officers and nobility to Russia. In Soviet Russia (1922–91), *Feldsher* was used to designate medical/health care professionals who mainly served rural areas.[85] Japanese *gunshin igaku* (military medicine) shared many features with the Prussian system, and *Feldsher* was one of them.[86] After Japan occupied Hokkaido in 1869, insurgents from garrison troops were converted to local health care providers who were subsidized by the government to open their own dispensaries. Like *kôi* in Taiwan, these practitioners in Hokkaido were allowed to charge a fee for treatment but still received a salary from the government as partial compensation for treating the poor and monitoring local hygienic conditions.[87] The German *Feldsher* system had been under careful consideration during the 1910s as a model for serving the poor in Japan. The term *hinmini* (doctor to the poor) was used to mean *Feldsher,* and in one source the origin of *hinmini* is traced to the Hokkaido experience.[88]

Gotô might have been inspired by the medical service in Hokkaido, since he promoted the similar *kôi* system in colonial Taiwan. The Japanese system predated the similar service promoted by the League of Nations in the 1930s as well as *chijiao yisheng* (barefoot doctors) in Communist China.[89]

Because of the financial difficulties and dangerous living conditions, Gotô could not attract enough qualified Japanese doctors to work at the public dispensaries in colonial Taiwan. Only the unqualified or the bravest were willing to work in such remote areas.[90] One way for the government to maintain public doctors' functions without increasing the its financial burden was to increase the number of private physicians. In 1897, medical education in colonial Taiwan became a factor that would fundamentally alter the development of Japanese colonial medicine.

In 1906, Gotô Shinpei left Taiwan and became president of Minami Mantetsudô Kabushiki (the South Manchuria Railroad Company, Mantetsu in Japanese) in Manchuria.[91] However, medical reform in Taiwan did not cease with Gotô's resignation. He had created a team that was pledged to carry out his medical reforms, with Takagi Tomoe and Horiuchi Takao as its leading figures. Moreover, Gotô had already established fundamental mechanisms and formal institutions that would carry on his legacy. At least two processes of medical reform were developing—monitoring policy goals and expanding medical resources. The institutions essential to those processes were the Taiwan Chûô eiseikai (Central Sanitary Committee of Taiwan), the police department, and the colony's medical school.

Takagi Tomoe: The *Eisei Sôtoku* (Governor of Hygiene) of Japanese Colonial Medicine in Taiwan

Although Gotô Shinpei had been in charge of the CBS for three years, he still faced hostility from the medical elite, which paid more attention to his poor family background and common education than his professional merit. The Sôma incident and his long conflict with the famous military surgeon Mori Ôgai underscored his continuing professional difficulties in Japan.[92] These difficulties followed Gotô to Taiwan. Mori criticized him as an unqualified doctor fit only to work as a middling politician. In one article, he scorned Gotô's mentor, Rudolf Virchow, and even claimed that Gotô was worse than Virchow because he had not received qualified training in medicine.[93] Despite these professional hurdles, Gotô still had Governor Kodama's full support and Takagi Tomoe's assistance in helping him rebuild his reputation in colonial Taiwan.

In sharp contrast to Gotô Shinpei, Takagi Tomoe (1885–1943) was unquestionably a member of the medical elite in Meiji Japan. He was born in Fukushima Prefecture and graduated from the Tokyo Imperial University Medical School in 1885. After eight years serving in hospitals, he worked at the famous Institute of Infectious Disease where he gained great respect for his research in bacteriology and serum studies,[94] which solidified his international reputation as a serum expert.[95] As already mentioned, Takagi won great acclaim after the success of his mass vaccination program against cholera and plague in Osaka and was rewarded with the post of Deputy Chief of the National Serum Academy. Despite Takagi's fame, the politics of academia would change his career. In the 1890s, the political pressure of merging the Private Institute of Infectious Disease into the governmental-owned Tokyo Imperial University caused many well-known researchers to resign, including Takagi, who had received Gotô's full authorization to establish medical services and public health administration programs in colonial Taiwan.[96] Takagi accepted the invitation from Gotô to serve as chancellor of the Hospital of the Governor-General's Government in Taipei and as dean of the medical school in 1902. Takagi was also asked to take charge of the epidemic prevention program, including plague prevention and the colony's antimalaria campaign.[97]

Takagi devised new sanitary systems and medical institutions, which Gotô had in place by 1906. As early as 1902, to reduce the threat of plague, the colonial government proposed the creation of a special institute staffed with medical experts. In 1903, the Ministry of Home Affairs approved a plan to establish the Rinji hôekyoku (Temporary Agency of Prevention or TAP). The TAP, a joint institute with the Sanitary Police Department, focused exclusively on anti-epidemic affairs and operated with Takagi as its first chairman. Takagi also helped the government organize the Temporary Committee on Prevention in his role as coordinator between the TAP and the police department.[98] In the years that followed, he designed a plague and cholera control program (1903–18) and pioneered an antimalaria campaign in 1910.

With the infrastructure of clinical medicine left by Gotô, Takagi extended the whole framework of medical services and sanitary works to keep them in line with trends in Japan. In 1907, he proposed the establishment of the Sôtokufu kenkyûsho (Research Institute of the Governor-General Government or RIGG) as a center for laboratory medicine.[99] To supplement the insufficient medical manpower and replace traditional practitioners, Takagi twice called on the medical school to provide at least sixty-five *igaku-senmongakkô* (vocational-level graduates of the medical college) annually.[100] Initially proposed in 1905, this plan was not fully implemented until 1916. Because of Takagi's efforts, a miniature Japanese version of *Staatsmedizin* appeared in colonial Taiwan complete with a research institute to satisfy the demands of laboratory medicine plus one medical school to educate practitioners in clinical medicine.

In 1919, Takagi resigned from sanitary affairs to take the leading position in the Taiwan Power Company. He appointed the military surgeon Horiuchi Takao as his successor. Horiuchi's career in colonial Taiwan reveals the extent to which clinical medicine was put at the center of Japanese colonial medicine. Born in 1873, Horiuchi, like Gotô, had only a high-school level of medical training before he became a surgeon in 1895 during the Sino-Japanese War. Following the occupation of Taiwan, he traveled extensively throughout the island with the military. According to an application he submitted to study in Germany, he admitted that he lacked training in laboratory medicine and relied instead on clinical observation for diagnosis and treatment.[101] To doctors such as Horiuchi, there was no way to gain a better position or win respect from the medical elite in Japan. However, with Takagi's full support, Horiuchi was able to study bacteriology in Germany for two years. Horiuchi returned to Taiwan to succeed Takagi and continue his mission of medical reform. He earned his doctoral degree from Todai in 1912. He held several important positions, including director of the Taihoku (Taipei) Red Cross Hospital and dean of the Taihoku igaku-senmongakkô (Taihoku Medical College) in 1916. He served at the medical college until 1947.[102]

The infrastructure for colonial medicine in Taiwan was completed in late 1910 and was maintained by Horiuchi, who seemed more devoted to training clinicians than educating laboratorists. Formal medical education began in colonial Taiwan in 1897 when Yamaguchi Hidetaka established the *Dojin ishi yôseisho* (Native Doctor Training Institute). What began as an intensive first-aid program expanded into a formal medical school after Takagi's appointment as dean in 1902; it became part of the Japanese imperial university system in 1928.[103] As a result, the majority of medical practitioners in Taiwan were graduates of either vocational high schools or medical colleges. Less than 5 percent of medical professionals before 1942 had received university or higher level training. The desire to be a doctor was common among the Taiwanese youth after 1910, and the total number of hospitals increased dramatically after the mid-1920s.[104] Although the number of public hospitals never exceeded 35, the number of private dispensaries, usually owned by Taiwanese physicians, grew to 263 by 1940.[105] Although Takagi and Horiuchi had training in laboratory medicine, they increased the influence of clinical medicine in Taiwan. The distinction between clinical and laboratory medicine in colonial Taiwan was maintained in the 1920s and 1930s. This will be discussed in detail in the following chapter.

Although the colonial government strongly emphasized the responsibility of the state to support medical students, in fact, income was the main incentive for Taiwanese in choosing a medical career.[106] The occupation of clinician, called *kaigyôi* (private clinician), was greatly envied by the Taiwanese for its easy money, as is suggested in the popular saying, "a clinician can earn money selling tap water."[107] Because of their wealth, Taiwanese clinicians were seen as leaders of local society. The dispensary was not only a place to obtain medical treatment but also a public space serving various needs in the surrounding community. Activities at dispensaries included hygienic education, cultural or social events, and even political gatherings.[108] Moreover, *honjitau* (a home visit to a patient) was an important part of the training of medical students in Taiwan.[109] Home visits fostered connections between clinicians and rich patients, which expanded the role of the dispensary in strengthening the clinician's socioeconomic network.[110] The dispensaries treated mostly poor people, and one Japanese physician characterized them as noisy environments, like brothels, motivated by greed and offering a *yaoya* (grocery store) type of treatment.[111] Although their profession was respected, Taiwanese doctors were not free from harassment by the police, and building ties with local police departments was an important survival strategy. Some doctors earned fortunes by selling various death or injury certificates to patients while the police could punish those who did not submit legal documents for funerals or lawsuits.[112] According to newspaper reports of the time, although many doctors were quite respectable, the Taiwanese public was concerned about the medical ethics of private clinicians.[113]

In general, while Gotô Shinpei paid particular attention to the health needs of the Japanese colonizers, Takagi Tomoe saw Taiwanese society as a whole and enlarged Gotô's plan into a comprehensive system in which, from a medical vantage point, the line between colonizer and the colonized became blurred. Taiwanese clinicians and their private dispensaries served local communities while altering Gotô and Takagi's original plan. The original plan stipulated that medical service should be provided by the state, but now it was in the hands of private practitioners, a group of Taiwanese elite. After 1910, Horiuchi accelerated the expansion of clinical medicine and produced a medical system that far surpassed anything Gotô would have imagined.

Knowing Taiwan: The Establishment of the Central Sanitary Committee of Taiwan and Investigations into Sanitary Conditions

"An island of ghosts" with a "prevalence of lethal malaria" was Japan's major impression of Taiwan before the 1900s.[114] While the harsh environment in Taiwan dampened the ambitions of military surgeons such as Mori Ôgai, it drove others deeper into investigation. The Central Sanitary Committee of

Taiwan was established just after the occupation. Unlike its counterpart in Japan, the CSCT was merely a technical institution meant to oversee the sanitary police system. Rather than being empowered with authority to command the police force itself, the CSCT was a scientific unit charged with investigating and identifying epidemics.[115] In 1896, the Taiwan Chihobyô oyobi densenbyô chousa iinkai (Committee for the Investigation of Endemic and Epidemic Diseases in Taiwan) became the first colonial institution with the same charge. Rapidly it became clear that the first priority of the colonial administrator was to grapple with epidemic crises, and address purely scientific interests second. In the following year,[116] the new Temporary Bureau of Prevention replaced the investigative committee. In 1903, its successor, the Temporary Committee of Prevention, served mainly as an investigative unit coordinating anti-epidemic campaigns with the police.[117] In fact, the Enforcement of Notifiable Diseases Act of 1896, not any scientific interest, served as a guide for the investigative work of these institutions.[118]

Aside from the strategic need to combat epidemics, the ability of Japanese modern medicine in the 1900s to cure certain diseases was the key consideration in designing related policies in Taiwan. For example, although malaria was a notorious endemic disease in Taiwan and recognized as such by early colonial officials, the government postponed its prevention campaign until 1910. Probably because the Japanese had experience dealing with outbreaks of plague in Hong Kong and Manchuria,[119] and because of Takagi's work on cholera in Japan, these two epidemics were chosen as the main targets of various anti-epidemic campaigns in the first decade of the twentieth century.

Medical professionals in colonial Taiwan advocated preventive medicine, especially a cowpox vaccination that had been successfully administered in Japan.[120] Meanwhile, even before modern bacteriology came to Taiwan in the 1920s most medical professionals there, unlike their Japanese counterparts, believed that there was nothing inevitable about sickness in the Taiwanese climate and much could be done to prevent it. The fact that one Japanese might be infected by a disease and another not was, for Horiuchi Takao, "proof that sickness is not an inevitable evil, but, in general, the consequence of inattention and mismanagement."[121] To the Japanese in Taiwan, cowpox vaccination seemed to be an effective means of preventing a smallpox epidemic. A mass vaccination program would not only protect Japanese colonizers but also should convince the Taiwanese to accept the advanced medicine that they brought in.

Promoting the cowpox vaccination was not easy. One obstacle was the vaccination itself. Subordinate staff involved in the vaccination program could not be trusted to produce accurate statements about their work and neither, it seems, could their superiors.[122] During the late Qing period (1880s), smallpox had been recognized as endemic in northern Taiwan,[123] but it was rarely treated in hospitals.[124] Finding medical facilities for the program became essential. Meanwhile, traditional Chinese medicine had a long history of smallpox variolation,[125] and it was used in Taiwan in opposition to government programs.[126] Therefore, only a small number of Taiwanese, those in cities, could benefit from the vaccination program in the beginning, and that number fell far short of Japanese expectations for comprehensively preventing an epidemic.

In 1896, with Gotô's advocacy, the Jennerian vaccination was extensively administered in Taiwan.[127] Although *kôi* were originally designated to carry out this vaccination program, their numbers were too small to complete the mission. In addition, it was difficult for them to win the trust of the Taiwanese. To compensate for that problem, in 1902 traditional practitioners were allowed to be licensed after passing an examination, and they assisted in the vaccination program under the supervision of *kôi*.[128] The coercive power of the sanitary police was applied to persuade the heads of the *ho-kô* to allow vaccinations to be administered in their offices (figure 2.2). The sanitary police had the right to arrest people who refused vaccination and to supervise the whole process.[129]

The combination of traditional practitioners and coercive powers established an important foundation for the mass vaccination program. In British India, a similar situation prevailed, and the colonial government adopted similar strategies to promote the Jennerian cowpox method.[130] It was as a result of compromise and government efforts, including coercion and education, not solely because of its efficacy, that the modern cowpox vaccine

FIGURE 2.2. Mass cowpox vaccination. Courtesy of Chung Chin-shui.

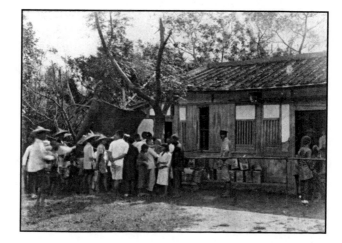

replaced traditional variolation in British India and Japanese Taiwan. The success of the mass cowpox vaccination in British India became a source of alarm, as continuing it would mean a large-scale financial commitment for the government.[131] Japanese-ruled Taiwan, on the contrary, turned the success of the program into a process to improve the accuracy of public health investigation—a key foundation for colonial rule and propaganda. Chart 2.1 plots the government's statistics on vaccination.

CHART 2.1. The relationship between smallpox vaccination and death in colonial Taiwan. (Data from Taiwansheng xingzheng zhangguan gongshu, *Taiwansheng wushiyinianlai tongjitiyao*, tables 49, 490, 491; pp. 76, 1272, 1274.)

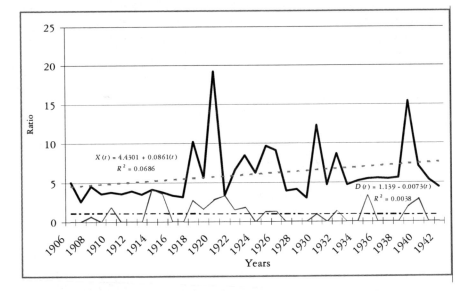

Note: Y axis was shown in $X'(t) = 100*X(t)$

$X(t) = C(t) /$ [total Taiwanese population (t)]

$C(t) =$ number of vaccinated cases in a given year

$D(t) = ds(t) /$ [total Taiwanese population (t)]

$ds(t) =$ deaths from smallpox in a given year

The comparison between $X(t)$ and $D(t)$ is important in determining whether or not the vaccinated cases are sufficient to eventually reduce the outbreak of smallpox epidemics in the following years.[132] Chart 2.1 shows an inverse relationship. The mathematical relationship also confirms our observation in the regressions. The regression of $X(t)$ is $X(t) = 4.4301 +$

0.0861t, and the regression of $D(t)$ is $D(t) = 1.139 - 0.0073t$. There was a sharp drop in $X(t)$ between 1921 and 1923 from 0.18 to 0.04. This situation could have been caused by the failure to import vaccine and enforce a reporting system. The smallpox vaccination produced lasting immunity. People beyond the initial point of contact would not be infected simply because there would be no one to transmit the virus.[133] The Taiwanese population during the colonial period was comparatively static, and it seemed clear that a major vaccination program should be able to break the cycle of infection. Unfortunately, the correlation coefficients (0.026) $X(t)$ and $D(t)$ show that the vaccination program was not extensive enough to break the infectious cycle, and so it did not produce the expected results before 1905. It is obvious that the colonial government could not rely on temporary units or intermittent action to deal with the permanent vaccination needs of an "unhealthy" Taiwanese population. Ultimately, without an accurate census of Taiwan's population the mass vaccination program would fail.[134]

Basically, the governor-general of Taiwan produced two types of public health investigation and statistical analysis during the colonial period: population censuses and investigations into causes of death and morbidity. Based on monthly returns from local governments via an information reporting system, the first census was conducted in 1905 and published in 1906 as *Taiwan jinkô tôkeisho* (Census of Taiwan).[135] To monitor the results of vaccination, data on vaccination and deaths from smallpox were shown in the census. These data, collected from monthly police department reports and individual household registrations, provided information on population size, age, causes of death, and birth and death rates for specific areas. However, the census data before 1910 were flawed in their recording of mortality rates for infants and children under age five.[136]

Although the colonial government launched the first census in 1905, the regular reporting system was not completed until 1910. During the period 1900–1910, the government had close administrative contact with local policemen and the heads of the *ho-kô* system, who reported deaths and outbreaks of major diseases to the local sanitation offices or the sanitary police.[137] There was evidence that the census takers had falsified some of the data: exaggerating or undervaluing cases, ascribing causes incorrectly, or accepting bribes to not report a case at all.[138] By using vaccination reporting for cross-examination, the corrected collection of vital data began in the late 1910s.[139] Basically, the field of medical statistics in Taiwan before the 1920s was still in its infancy, although some data on urban Japanese citizens and troops can be considered relatively sophisticated.

Due to the deficiencies mentioned previously, vital data before 1905 do not back up government claims about serious diseases in Taiwan.[140] The fatality rate from smallpox in the Taiwanese cases is also most likely understated.[141] Beginning in the 1920s, Taiwan stood on firmer statistical ground. The reporting system first included private and charity hospitals (public hospitals were included from the beginning) to aid in the identification of diseases being carried out by local police and heads of *ho-kô*.[142] After 1923, all hospitals took full responsibility for identifying cases of smallpox, as well other diseases, and left it to the police to fill out the reporting forms correctly.[143] Because of cooperation in the identification of diseases and the ubiquitous police system, the data were more accurate than before. Moreover, private dispensaries began to flourish after the mid-1920s (see chapter 3). All public dispensaries, and even some private dispensaries in the countryside, were charged with providing disease identification. After 1920, the colonial government decided to appoint well-equipped private dispensaries to serve as reporting agents.[144] With the rapid growth of private dispensaries in the 1930s, a comprehensive public health reporting system evolved through cooperation among the sanitary police, the *ho-kô* system, and various medical facilities.

With the rapid extension of vaccination to Taiwanese children enrolled in schools after 1910, the Japanese population became less vulnerable to smallpox than to diseases that were less predictable, particularly cholera and dysentery. However, declining susceptibility to smallpox did not mean that it ceased to be a matter of Japanese concern.[145] The vaccination policy was at least partly initiated to protect the health of the Japanese. Careful watch was kept in major cities and seaports to minimize the potential risk of serious epidemics, including smallpox. Following the development of the public health reporting system, surveillance for outbreaks of smallpox ended after the 1920s.[146] Where cowpox vaccinations were introduced with the cooperation of new Japanese-supported and -trained leaders, resistance to the vaccination program was overcome in time.

The reporting of smallpox cases in Japan after 1901 was more accurate and the data more reliably organized.[147] Moreover, administrators of the vaccination program seemed surprisingly optimistic in view of the considerable opposition vaccination had encountered in Japan.[148] Although nationwide public health investigations and household registration were both implemented in Japan around the turn of the twentieth century, a population census was postponed until 1920 for various reasons, including technological difficulties.[149] Between 1905 and 1920, colonial Taiwan had held two censuses (1905 and 1915) and jointly launched the third one with Japan in 1920. All necessary modifications and adjustments for a successful census had been tried in Taiwan before the First Census of the Japan Empire was taken in 1920.

In this case, medicine was not a tool of empire used to control the colony. From promoting the vaccination program to improving census-taking and investigative skills, Taiwan was essentially a laboratory.

Based on better population data, authentication of causes of death and epidemiological statistics also improved. The improvement in the reporting system and sanitary investigations after the 1920s laid a better foundation for the colonial government to work on the two core questions in Tsuboi's report. The first of these—the "acclimatization question"—was of great political significance because it cast doubt on the long-term efficacy of the health environment of the Japanese in Taiwan. The second—the question of medical practices—led the Japanese to consider the utility of medical knowledge imported to Taiwan and to assess their lifestyle in relation to that of their subjects. The coincidence between Tsuboi's conclusion and many European physicians' worries about sanitation in the tropics implies that European tropical medicine would be a major source of medical reform in colonial Taiwan.[150]

From 1910 through the 1920s, public health investigations were extended from general observation to specific studies, from supervising living habits to physical measurements of population. Certainly, these investigations were prompted by medical standards for public health development that were based on Japanese and European contexts. These investigations were usually small scale and centered on one or two areas. The subjects were usually selected in designated Japanese residential areas or government-owned plantations where a limited survey of morbid conditions was conducted; others who could be expected to have medical problems were forced to participate and therefore were not representative of the population.

With better sanitary measures and statistical data on the population, the colonial administration could also pinpoint medical problems and even calculate the monies lost to public health crises. As the third dean of the Governor-General Government Medical College, Horiuchi Takao, explained in 1935:

Each mortality equals thirty-four sick persons, and sick persons on average have to rest for twenty days in a year. Assuming that the daily medical expense for each patient is 0.5 yen, and the financial loss for each person's sick leave is 0.333 yen per day, then whenever there is one fatality it means that we lost 566 yen [(0.5 + 0.333) × 34 × 20]. Take the year 1930 as an example. In this year, the total population [of Taiwan] was about five million. If the mortality rate remained as high as that in 1905, then total mortality in the population would increase to about eighty thousand. That is to say, we would have lost an extra 45,310,000 yen.[151]

Horiuchi's assessment of human life in terms of monetary value shows that the real purpose of Japanese colonial medicine in Taiwan was economic rather philanthropic.

Although those conducting public health investigations encountered major problems, the Governor-General Government in Taiwan thoroughly supported it. The investigations reached their peak in the 1930s when the government promoted more extensive investigations. Publications such as *Eisei chôsa* (Public Health Investigation), a series of books including *Volume of Diseases*; *Statistics of Causes of Death in Taiwan*; *Volume of Infants and Children by Age Group*; *Tuberculosis in Taiwan*; *Statistics of Malaria in Taiwan*; also *Lepoto: Eisei chôsa* (Reports of Public Health Investigation); *Ahen kankei chôsa* (Opium-related Investigations); and *Eisei Gaiyo* (The General Sanitary Situation) were all government supported and promoted.[152] Influenced by the attitudes of the colonial administration, local governments published the results of their own public health investigations.[153]

Government statistics from censuses and sanitary surveys are available for the years 1906–40. The results were reliable and helped the colonial government discover such interesting patterns as differences in causes of death between the Japanese in Taiwan and the Taiwanese (see chart 2.2).

CHART 2.2. Causes of death among Taiwanese and Japanese in Taiwan.

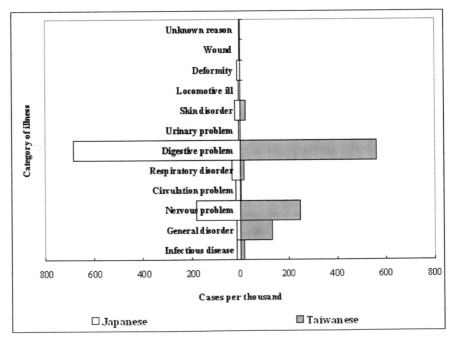

As shown in Chart 2.2, the Japanese in Taiwan obviously suffered from more digestive problems while the Taiwanese had more nervous problems and, especially, general disorders. Compared to well-defined health problems such as locomotive disorders, skin disorders, and digestive problems, the categories nervous problems and general disorders subsumed most deaths that lacked an accurate diagnosis. This presumed misclassification of causes of death among Taiwanese was significant before the mid-1920s and led to inaccuracies in the census.[154]

The classification by race in government statistics on sanitary affairs provided a firmer ground on which the colonial authorities could distinguish treatment and vaccination targets and decide priorities. Moreover, in the 1920s the CSCT and other sanitary agencies of the government conducted a series of investigations into health conditions in Taiwan. These surveys succeeded in achieving the original mission of the epidemic investigations in the 1900s. However, the goals and items under investigation in the later surveys were clearly beyond the limits of the Enforcement of Notifiable Diseases Act of 1896 and the amendatory acts passed thereafter. Sanitary conditions, endemic diseases, and comparisons between the Japanese in Taiwan and the indigenous Taiwanese were the major concerns of these surveys.[155]

Colonial Medicine: Tool of Empire?

The health of the Japanese in Taiwan was the most important concern of the colonial government. Before the government invested heavily in public health and medical infrastructure, encouraging self-discipline in personal hygiene was a logical step to prevent Japanese from picking up "unhealthy" habits from the Taiwanese.[156] However, physical isolation was not the way to acclimatize the Japanese to colonial life. *Taiwan eisei kaiyô* (Summary of Sanitation in Taiwan),[157] published by the colonial government in 1913, drew heavily but selectively on Chinese dietary habits. Its authors suggested that discriminating Japanese might glean useful knowledge from the "absurd" customs of the Taiwanese, for example, drinking only boiled water.[158] The colonial government's sentiments were echoed by medical professionals in Japan. One professor, Minasaki Takena, believed that the consumption of *sashimi* (raw fish and meat) was the root of many of the digestive ills among the Japanese and suggested that they consume well-cooked meat and boiled water as the Taiwanese did.[159] Attention was focused on dietary habits for an obvious reason: there had been repeated waterborne epidemics of cholera.[160]

Gotô's top reform priority was improving medical and sanitary work in urban areas. Carrying out his plan, Japanese medical professionals used the sanitary police to execute reform measures within the urban environment and used city hospitals as their technical base. While hygienic conditions improved in urban areas, Taiwan's immense rural population remained "unsanitary" and "uncivilized" in the opinion of most colonizers. Gotô had little time to address medical problems in the countryside, and until the 1920s medical and public health reforms were limited to urban areas, following the European model of public hygiene in the nineteenth century.

Building Healthy Cities for the Colonizers

Japanese doctors believed that Taiwan's warm, humid climate was the major cause of its people's deteriorating health and civilization. Thus, many early efforts concentrated on reducing temperature and humidity; for example, a "healthy" house should be built of bricks, with windows to increase airflow, so as not to retain unwanted heat and foster disease.[161] With full authorization from Governor Kodama, Gotô first appointed Takagi to tackle the "acclimatization question." In the 1890s, immediately after his appointment as *shigai kaisei komon*, the first consultant on urban reform, Takagi and his subordinates accepted Tsuboi's report and divided Taiwan into "healthy" and "unhealthy" zones based on Japanese standards. Underlying this division was a belief that over time the Japanese might gain immunity to the vicissitudes of climate and disease in Taiwan.[162]

The belief in the adaptability of physical constitutions was derived from popular notions of environmental influence,[163] which reached a high stage of sophistication in the hygienic studies produced during the Meiji period.[164] Despite Todai's goals of increasing medical facilities throughout Taiwan, Takagi and his colleagues chose city planning as their first priority as a means of increasing the "healthy" residential areas for Japanese colonizers.[165] Gotô recruited people outside the Todai group to execute his medical reforms and relied on military surgeons, who had hands-on experience. The concepts of urban sanitation reform employed in Europe were essential to Taiwan's urban reform movement.[166]

A key element in the plan to create "healthy" zones—areas without industrial pollution but with sporadic outbreaks of cholera—was a comprehensive water system. The first water system was established in 1896 for Taipei City, and the population it served increased substantially over time (table 2.1), from less than 1.5 percent before 1905 to nearly 16.1 percent by 1942.

Between 1905 and 1942, the rate of increase proceeded at 0.6 percent per year with three construction peaks: 1908–9 witnessed an increase of 3.7 percent due to construction of a water supply system around and within Taipei City; from 1921 to 1922, the rate increased by 2.6 percent; and from 1930 to 1931 the rate increased by 3.2 percent.[167] The timing of the increases matched the establishment of a political center (before 1900), agricultural modernization (1920s), and industrialization (1930s).[168] Most prominent, the timing and pace of these developments underscored Gotô's argument that improvements in hygiene would lead to increased productivity among the population.

TABLE 2.1. Increases in Water Supplies in Taiwan and the Population Served

Years	Number of Water Systems	Total Population	Population Served		Rate of Population Served	
			Expected	Actual	Expected (%)	Actual (%)
1905	2	3,123,302	43,000	no record	1.4	no record
1906	2	3,156,706	43,000	no record	1.4	no record
1907	3	3,186,373	59,000	no record	1.9	no record
1908	3	3,213,996	59,000	no record	1.8	no record
1909	4	3,249,793	179,000	no record	5.5	no record
1910	6	3,299,493	185,300	no record	5.6	no record
1911	8	3,369,270	190,600	no record	5.7	no record
1912	12	3,435,170	211,100	no record	6.1	no record
1913	16	3,502,173	255,400	no record	7.3	no record
1914	18	3,554,353	290,175	no record	8.2	no record
1915	18	3,569,842	290,175	no record	8.1	no record
1916	21	3,596,109	321,675	no record	8.9	no record
1917	21	3,646,529	321,675	no record	8.8	no record
1918	22	3,669,687	358,175	no record	9.8	no record
1919	22	3,714,899	358,175	no record	9.6	no record
1920	22	3,757,838	368,050	no record	9.8	no record
1921	25	3,835,811	385,925	no record	10.1	no record
1922	28	3,904,692	496,425	no record	12.7	no record
1923	34	3,976,098	504,775	no record	12.7	no record
1924	35	4,041,702	508,775	no record	12.6	no record
1925	45	4,147,462	543,095	no record	13.1	no record
1926	48	4,241,759	588,715	no record	13.9	no record
1927	54	4,337,000	637,965	no record	14.7	no record
1928	57	4,438,084	678,465	no record	15.3	no record
1929	63	4,548,750	745,765	no record	16.4	no record
1930	72	4,679,066	788,465	432,435	16.9	9.2
1931	73	4,803,976	966,465	459,999	20.1	9.6

TABLE 2.1. Continued from previous page

Years	Number of Water Systems	Total Population	Population Served		Rate of Population Served	
			Expected	Actual	Expected (%)	Actual (%)
1932	76	7,929,962	1,065,265	473,088	21.6	9.6
1933	77	5,060,507	1,067,865	511,979	21.1	10.1
1934	84	5,194,980	1,100,021	548,370	21.2	10.6
1935	91	5,315,642	1,118,621	581,531	21.0	10.9
1936	93	5,451,863	1,140,221	631,180	20.9	11.6
1937	98	5,609,042	1,272,221	739,874	22.7	13.2
1938	123	5,746,959	1,273,292	786,230	22.2	13.7
1939	123	5,895,864	1,326,321	848,208	22.5	14.4
1940	123	6,077,478	1,349,240	889,106	22.2	14.6
1941	123	6,249,468	1,359,975	979,842	21.8	15.7
1942	123	6,427,932	1,414,525	1,035,957	22.0	16.1

Source: Taiwansheng xingzheng zhangguan gongshu, *Taiwansheng wushiyinianlai tongjitiyao*, 1281.

Note: In the colonial period, the construction and management of the water supply system was the local government's responsibility. Therefore, the numbers served by the water system were counted by each headquarters unit. For example, although the Erlin water system merged with the Changhua system after 1928, I count them as two systems because the Erlin water management board still existed after that merger and functioned independently.

Interestingly, the colonizers' argument that a better water supply system in colonial Taiwan would reduce the risk of epidemics has been interpreted by some scholars as a sign of the modernization brought by the Japanese.[169] Indeed, the greater total length of the water supply system seems to strongly support the idea of Japanese colonization as an agent of modernity and the postwar argument that medicine was a "tool of empire." Ostensibly, the water supply system served the Japanese residential areas in the cities, Japanese-owned plantations, and immigrant villages of eastern Taiwan, but in fact its main purpose was industrial and economic, and any positive impact on health conditions was a random side effect. The links among sanitary engineering, city planning, and colonial rule are especially clear when we consider the geographic distribution of the water supply system (see table 2.2).

TABLE 2.2. Populations Served by the Taiwanese Water Supply System

District	Region	Population at the End of 1940	Population Served	Rate of Population Served (%)
Taipei	Northern west	1,192,664	593,875	45.27
Hsinchu	Northern west	815,592	78,400	9.61
Taichung	Middle west	1,352,410	185,300	13.70
Tainan	Southern west	1,524,860	262,000	17.18
Kaohsiung	Southern west	888,869	193,800	21.80
Hualien-kang	Northern east	146,847	49,000	33.37
Taitung	Southern east	88,472	38,227	43.21
Penghu	Isles	67,764	10,000	14.76
Total		6,077,478	1,356,602	22.32

Sources: Taiwansheng xingzheng zhangquang gongshu, Taiwansheng wushiyinianlai tongjitiyao, 1281; Taiwan suidôji (Taiwan's Water System) (Taihoku: Taiwan suidô kenkyûkai, 1941), 619, 653, 677–82.

Note: The romanization of each place-name follows current usage in Taiwan.

As shown in table 2.2, eastern Taiwan (Taitung and Hualien-kang) enjoyed the highest percentage of population served by the water supply system, 38.29 percent. After 1897, the colonial government developed Taihoku (now Taipei) as the political center of the colony and began city planning efforts to create a "healthy" environment for its dense Japanese population.[170] If we subtract the rate in Taipei from the numbers in the table, the average percentage of population served by the water supply system in western Taiwan (Hsinchu, Taichung, Tainan, and Kaohsiung), with nearly 75 percent of the total population, is only 15.27 percent, well below the islandwide average of 22.32 percent.

In contrast, eastern Taiwan, despite its low population density, enjoyed the highest percentage of people with access to the water supply. In 1910, the colonial government adopted a policy of encouraging Japanese to settle in eastern Taiwan by building villages for them. Each village had public schools, government offices, public transportation, a water supply system, and a sewage system.[171] The government-owned sugar refineries in eastern Taiwan also built water supply systems for both industrial needs and workers' daily use.[172] In aboriginal areas, the Japanese built a water supply system before they officially declared sovereignty over these lands.[173]

Pure water and effective sewage systems were the core elements of medical reform and public health policies in colonial Taiwan. They were expensive to construct and maintain, and their success in preventing disease was unclear, as demonstrated by the morbidity rates for several waterborne diseases.[174] For instance, the morbidity rate from diarrhea-like illnesses declined from 0.79 per thousand in 1905 to 0.15 in 1942, but the morbidity rate from typhoid increased from 2.37 per thousand in 1905 to 5.18 in 1942 (see chart 2.3).[175]

CHART 2.3. Morbidity rates from diarrhea-like illnesses and typhoid, 1905–42

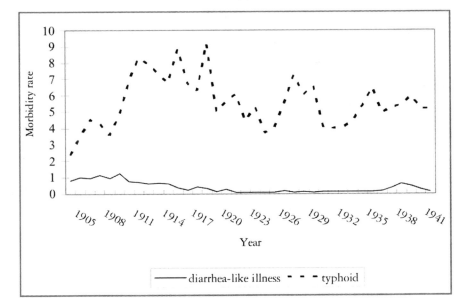

Source: Taiwan Sôtokufu Statistical Books, various issues, (Taihoku: Taiwan Sôtokufu Togeka) 1905–42.

Note: The morbidity rate is defined as the number of cases in a given year divided by the number of people in the population at the end of that year. Usually, the rate is incidence per one thousand persons.

There are two possible explanations for the difficulty of charting a correlation between the changing morbidity rates of waterborne diseases and the expansion of the water supply system. First, most of the water systems were built for industrial not household use. Second, because of the expense, maintenance of water systems always lagged behind need.[176] Even though local governments could not afford the maintenance costs, the governor-general transferred the ownership and management of water systems to local administrations in 1930,which eventually led to a decline in quality.[177]

Todai's policy of increasing facilities benefited only the Japanese population in cities, on several government plantations, and in immigration villages. However, as a Japanese who lived in the filthy environment of Taiwan, Takagi obviously understood that any colonizer's residence would be impossible to isolate from these problematic surroundings either socially or biologically. Although Tsuboi's investigation set guidelines for Takagi's plan to build a "healthy zone" for the Japanese in Taiwan, Takagi's effort in the end was appreciable for its multiple functions, sanitary and economic, which served the whole colonial population, including the colonized Taiwanese.

The results of the sanitary work were not always predictable. For example, the same technology did not produce the same results in Taipei City and immigrant villages. Therefore, the water system cannot be seen as a simple explanation for the reduced incidence of many diseases. Furthermore, the lower percentage of the population served by the water supply system in western Taiwan does not correspond to lower mortality rates there. The improvement could have been the result of increased economic growth, a side effect of the water system. In general, in Japanese residential areas medicine could be seen as a tool of empire. But the meaning of *empire* varied depending on who or what was serving the empire's interests, and there was no guarantee as to outcome.

Rural Taiwan: A Pit of Disease

Although the colonial government in Taihoku had the power to issue directives as early as the 1920s, the organizational machinery did not always exist to ensure that they were implemented efficiently.[178] Manpower shortages could be compensated for somewhat by recruiting local practitioners, but recruitment had to be kept below the level that would threaten the centralization of colonial rule. Application of public hygiene to rural Taiwan was financially impossible, and the sanitary budget for rural needs remained low even between the 1920s and 1940s, a period of economic growth in colonial Taiwan. The expenditures on health in Taiwanese cities usually accounted for more than 75 percent of the government budget for sanitary affairs. This meant that urban residents enjoyed at least three times the per capita expenditure of those in rural communities (see table 2.3).

In contrast to the "healthy zones" in urban areas, the countryside remained the preserve of the "uncivilized" Taiwanese and was seen as a reservoir of disease. Lack of money and Taiwanese hostility to these initiatives posed major problems. Like other colonial designs, the relationship between the

TABLE 2.3. Health Expenditures by the Colonial Government in Urban and Rural Areas

	Colonial Government			Health Expenditures			
Year	Total Expenditures (A)	Health Expenditures (B)	(B/A) (%)	Urban Areas (C)	(C/B) (%)	Rural Areas (D)	(D/B) (%)
1920	119,148,064	750,736	0.63	750,519	99.97	217	0.03
1921	112,035,565	2,446,189	2.18	1,719,291	70.28	726,898	29.72
1922	113,420,521	3,096,200	2.73	2,143,917	69.24	952,283	30.76
1923	111,097,561	2,871,514	2.58	2,098,455	73.08	773,059	26.92
1924	113,614,797	2,905,267	2.56	2,010,637	69.21	894,630	30.79
1925	119,559,876	3,574,774	2.99	2,705,493	75.68	869,281	24.32
1926	131,778,004	3,376,515	2.56	2,466,423	73.05	910,092	26.95
1927	138,626,830	3,708,477	2.68	2,597,709	70.05	1,110,768	29.95
1928	147,523,811	4,125,619	2.80	2,833,783	68.69	1,291,836	31.31
1929	150,240,607	4,104,894	2.73	3,017,166	73.50	1,087,728	26.50
1930	129,757,760	4,266,353	3.29	3,364,959	78.87	901,394	21.13
1931	115,972,147	3,847,081	3.32	3,080,339	80.07	766,742	19.93
1932	120,303,279	3,842,162	3.19	3,042,234	79.18	799,928	20.82
1933	130,812,153	3,603,978	2.76	2,661,693	73.85	942,285	26.15
1934	141,617,595	4,264,223	3.01	3,157,610	74.05	1,106,613	25.95
1935	156,549,367	4,499,220	2.87	3,498,853	77.77	1,000,367	22.23
1936	175,771,837	4,673,200	2.66	3,505,930	75.02	1,167,270	24.98
1937	202,836,543	5,734,895	2.83	3,750,044	65.39	1,984,851	34.61
1938	233,817,394	5,711,010	2.44	3,686,960	64.56	2,024,050	35.44
1939	288,498,326	5,693,376	1.97	3,659,261	64.27	2,034,115	35.73

Source: Taiwansheng xingzheng zhangguan gongshu, *Taiwansheng wushiyinianlai tongjitiyao*, 982, 1017–20.

CSCT and local sanitary services was by no means a simple chain of command. Because of the difficulties in finance and transportation, it was impossible for the CSCT to treat individual cases in rural areas. Although decentralization of the medical administration might have eased the immediate medical needs of rural areas, it would have left too much power and responsibility in the hands of the local Taiwanese gentry, a prospect viewed negatively in colonial Taiwan.

Unlike the urban model, the sanitary police system in the countryside was designed for integration with the traditional *ho-kô* system to promote health-related measures on a household basis.[179] This integration helped the colonial government link the traditional Taiwanese social structure (*ho-kô*) to a new colonial institution (the police force) through a mechanism of regular reports and checkups. This meant that without the cost of building a brand new administration the colonial government had a way to reach every resident in Taiwan. The government also permitted some members of the sanitary police (the *keisatsu i* or "police physicians") to practice medicine in rural areas and paid them a bonus for their efforts.[180] The training of police physicians was relatively meager, similar to that of the medical corps in the army. Their major task was similar to forensic medicine and allowed them to practice in areas with no medical resources. Police physician in Taiwan was merely a part-time position, and there were never more than fourteen of them.[181] As the number of private physicians increased after the mid-1920s, the functions of police physicians were restricted. In 1944, their title was changed to "sanitary engineer" and their role restricted to forensic work.[182] The institution of police physicians was thus merged with the public dispensary system in Taiwan and became the main purveyor of major medical relief in the countryside.[183] To a certain extent the sanitary police might be seen as watchdogs guarding health conditions in the cities while in the countryside they served as state agents of medicine.

The concept of police physicians was an extension of the earlier emergency medical teams. Its objectives were twofold: first, the Japanese immigrants would carry out the function of emergency teams charged with prevention and government hygienic discipline, and second, they would educate or "civilize" the Taiwanese, in the words of Takagi, and promote a "healthy and civilized" society by any medical standard.[184] However, the government found it difficult to recruit sufficient manpower from Japan. Therefore, colonial administrations had to rely on Taiwanese physicians and sanitary police to relieve the shortage of manpower and execute hygienic policies in rural areas.

During the early stages of the occupation, the Japanese relied on traditional physicians and police to deal with epidemics.[185] However, the colonial government was reluctant to include Taiwanese physicians in the formal system of medical care in the countryside. If Japanese settlers were to avoid being infected by the Taiwanese community, it was obvious that the team of medical professionals had to be expanded and local Taiwanese recruited. In 1897, Yamaguchi Hidetaka's proposition that a *dojinishi yoseishô* (medical training program) be established for indigenous people received strong support from Gotô.[186] Although the medical school changed its name to Taiwan Sôtokufu Medical School in 1899, Taihoku Medical College in 1918, and the Medical School of Taihoku Imperial University in 1936, its main goal never changed: to train medical professionals drawn from the Taiwanese population who would support colonial rule.[187] Because of the number of local students enrolled in the medical education system, the number of doctors trained in Western medicine dramatically increased after the 1920s. By the end of the 1930s, more than 90 percent of all doctors in Taiwan practiced Western medicine while only 2 percent treated their patients using traditional remedies. The increase of manpower in Western medicine was finally extended to the countryside after the mid-1920s, after the framework was in place in urban areas.

The compromise that absorbed the traditional *ho-kô* system into the sanitary police force and recruited Taiwanese to rural dispensaries modified Gotô Shinpei's original ideas but successfully adapted Takagi's public hygiene design to create a healthier environment in rural areas. The changes reversed the image of the Taiwanese countryside from a notorious "reservoir of diseases" to a "wonderland for immigrants" after the mid-1920s.[188] A new generation of Taiwanese doctors and their acceptance of Japanese colonial medicine completely changed Taiwanese attitudes toward modern medicine. In the 1930s, vaccination was still culturally unacceptable to some Taiwanese, although their numbers were probably not significant. Where vaccination was introduced with the cooperation of new Japanese-supported and -trained Taiwanese elites, it seems evident that any amount of resistance would have been overcome in time.[189]

In summary, after nearly a decade of chaos—military resistance, epidemics, and financial difficulties—the Japanese excitement over having a colony turned to bitterness. Harsh conditions in Taiwan scared off many Japanese and extinguished their ambitions. The arrival of Gotô Shinpei in 1902 was a watershed moment in Japanese colonial rule. Gotô, an excellent administrator but a mediocre doctor in the view of some Japanese, developed a theory of colonial medicine by modifying the ideas of German *Staatsmedizin*—a theory he did not have chance to apply in Japan. More important, he seized the opportunity afforded by the friction between Kitasato's team and Todai, inviting

Takagi Tomoe to Taiwan to lead the medical reform efforts there. Without Gotô Shinpei, colonial medicine in Taiwan would have been merely a series of temporary strategies for dealing with medical emergencies and interminable diseases. He laid out a theory that combined existing medical functions as well as creating new infrastructures to systematically promote medical services and public health regulation. In addition, he always asserted that colonial medicine in Taiwan had been well planned, and contemporary scholars have indiscriminately assumed a causal relationship between the establishment of medical services and many health improvements. Both assertions support the "tools of empire" discourse. However, health improvement actually occurred rather late due to the need for compromise and trial and error procedures.

Public hygiene guided Gotô and Takagi's city planning to create a "healthy" environment for the Japanese ruling class. Under a centralized administration, the sanitary police were charged with investigating all potential threats in the local community and the CSCT with playing the role of technical consultant. With these efforts, new medical institutions were established in Taiwan by the 1920s, marking the beginning of innovations in medical reform. Public health reform in colonial Taiwan served to legitimize colonization and improve the surveillance capacity of the colonists. David Arnold claims that colonial medicine in British India also played a key role in colonial ideology and ruling technology.[190] However, before the 1920s only urban areas experienced health improvements, and analysis shows that the relationship between an improved water supply system and reduced mortality rates was not causal but random. While the water system might be seen as a "tool of empire," its impact on public health remains unclear.

The colonial government nevertheless worried that disease among Taiwanese communities would create long-term risks. A low-cost health care system was first adopted by the colonial government. Initially, *kôi* and police physicians were added to the system. However, the difficulties encountered in promoting cowpox vaccination suggested that the system needed native mediators, and Taiwanese clinicians were trained to play that role. In the end, various health care elements, such as private dispensaries, *kôi,* and police physicians, were introduced into the Taiwanese urban and rural environments. Practitioners not only provided treatment without spending more government money, but, most important, they effectively kept Taiwanese sanitation under constant government surveillance. On the surface, this may look like another case of "tools of empire," but private dispensaries grew rapidly and eventually assumed the functions of *kôi* and police physicians. The Japanese could use medicine as a "tool of empire," but avoiding government interference became a tool of Taiwanese clinicians. This phenomenon was somewhat blurred in the

1920s, but in the 1930s it became clear. In the end, the separation of laboratory medicine and clinical medicine had racial meaning in 1930s Taiwan. Generally speaking, sanitary work in the cities initiated before the 1920s—for example, the introduction of vaccination programs and dispensaries and the expansion of public health reporting—later became part of colonial life in rural Taiwan. The improvement of medical care in rural Taiwan was in fact a sign of essential change in Japanese colonial medicine, which, after the 1920s, could no longer be adequately explained by means of the "tools of empire" theory.

3

The 1920s
Revising *Staatsmedizen* for the Colony

Gotô Shinpei left Taiwan in 1906, but the construction of medical services in colonial Taiwan did not cease after his resignation. Gotô had already created a team to continue his medical reforms, and Takagi Tomoe and Horiuchi Takao were its leading figures. Moreover, Gotô installed some fundamental mechanisms and institutions before leaving. Takagi's modifications to Gotô's foundation in the 1910s were far reaching, and vital components were added to colonial medical services. By the 1920s, it was commonly accepted in governmental propaganda that Japanese colonial rule had "civilized," and its medicine "sanitized," Taiwan. As a result, China was now counterpoised against Taiwan, portrayed as a filthy neighbor carrying lethal diseases. Only several health problems (e.g., malaria and opium smoking) in the native society served as medical remnants of Taiwan's Chinese past.

At least two processes of medical reform were developing in the hands of Takagi and others. Important new institutions—the Central Sanitary Committee of Taiwan, the police department, and the medical school—monitored policy goals and expanded medical resources. By the end of the 1910s, at least, two major characteristics of reform activity had appeared in the emphasis on laboratory medicine and clinical practice. Laboratory medicine represented the academic interests of Japanese medical scholars while clinical practice would alter Taiwanese attitudes toward Western medicine with a significant social impact.

During the first half of the twentieth century, bacteriology and related laboratory discoveries were essential features of German medicine, and thus for Japanese medicine as well. In Japan, the development of clinical medicine preceded that of laboratory-based medicine, although the laboratory and clinical practice were connected in education. However, colonial Taiwan lacked sufficient funds and facilities to support laboratory development. In addition, because of the sanitary and medical conditions in Taiwan, the immediate health need was patient care, and it was the demands of emergency treatment that stimulated the rapid development of clinical skills.

After the 1920s, the separation between laboratory medicine and clinical practice—in research, education, and practice—became a pressing concern. The number of Taiwanese medical practitioners quickly increased when the formal medical education system was established in the mid-1920s. Private dispensaries eventually replaced public hospitals in providing medical services to the Taiwanese population. Most important, the target of medical service switched from epidemics such as cholera and plague to endemic diseases such as malaria and social ills such as opium addiction. Generally speaking, colonial medicine in Taiwan after the mid-1920s was a hybridized and compromised system that mixed Japanese demands for the colonizers' survival and efforts to meet indigenous needs.

Quarantining Epidemics from China

Gotô's reforms initially concentrated on improving the island's general sanitary conditions. With the exception of smallpox in certain areas, no specific disease was chosen as a target of reform before the 1900s. Following the expansion of medical reform and diminished social unrest, the elimination of major diseases and the control of health problems became a policy goal in colonial Taiwan.[1] In different stages of the reform, Japanese experts targeted different diseases and problems, their focus shifting from major transcontinental epidemics to endemic health problems.

Diseases from a "Filthy" Neighbor: China

Not all of Taiwan's diseases were a product of its unsanitary environment. Cholera and plague, for instance, were determined by colonial administrators not to result from Taiwan's climate or its environment, and smallpox, as discussed in the previous chapter, was also understood to be largely independent of environmental influences. But the great majority of health problems—"malarial fever" and "unsanitary behaviors," which came under the designation *fûdobyô* (illness caused by local characteristics)—were believed to be affected to various degrees by the environment of Taiwan and the "uncivilized" behavior of the Taiwanese.

Cholera and plague invaded Taiwan frequently before the 1920s, causing several crises. Japanese troops were the first victims of cholera during the military action of 1895, and cholera epidemics threatened the lives of Japanese in Taiwan in 1916, 1919, and 1920.[2] In 1896 and 1898, plague caused great panic in the colonial government and a huge loss of life.[3] It must be pointed out that, while these epidemics did not have a significant impact on long-term mortality rates for the whole colonial period, they did cause high mortality over the short term (see table 3.1).[4]

TABLE 3.1: Mortality from Cholera and Plague in Taiwan, 1896–1921

Year	Cholera			Plague		
	Number of Patients	Number of Deaths	Mortality Rate (%)	Number of Patients	Number of Deaths	Mortality Rate (%)
1896				258	157	60.85
1897				730	566	77.53
1898	1		0.00	1,233	882	71.53
1899				2,537	1,995	78.64
1900				1,097	809	73.75
1901	1	1	100.00	4,496	3,670	81.63
1902	746	611	81.90	2,308	1,853	80.29
1903	1	1	100.00	886	709	80.02
1904	1	1	100.00	4,500	3,374	74.98
1905				2,398	2,100	87.57
1906				3,272	1,609	49.17
1907	3	2	66.67	2,592	2,241	86.46
1908				1,270	1,059	83.39
1909				1,026	848	82.65
1910	13	8	61.54	19	18	94.74
1911				308	334	108.44
1912	333	256	76.88	222	185	83.33
1913				136	125	91.91
1914				567	488	86.07
1915				74	56	75.68
1916	34	16	47.06	5	4	80.00
1917	2	1	50.00	7	7	100.00
1918	1	1	100.00			
1919	3,835	2,696	70.30			
1920	2,570	1,675	65.18			
1921	1		0.00			

Sources: Taiwansheng xingzheng zhangquang gongshu, ed., *Taiwansheng wushiyinianlai tongjitiyao* (A Statistical Summary of Taiwan over the Past Fifty-one Years) (Taipei: Taiwansheng xingzheng zhangquang gongshu, 1947), table 490, 1271–73; Taiwan igakukai, ed., *Taiwan eisei gaiyô* (Summary of Sanitation in Taiwan) (Taihoku: Taiwan igakukai, 1913), 139.

Note: The accuracy of records of causes of death was questionable before 1910. However, because of governmental concern and military regulation, records for cholera and plague were more accurate than for other causes of death between 1900 and 1910.

The medical experts of the colonial government identified both epidemics as diseases emerging from an "unhealthy China."[5] This position reflected the same attitude that characterized Tsuboi Jirô's report on Taiwan's sanitary conditions in 1899, the only difference being that Tsuboi's reference to "Taiwan dewa fukenkô no jitai" (unhealthy conditions in Taiwan) was replaced by "epidemics from unhealthy China" in various government reports produced after the 1910s.[6] Prior to 1915, two epidemics caused high mortality rates in Taiwan. Doctors such as Mori Ôgai believed that the diseases had been brought from unhealthy China to healthy colonial Taiwan, and thus the eradication of these diseases would reveal the superiority of Japanese medicine and colonialism.[7] With support from colonial authorities, medical professionals chose cholera and plague as targets for prevention.

Major diseases such as cholera and dysentery had long existed in Japan, and contact with the West brought new ones.[8] During the Meiji Restoration, the development of a public health and sanitation program played a major role in improving health and reducing mortality.[9] Although the improvement in general health is difficult to evaluate and some significant health hazards remained, the Japanese were very optimistic as a result of their victory over cholera and their smallpox vaccination program.

Physicians and sanitary officials in the colonial government borrowed from the Japanese experience with cholera control and antiplague campaigns to formulate their policies. Most sanitary officials in Taiwan, confident in the strength of laboratory medicine in Japan, believed that it would help create the healthy conditions needed for survival. Two experiences indicated that the Japanese were capable of incorporating laboratory discoveries into the sanitary administration: the battle to control cholera epidemics in Meiji 19 (1886) and Kitasato's antiplague campaign in Manchuria in the 1910s.[10] The latter particularly demonstrated confidence of the international medical community in Japanese medicine, especially bacteriology, when Kitasato was elected president of the International Plague Conference at Mukden in 1911.[11] It was a common conviction among the Japanese that their medicine had matured enough to be ready for export. For the sanitary officials of the colonial government, the importation of such medical knowledge was practically and logically necessary.

Cholera. To ensure the health of colonial personnel, medical professionals had to reduce the impact of epidemics. Japanese observers of the 1902 cholera epidemics noted one aspect of the disease that was of particular significance for the subsequent history of cholera in Taiwan: its predilection for infecting the indigenous poor. Although Japanese residents were at first alarmed by the disease's spread, most were saved by their comparatively healthy living conditions and superior diet. Japanese mortality on average was half that of the indigenous poor.[12] However, the huge loss of life among Japanese soldiers in 1895 was a reminder that there was no absolute immunity, and there was concern that Japanese might succumb to the disease.[13]

Before the establishment of well-equipped laboratories, the government tended to see cholera epidemics as a problem caused by climate and to leave the solution to the "reform of unsanitary living conditions and the polluted water supply in urban areas" (see figure 3.1).[14]

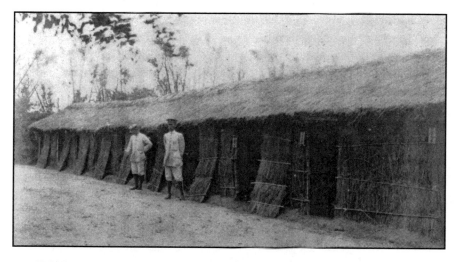

FIGURE. 3.1: Isolation ward for cholera patients. Courtesy of Chung Chin-shui.

Preventive measures were primarily restricted to quarantine laws in Keelung Harbor, through which the disease was imported.[15] While no significant mortality was reported from epidemic cholera between 1903 and 1911, medical professionals influenced by germ theory were still critical of government measures. For example, Horiuchi Takao, who believed that previous measures were incapable of totally eradicating epidemic cholera in the colony, asserted that the former preventive strategies lacked a bacteriological basis. He encouraged the development of experimental medicine in the colony and hoped to set up a bacteriological laboratory that would operate at the center of the anti-epidemic campaigns.[16] Horiuchi's article expressed strong confidence in the laboratory medicine prevalent among medical practitioners in colonial Taiwan. This confidence continued even during the devastating cholera epidemics of 1919 and 1920. The government insisted on the important role of the Research Institute of the Governor-General Government (RIGG) in controlling the disease, and he used this as a reason to upgrade its status and rename it the Chûô kenkyujyo (Central Institute of Research or CIR) in 1921.[17]

Plague. The antiplague campaigns followed a similar course. The government first issued regulations on the prevention of major epidemics, especially bubonic plague. In Taiwan prior to 1910, the mortality rate for plague was 80 percent or above.[18] In fact, between 1896 and 1900 medical professionals in Taiwan had not formed any clear opinion on how best to treat or prevent the disease. Uncertain of how to respond to the threat, medical professionals and colonial administrators implemented quarantine laws, on the one hand, and asked for medical assistance of experts and supplies from Japan on the other. In order to identify the etiological features of the disease, the famous bacteriologist Onogata Seiki visited Taiwan in 1896.[19] Both Shiga Ketsu, a researcher at the Private Institute of Infectious Disease, and the surgeon Okada Kotaro conducted fieldwork there in 1898.[20] On the basis of their suggestions, government medical officers, most of them sanitary policemen themselves, opted for compulsory segregation and sanitary cordons over voluntary and other more general sanitary measures. Their zealous approach probably owed much to the enthusiasm for bacteriological theory and the preventive methods of laboratory medicine. Horiuchi's works on etiology and the diagnosis of plague exemplify the prevalence of such attitudes among Taiwan's medical community.[21]

Without proper equipment and expertise, by 1900 the colonial government could only strengthen general sanitary measures and the executive power of sanitary policemen.[22] To reduce the threat of plague, the colonial government encouraged the Taiwanese to catch rats by paying half a yen per rat. However, some people began raising rats to get the money, which exhausted the limited budget for plague prevention. In addition, for the Taiwanese there were negative side effects to the rat control program for reporting the discovery of dead or infected rats resulted in examinations and possibly quarantine. People could be arrested and sent to an isolation ward merely because an infected rat was caught in a neighbor's home.[23] The rat control program was discontinued in the 1900s when the plague campaign began targeting patients rather than the animal vector.[24]

The plague epidemic provided a testing ground for specific methods of prevention based on the principles of bacteriology. In October 1897, the government set up a committee to inquire into the epidemiological features of the disease. Based on the discoveries and suggestions of the committee, the government appointed a physician, Chikuyama Kiichi, to preside over an inoculation program. Inoculation was introduced into the local community on an experimental basis first in the southern city of Tainan and then in military compounds elsewhere in the colony. There was no philosophical contradiction between sanitarianism and inoculation in early-twentieth-century Japan because both were based on the germ theory of disease. However, financial constraints were an impediment to instituting costly sanitary engineering while immunization proceeded among Japanese troops and the surrounding population.[25] Plague serum was produced in colonial Taiwan in much the same way as the well-known Haffkine's plague vaccine was produced in India. Plague bacillus was sent down characteristic stalactite cultures for four to six weeks, and then the microbes were killed by heating the flask to 65°C for one hour. The finished product contained not only the bacilli but also their metabolically produced toxins, which meant that the serum was not only a preventive but also a therapeutic treatment.[26]

Despite positive results in Tainan, the government did not continue the program after 1901. Government reports revealed that the inoculation program was limited to a small group of people in six southern regions.[27] Chart 3.1 shows the benefits of the inoculation program. One factor in the suspension of the program was that the supply of serum from Tokyo's National Serum Academy was not stable.[28]

CHART 3.1: Benefits of plague inoculation in Taiwan, 1901.

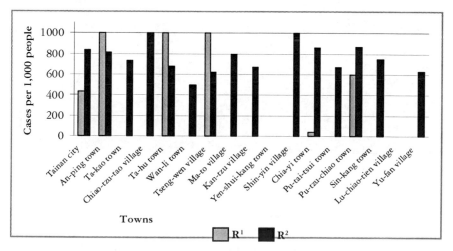

Note: The romanization of each place-name follows current usage in Taiwan.

R^1 = plague deaths per thousand people inoculated.

R^2 = plague deaths per thousand people not inoculated.

However, opposition from the Sanitary Police Department is the main reason why the program was eventually abandoned. The department believed that the inoculation program was inefficient and insisted that plague was a disease hidden in the "filthy environment."[29] According to their line of thinking, an "environmental disease" should be controlled by cleaning up transmission agents such as contaminated dirt and animals not by focusing on the human body. This attitude prevailed until the appointment of Takagi in 1902.[30] The department cited the unreliability of the plague inoculation program and expressed confidence in theories about environmental sanitation that were common in the early twentieth century before the development of bacteriology and the discovery of antibiotics. For the ill and the suspected ill, strict isolation was enforced. Sanitary policemen and *keisatsu i* (police physician)[31] actually had more power to identify diseases than licensed doctors.

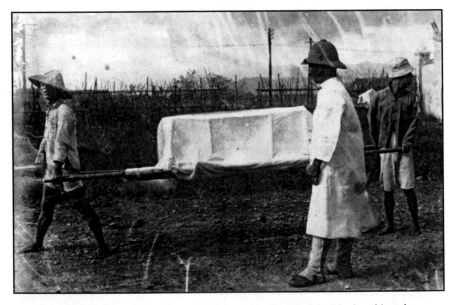

FIGURE 3.2: Taiwanese carriers and a *keisatsu i* (police physician) in the white robe moving a body infected with plague. Courtesy of Chung Chin-shui.

Those who favored inoculation to combat epidemics early on included staff members in public and military hospitals. The majority of medical officials—nearly one thousand sanitary policemen—instead placed greater emphasis on general sanitary improvement and evacuation of infected areas.[32] This bias in Taiwan's medical community dominated attitudes from the time that Gotô and Takagi first raised the issue of medical reform in 1902.

Expenditures for inoculation and building quarantine wards exhausted the government budget in 1895–96 when a deficit of 18,021 yen for plague elimination equaled almost half the budget for sanitary expenditures.[33] Obviously, the colonial government needed a way to share the burden of plague prevention with the Taiwanese population. Traditional sanitarianism— a concept that aimed to reduce environmental pollution through sanitary engineering—was a possible a solution.

To reduce the threat of plague, in 1902 the government issued a comprehensive plan that included the founding of a special medical institute. As mentioned in the previous chapter, Takagi Tomoe founded and chaired the Temporary Agency of Prevention (TAP) in 1903 to coordinate medical activities with police action. Adopting an attitude of compromise, he insisted that inoculation be used only in addition to a general sanitation program. He was equally opposed to compulsory segregation, preferring a combination of medical inspection and evacuation of infected areas.[34] Takagi's position was not simply an accommodation to the sanitary police; it also reflected concerns about the possibility of a hostile reaction to the inoculation program among local Taiwanese.[35] The target of prevention shifted from the human body to the rat. The rat destruction program became the hub of a more general strategy, which continued in most Taiwanese towns and cities after 1902. However, in 1905 TAP declared that, while complete extermination of rats within a locality was impracticable, such tactics might "materially diminish" the effect of plague within a given area.[36] Because of the establishment of RIGG, Paul-Louis Simond's theory of plague transmission began to gain ground in Taiwan.[37] The acceptance of this theory resulted in a more realistic approach to plague prevention, which focused on the extermination of rats on commercial and domestic premises. It was thought that such a campaign would have to go hand in hand with the colony's urbanization program.[38] As urbanization increased, the government could send more agents to enforce the coercive inoculation program in appointed areas.[39]

Although it is difficult to estimate how much the government saved by adopting sanitarianism, Fan Yanqiu believes that it not only helped to eliminate plague but also helped to reduce the burden on the budget, unify the sanitary surveillance system, and promote a healthy environment for the colonizer.[40]

In addition, there was some evidence to suggest that inoculation was slowly gaining support among the Taiwanese. Previously, they suspected that the inoculation program was prompted by sinister government motives. Rumor had it that inoculation would lower reproduction rates and reduce the Taiwanese population.[41] Taiwanese medical graduates played an important role in persuading the local population of the importance of inoculation and the improvement in survival rates for the inoculated.[42] As the plague threat declined, the government decided to close TAP and in 1909 transferred its duties back to the Sanitary Police Department.

After struggling to eliminate plague epidemics between 1902 and 1910, the government declared that the indigenous form of the disease was finally under control. However, new cases were reported in 1911, and the government had to reestablish TAP at the end of that year. The epidemic of 1914 brought another three-year panic. Unlike previous cases, TAP announced, the epidemic of 1914 came from outside Taiwan. As with the cholera epidemic, medical professionals tended to identify the plague as a "disease from unhealthy China."[43] The epidemic of 1914 ended in 1917. After that year, the number of cases of plague quickly dropped, but the disease did not fully disappear until after 1945.

Generally speaking, after the 1920s deaths from cholera in Taiwan never approached the peak of 2,693 in 1919; the annual cholera death rate from 1920 on was below two digits. Cases of plague also dropped from 30,101 (including 24,104 deaths) to zero in 1918.[44] The cases of cholera and plague control reflect two facets of medical reform policies during the expansion period. First, under the influence of laboratory medicine imported from Japan, medical practitioners in Taiwan were confident in the powers of bacteriology and other new medical sciences. Second, in the cases of cholera and plague, Gotô's main goal became to maintain healthy conditions in Taiwan. "Unhealthy China" therefore had to bear responsibility for all serious epidemics in the Japanese colony.

Expanding Medical Resources in Colonial Taiwan

The successful campaign against epidemics in the 1910s laid a foundation for the colonial government in its search for better strategies with which to address future crises. As the major threat of epidemics virtually disappeared, more efforts were invested in building a comprehensive system of medical service in Taiwan. Laboratory and clinical medicine coexisted during the period of expansion of medical services, 1900 to the 1930s. As the Meiji government embraced German *Staatsmedizin* in the late 1870s, medical practitioners incorporated its other aspects, including laboratory medicine, into Japanese state medicine. The essential characteristics of *Staatsmedizin* were the proliferation of laboratory techniques, the licensing of physicians, the training of physicians in state schools, and the standardization of medical treatment. The proliferation of laboratory techniques first enlarged the capability of biological medicine and later determined the processes for licensing and standardization.[45] By the end of the nineteenth century, before the Japanese occupied Taiwan, a dual medical system had developed in Japan. On the one hand, there was a large body of primarily government-supported medical researchers who made new laboratory discoveries and set scientific standards that became the foundation for government regulation. On the other hand, a growing body of urban-based licensed physicians—trained at major medical schools, licensed by the state, and practicing "legal medicine" according to the performance standards set by the government—relied increasingly on the laboratory.

The Koch Institute in Berlin had been the inspiration for several Japanese civilians acting in a nonofficial capacity to promote laboratory medicine in their own country. Beginning a fund-raising campaign when Kitasato returned from Germany in 1892, Fukuzawa Yukichi donated land and money to open the Shiritsu Densenbyô Kenkyujyo (Private Institute of Infectious Disease) in Tokyo. Modeled on the Koch Institute, it was concerned primarily with antiplague treatment and the production of antiplague serums. It also conducted routine bacteriological analyses of water and food together with original research into the nature of disease.[46] During the early stages of the occupation, the institute helped identify the chief sanitary problems in Taiwan and provided assistance to colonial officers.[47] After the 1900s, growing support among Japanese intellectuals for state sponsorship of medical science provided a climate in which medical research was looked on more favorably by the government. This trend finally produced the *kokuyokai* (nationalization) policy.[48]

The Establishment of Laboratories in Colonial Taiwan

In response to the nationalization policy, in 1907 Takagi proposed that the colonial government establish the Sôtokufu Kenkyujyo (Research Institute of the Governor-General Government or RIGG) in line with a similar trend in Japan.[49] According to his original proposal, the department's major duty would be to assist in economic development and sanitary improvement.[50] Records show that bacteriology and biochemistry were the real foci of RIGG, for which Takagi was the first deputy chief. The institute had two divisions, hygiene and chemistry. The Division of Hygiene began operations in 1909, taking responsibility for research on epidemic and endemic diseases, local climate, and public health. Its research findings became an important basis for government policy. The division included laboratories specializing in seven major areas: bacteriology, protozoology, pestilence, parasitism, animal pestilence venin, and aquachemistry. The institute expanded to twelve laboratories and merged with other institutes to form the Chûô Kenkyujyo (Central Institute of Research or CIR).[51] In addition to the important contributions to medicine made by the faculty of the Sôtokufu medical school, the CIR continued to operate after 1945.

The administrative structure and research subjects of RIGG and CIR followed the model of the Private Institute of Infectious Disease and, after 1899, the Kanritsu Densenbyô Kenkyujyo (National Institute of Infectious Disease).[52] The establishment of the institute clearly echoed domestic developments unfolding in Japan. Annual reports of RIGG and CIR through 1940 indicate that researchers in both institutes were primarily concerned with medical experimentation rather than therapeutic skill. In addition, the Taiwan scholar Ôda Toshiro claims that the academic interests of Japanese medical practitioners drove the development of medicine in Taiwan.[53] Japanese were in the majority on the staffs of RIGG and CIR; only three Chinese names appear on annual reports during the total thirty-year history of the institute.[54] In short, RIGG and CIR were research centers for Japanese medicine operating in colonial Taiwan. Japanese researchers controlled the agenda and expressed the same interest in experimental medicine as their domestic colleagues did.

The government not only established RIGG and CIR but fixed them at the top of the medical system in the colonial bureaucracy. Before 1909, CSCT was the main institution in the system charged with providing experimental findings for the practical needs of the Sanitary Police Department. However, it had only limited capabilities in undertaking biological research. The experimental basis of CSCT was research being accomplished in affiliated laboratories at public and military hospitals, but these laboratories lacked the proper equipment and stable budget needed to accomplish CSCT's goals.[55] During pandemic crises, the colonial government usually had to seek help from Japan. The situation changed after 1909, however. RIGG and CIR were given a stable budget—between 2 and 8 percent of the total health budget—by the colonial government, which enabled them to maintain sufficient equipment and manpower.[56] They topped the medical system and led the experimental function of CSCT. Moreover, while CSCT was only a civilian organization established by government order, RIGG and CIR were government institutions with the legal power to execute policy.[57] From an administrative standpoint, they had greater support from the government and a closer connection with the Sanitary Police Department.

As mentioned previously, Tsuboi's sanitary survey in 1899 occasionally revealed an attitude similar to that of many European physicians, who worried about sanitation in the tropical colonies. Before 1895, some Japanese physicians had already noted medical developments undertaken by colonial administrators in India and East Africa. Following the rise of germ theory and the occupation of Taiwan, these physicians' concerns led to a broader and more pervasive system of state medicine and public health in colonial Taiwan. Various research reports and publications from RIGG and CIR revealed the establishment of a new tropical medicine discipline in Taiwan based on germ theory and a corresponding intensification of environmental control. These changes were epitomized by the public health measures and medical research that emerged between 1900 and 1920.[58]

Although the activities of RIGG and CIR revealed the academic interests of Japanese medical practitioners in the colony and echoed unfolding trends in Japan, this did not mean that the government lost its concern for colonial medical problems. In the case of colonial Taiwan, it is misleading to claim that the colonial government chose to burrow into medical research as a way to avoid further commitment to medical and sanitary reform.[59] As early as 1905; the colonial government sent a team of physicians to investigate the endemic plague in Taiwan. Some members of the team suggested looking at the environment rather than searching for a specific contagion. However, the intention to introduce tropical medicine into laboratory research in colonial Taiwan was very practical. Japanese experts primarily aimed to stop the epidemics rather than studying the diseases in a laboratory. The expansion of laboratory resources into educational institutions was begun only in the 1930s by a few Japanese doctors working at medical schools and later at the Institute of Tropical Medicine in Taipei.

The appearance of RIGG and CIR also meant that the primitive "emergency" medical reforms of Gotô Shinpei had expanded and become comprehensive in the field of experimental medicine and were supported by both academic interests and the colonial government. Laboratory medicine—the third element of medical reform previously lacking in Taiwan—was put in place and the transfer of Japanese medical organizational models into the colony was completed.

Medical Education in Colonial Taiwan

Compared to its design in Japan, medical education in colonial Taiwan was essentially vocational from the beginning. The Japanese system was divided between the elite education of university graduates and vocational training for college students, which together made up a comprehensive process supporting the whole range of medical services, both research and clinically based. Tsuneo Ozeki, who has studied the career patterns of graduates from Tokyo University, finds that most university graduates before the 1920s became practitioners in public hospitals and government research facilities while doctors of lower rank (below college level) practiced in private dispensaries.[60] Although the standards of teaching in the universities did not change with the rapid increase in the number of medical graduates in Japan in the first decade of the twentieth century, even university graduates had to work in private dispensaries due to the tight job market. For example, by 1902, among 709 living university graduates of medical universities in Japan, 195 had already become *kaigyôi* (private clinicians).[61] Because of the surplus of university graduates, not surprisingly, in Taiwan the research institutions RIGG and CIR were dominated primarily by Japanese nationals while Taiwanese practitioners worked at hospital bedsides or in dispensaries.

As medical research laboratories merged with the colonial bureaucracy, the government initiated formal medical education programs in line with the establishment of state medicine. Formal medical education began in colonial Taiwan in 1897 when Yamaguchi Hidetaka established the Dojin ishi yôseisho (Native Doctor Training Institute). What began as an intensive program in first aid expanded to become a formal medical school, a Sôtokufu igakô (vocational high school), in 1902. It was upgraded to Taiwan Sôtokufu igaku-senmongakkô (college level) in 1918, with the title changed to Taihoku igaku-senmongakkô in 1922, and eventually became part of the Japanese imperial university system in 1936.

In the beginning, Takagi and Yamaguchi were concerned about how to balance medical needs and maintenance of the centralized structure of the sanitary administration, especially the best way to resolve the shortage of medical practitioners.[62] Two solutions for the shortage were the settlement of Japanese medical practitioners in the countryside and the expansion of the Japanese medical education system to train Taiwanese. When the recruitment of public doctors from Japan failed (see chap. 2), after 1897 two categories of medical practitioners were produced from intensive government medical courses. One was the *keisatsu i* (police physician). The other was the *genji i* or *otsushô ishi* (B-class doctor with a limited practice), former first-aid helpers in villages and townships.[63] Before the colonial government raised enough manpower to provide adequate medical services in colonial Taiwan, B-class and police doctors played an important enforcement role for various hygienic regulations in rural society.[64] Although their status was different, they were both executors of regulations and practitioners of medicine with official authority.

The establishment of formal medical education in Taiwan greatly impacted the centralized sanitary administration of the government. It allowed private Taiwanese physicians to share administrative power with government medical personnel such as sanitary policemen, *ko i* (public doctors), B-class doctors, and police doctors, all of whom represented the power of the colonial government. The change began in 1899 when the government first upgraded the first-aid training program to intensive training in a medical school. This meant that Taiwanese could begin to practice medicine rather than only working as medical assistants. According to school regulations, the training program only accepted Taiwanese students. Segregation may not have been the main reason for rejecting Japanese students. The training program mainly concentrated on clinical skills, and to maintain the prestige of Japanese medicine in the colony the government had strong reasons to keep Japanese students away from such "low-level" training, which did not provide sufficient opportunities for laboratory internships. Furthermore, students of the medical school received government subsidies and could accept official appointments for five years after graduation. The appointments were usually for therapeutic work in public dispensaries not laboratory positions.[65] On completion of their appointments, medical graduates seldom rose to high-level positions in public hospitals and tended to work in private dispensaries. Thus, the colonial government ensured that the Sôtokufu igakkô, by the educational standards of the time, would be a second-tier school from the very beginning.

The establishment of the Sôtokufu medical school did not immediately solve the medical manpower shortage as the government had hoped. In its first six years, the medical school had an average graduation rate of only 10 percent and a withdrawal rate of more than 30 percent.[66] The situation changed after the 1905 primary education reform, however, which improved the Japanese primary school curriculum and encouraged Taiwanese to study modern medicine after graduation. The Japanese colonial education system was entirely in Japanese, so by 1905 the first generation of students that had been schooled entirely in Japanese would have been entering the Sôtokufu medical school. The improvement in Japanese-language fluency among Taiwanese medical students reduced the withdrawal rate and increased the number of graduates. Meanwhile, beginning in 1905 medical students could decide whether to accept or refuse the government subsidy. This resolved the problem of Taiwanese students' reluctance to work for the colonial government.[67]

Later the medical school entrance examination became very competitive, and the number of graduates increased. The percentage of students passing the entrance examination dropped from 72 percent in 1905 to an average of 12 percent after 1919.[68] However, to supplement the insufficient medical manpower and replace practitioners of traditional medicine, Takagi suggested that the Sôtokufu medical school provide at least sixty-five graduates annually in 1905 and 1906, but this goal was not reached. In 1918, the Sôtokufu igakkô was reorganized as the Taihoku igaku senmon gakkô. Under the new medical college regulations, tropical hygiene and tropical epidemiology became essential courses for students.[69] After 1918, the number of graduates rapidly grew, although the majority was still Taiwanese until the mid-1930s.[70] While the major course work was still in clinical skills, with the new additions to the curriculum graduates stood a better chance of receiving higher-level training in experimental medicine.

As the number of Taiwanese medical graduates increased and their training improved, they began to take over the former functions of public and B-class doctors. In addition, as the number of civilian physicians increased the functions of the *keisatsu i* (police physicians) were reduced to simple birth and death registration duties.[71]

From table 3.2, we are able to easily identify 1924 as the turning point when the number of doctors exceeded the level in 1902 and the majority was obviously working in private dispensaries. Moreover, as police physicians, public doctors, and B-class doctors did not represent a significant segment of total medical manpower, the newly created private dispensary doctor had to play the role that the government had originally designed for official medical practitioners. It is worth noting that the sharp decline in traditional practitioners was only among licensed practitioners. Without a second licensing examination, over time there was a significant decline in legal practitioners of Chinese medicine.[72] In the 1930s, botanical drugstores served the therapeutic needs of those who practiced illegally, primarily in rural areas.

TABLE 3.2: Numbers of B-Class Physicians, Private Dispensary Doctors, Police Doctors, and Traditional Physicians in Taiwan, 1897–1942

Year	Public and B-Class Physicians	Private Dispensary Doctors[a]	Police Doctors[b]	Sub total[c]	Traditional Physicians	Total Physicians
1897	94	76	0	259	no record	no record
1898	73	65	0	211	no record	no record
1899	72	64	0	208	no record	no record
1900	68	73	0	223	no record	no record
1901	69	74	20	226	1,223	1,508
1902	73	83	20	250	1,903	2,215
1903	71	78	20	238	1,853	2,156
1904	71	85	20	251	1,742	2,064
1905	74	94	20	275	1,671	2,041
1906	73	106	20	298	1,506	1,904
1907	75	120	20	331	1,458	1,963
1908	77	140	4	375	1,418	1,872
1909	77	154	12	351	1,314	1,791
1910	80	179	12	383	1,266	1,823
1911	84	197	12	388	1,223	1,801

1912	85	224	12	423	1,161	1,830
1913	89	251	12	458	1,100	1,850
1914	92	287	12	509	1,041	1,878
1915	94	329	12	578	979	1,941
1916	105	369	12	583	927	1,887
1917	103	399	12	610	887	1,912
1918	105	414	12	667	830	1,989
1919	104	462	12	721	786	2,007
1920	99	508	13	763	732	2,041
1921	101	542	14	816	674	2,084
1922	123	543	14	821	632	2,026
1923	132	570	14	882	583	2,036
1924	162	601	14	927	558	2,596
1925	169	649	14	972	522	2,676
1926	187	666	14	1,019	486	2,790
1927	188	717	14	1,112	456	2,861
1928	192	724	14	1,101	422	2,948
1929	209	805	14	1,185	384	3,081
1930	209	857	14	1,272	354	3,261
1931	225	897	14	1,322	325	3,416
1932	233	965	14	1,403	305	3,618
1933	241	1,017	14	1,466	281	3,723
1934	249	1,012	14	1,549	256	3,878
1935	248	1,103	14	1,674	233	4,062
1936	261	1,201	14	1,817	204	4,234
1937	272	1,240	14	1,845	181	4,365
1938	272	1,321	14	1,983	163	4,562
1939	279	1,328	14	2,018	141	4,647
1940	291	1,537	14	2,401	133	4,345
1941	293	1,513	14	2,228	119	4,397
1942	284	1,665	14	2,441	97	5,619

Source: Taiwansheng xingzheng zhangquang gongshu, ed., *Taiwansheng wushiyinianlai tongjitiyao* (A Statistical Summary of Taiwan over the Past Fifty-one Years) (Taipei: Taiwansheng xingzheng zhangquang gongshu, 1947), 1249–50.

[a] Numbers before 1909 are estimated on equation: 0.47 × (subtotal of public doctors). The coefficient 0.47 comes from average mean of official estimated numbers in 1899, 1902, and 1906.

[b] Police doctor was a part-time position before 1908; the title was changed to *eisei gishi* or *gishō* (hygiene mechanic) in 1944.

[c] Numbers include physicians working at hospitals in urban areas.

Unlike the proposal to establish RIGG and CIR, the colonial government established the Sôtokufu medical school to teach clinical medicine for treating practical problems rather than to produce university graduates for laboratory work, as in Japan. Medical education bylaws in colonial Taiwan restricted enrollment to local students until 1936, and public hospitals refused to provide internships for graduates for reasons of race as most of their patients were Japanese.

Without an internship, clinical training was incomplete. In 1905, only the Japanese Red Cross hospital in Taipei could provide internship training to Sôtokufu medical graduates. Even so, this meant that medical training for Taiwanese would merely range from emergency curative to reliable therapeutic work.[73] Although discrimination existed,[74] twelve public hospitals opened internships to graduates of the medical school by 1940. Internships in major hospitals improved the social status of indigenous physicians by enhancing their credibility and creating a network of medical care that operated through private dispensaries and public hospitals.[75]

Table 3.3 shows a very different distribution for Taiwanese medical graduates than for their Japanese counterparts.[76] Because of the success of the school in providing medical education, the number of hospitals increased dramatically after the mid-1920s. However, while the number of public hospitals never exceeded 35, the number of private hospitals or dispensaries owned by Taiwanese physicians increased to 263 by 1940.[77] While public hospitals had better equipment and medicine, the average cost of treatment was much higher than in private hospitals.[78]

In addition, Japanese physicians, most of whom were trained in Japan, still held the majority of positions as residential physicians in public hospitals and the high-level administrative positions in public hospitals. Between 1902 and 1940, 81.87 percent of medical practitioners in public and private facilities were graduates from Taiwan, but only 12.66 percent had received training in public hospitals. A mere 5.46 percent of these were able to continue to practice in the hospital after their two years of resident training.[79] That is, despite the considerable Japanese investment in building public hospitals, the main contribution was not from Japanese doctors in well-equipped public hospitals but from Taiwanese practitioners in private dispensaries.

To maintain education in clinical medicine, in 1935 the government established the medical school of Taihoku Imperial University as a part of the imperial university system. Unlike what had happened in Japan, the Taihoku medical college was not converted into a medical university but coexisted with the medical school at Taihoku Imperial University.[80] A comparison of the curriculum and graduates shows that the Taihoku Imperial University

TABLE 3.3: Occupational Distribution of Medical Graduates in Taiwan according to a 1921 Survey

Year of Graduation	Doctor in Private Dispensary	Public Doctor	Doctor in Government Institution	Advanced Student	Unknown
1902	1	no record	no record	no record	no record
1903	no record	no record	no record	no record	no record
1904	5	1	no record	no record	no record
1905	6	no record	no record	no record	no record
1906	14	2	no record	no record	no record
1907	16	4	no record	no record	no record
1908	15	1	no record	1	no record
1909	14	3	1	no record	no record
1910	19	3	3	no record	o record
1911	23	2	1	no record	no record
1912	26	no record	no record	no record	1
1913	34	1	no record	no record	no record
1914	23	4	no record	no record	no record
1915	37	1	2	no record	no record
1916	27	1	1	no record	1
1917	32	1	3	no record	no record
1918	31	no record	4	no record	no record
1919	26	1	9	no record	no record
1920	22	no record	15	no record	2
1921	4	no record	19	no record	12
Total	374	25	53	1	16

Source: Taiwan Sôtokufu igaku senmon gakkô, ed. *Sôtokufu igaku senmon gakkô ichiran* (Overview of the Sôtokufu Medical College) (Taihoku: Sôtokufu igaku senmon gakkô, 1922), 162.

Note: "No record" indicates either zero or lack of data. For example, from the class of 1909 fourteen graduates went to work in private dispensaries, three became public doctors, and one went to work in a government institution. For the rest, there is no record.

medical school had more courses and better training in laboratory medicine, and the number of Japanese students also increased.[81] Thus, it is reasonable to conclude that nationalism and political considerations affected the development of medical education in colonial Taiwan.

A Hybrid Medical System that Favored Physicians

In the early 1920s, there were many signs that a sanitary and medical infrastructure of colonial medicine had been established in Taiwan. Gotô's original plan was nevertheless compromised by its integration into the colonial context: the need to cooperate with the local elite, to depend on local resources—people's support and economic funding—and to address the medical problems of Taiwan's tropical environment. Miriam Ming-cheng Lo calls this transition of Gotô's ideal into colonial reality "the history of hybridization."[82]

Training private practitioners was meant to reduce the financial burden on the government budget. In fact, finances were a key issue when the colonial government designed Taiwan's medical care system. The government only offered comparatively low-cost medical care services. Chart 3.2 shows that the proportion of public health and medical expenditures in the colonial governmental budget was lower than that of Japan. The proportion was even lower after private dispensaries began to provide more medical services to Taiwanese society. Even so, despite the increase in graduates and their achievements in clinical medicine, the distribution of the government budget still favored the RIGG and CIR research institutes.[83]

As discussed earlier, the number of private dispensaries increased as the number of medical graduates grew. The therapeutic functions of public doctors were soon being provided by private physicians. By 1940, the total number of medical doctors in Taiwan was 3,426, only 291 of whom were public doctors; 2,173 were Taiwanese, and 1,253 were Japanese. The changing ratios also show how Taiwanese public doctors began to replace Japanese public doctors over time. The statistics from 1913 show that the ratio of Japanese to Taiwanese public doctors on the whole island was 69 to 20. However, by 1940 Taiwanese public doctors had become the majority (a ratio of 167 to 124).[84] Only in Taipei (the political center) and eastern Taiwan (the immigration areas) was there a higher ratio of Japanese public doctors compared to Taiwanese public doctors, namely, 25 to 19 in Taipei and the eastern areas, 24 to 1 in Taitung, 17 to 10 in Hualienkang, and 5 to 1 in the Penghu Islands; in the western areas, the ratios were 10 Japanese public doctors to 35 Taiwanese in Hsinchu, 16 to 31 in Taichung, 15 to 36 in Tainan, and 16 to 30 in Kaohsiung.[85] In short, the graduates of Taiwan's medical school and college, most of them

Taiwanese, eventually took over government medical functions, including such positions as public doctor, B-class doctor, and police physician.

CHART 3.2: Public health expenditures as a percentage of total governmental spending in Taiwan and Japan, 1911–38. $E(t)$ = health expenditures; s.e. = standard error. (Data from *Taiwan Sôtokufu Statistical Books;* and Koseisho ed., *Isei hyakunenshi furo,* 32–33, for the years 1910–41.)

A. Taiwan

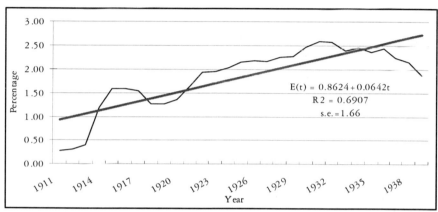

B. Japan

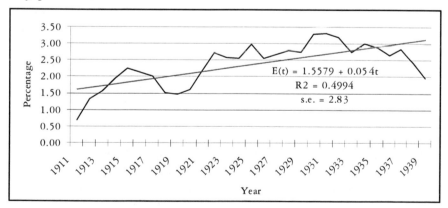

Doctors' Monopoly in the Medical Services Market: The Relationship between Doctors and Pharmacists

Besides the discrimination in government facilities, the mechanism of Japanese colonial medicine in Taiwan favored a privatized medical services market, especially for doctors. It was impossible for the colonial government to share political rights with Taiwanese doctors, but sharing the economic benefits of a privatized market for medical services was acceptable. Compared to the status of pharmacists, midwives, and nurses, doctors in Taiwan were the only medical professionals trusted by both the colonial government and the indigenous society. The colonial government thus never set any training standards for the other professions. Pharmacists and doctors both played important roles in developing modern medical services, and the following discussion addresses the relationship between those two professions in colonial Taiwan as a means of illuminating features of Japanese colonial medicine.

Based on the revision of Ise (Medical Regulations) in Japan in 1884, the colonial government issued the Taiwan igyôkisoke (Regulation of Medical Practice in Taiwan) following the occupation and quickly issued the Taiwan yakuzaishi yajusho seyakusha torishimarikisoke (Regulations for Pharmacists, Drug Sales, and Drug Manufacturing) in 1896.[86] According to the 1884 revision, the government allowed private practitioners to open dispensaries.[87] There the functions of prescribing and dispensing would be combined under the supervision of dispensary clinicians.[88] Both regulations in Taiwan were almost the antecedents of the 1884 revision in Japan, which gave doctors the privilege of selling medications.[89] The Taiwanese documents differed from the Japanese in only two respects: the geographic restriction—doctors were licensed by the colonial government to practice only in Taiwan—and the lack of pharmaceutical education provided to the colonial population.[90]

Besides the legal protection guaranteed by the 1884 revision, colonial policies also helped Taiwanese private doctors gain a monopoly in the market of medical services. In one way, the colonial government attempted to suppress the practice of Chinese medicine, which reduced the competition from Western doctors, especially private ones. In 1897, there were 1,070 dojin i (indigenous physicians), including 29 ryô i (expert physicians), 97 se i (hereditary practitioners), 91 jû i (Confucian physicians), 829 ji i (current medical practitioners), and 24 yô i (Western physicians).[91] The licensing examination for Chinese medicine practitioners in 1902 was the only one of its kind during the colonial period. The number of licensed traditional practitioners dropped rapidly from more than 2,000 in 1902 to fewer than 40 in 1945.[92] However, despite the increase in private dispensaries, the decrease in traditional practitioners, and dramatic population growth, the ratio of people served per doctor never exceeded the level of 1902. By the end of the 1930s, more than 90 percent of the doctors in Taiwan were practicing Western medicine while only 2 percent—and fewer legally—were treating their patients with Chinese medicine.

To further support doctors' monopoly in the market of medical services, no pharmaceutical education or licensing examinations were provided for pharmacists; formal pharmaceutical education was never even considered in colonial era Taiwan. Without such training and licensing, it was difficult for pharmacists to maintain a professional image, and, indeed, they were often considered medical salesman.[93] This situation deeply harmed the profession; pharmacists had no power to balance against that of doctors. Chart 3.3 shows the career relationships among the three major medical professions.

CHART 3.3: Careers of Taiwanese medical and pharmaceutical professionals. Shaded areas indicate the main body of each profession.

Profession and Training	Medicine	Pharmaceuticals	Botanical Pharmacognosy
Professional/elite (university)	Some in government facilities and private dispensaries	None	Few in government institutes
Vocational (college)	Majority in private dispensaries	Few in commercial pharmacies	None
Lay practitioners and others	Private dispensaries	Majority in drugstores	Botanical drugstores

Source: Fan Zuoxun ed. *Taiwan yauxue shi*, pp.73 and Taiwansheng xingzheng zhangquang gongshu ed., *Taiwansheng wushiyinianlai tongji tiyao*, Table 529.

The number of legal pharmacists in Taiwan increased from 13 in 1912 to 257 in 1942. The increase in pharmacists shows a trend less dramatic than but similar to that for persons practicing in private dispensaries.[94] To respond to economic growth and the increased need for medical services in Taiwan, the colonial government announced the Yakuzaishihô (Regulation of Pharmacists) in 1925, in which it accepted pharmacists' licenses issued in Japan.[95] However, the government still refused to open up pharmaceutical education programs in Taiwan, even on a vocational level.

An accelerated population increase and slower growth in licensed doctors after the mid-1920s stimulated the need for health care and eventually expanded the market for medical services. Also major medical facilities, including private dispensaries and pharmacies, were usually located in cities and their outlying areas. Due to the difficulty of accessing these facilities, traditional medicine and botanical materials, with their convenience and cheaper price, came to replace Western medicine in rural areas. In 1921, there were 2,666 shyôyakuten (botanical drugstores) in Taiwan, including yakuten (drugstores) and botanical over-the-counter (OTC) vendors, while there were only 2,782 yakkyoku (pharmacies). The cost of opening a drugstore was much less than the cost of opening a dispensary or pharmacy. According to the regulations, only licensed pharmacists could open a pharmacy while drugstores had no such requirement. The investment in pharmaceutical training and licensing examinations had to be included. In addition, the main business of botanical drugstores was the sale of kanbôyaku (Chinese medicine).[96] Pharmaceutical manufactories in colonial Taiwan were small and home styled.[97] The major benefit in terms of market competition was the cheaper price. For example, in 1938 a tablet of aspirin-based antipyretic cost 1.2 yen and the kagaku kanbô (scientific Chinese medicine) Saliso Karuchikoru, used for the same purpose, was 0.6 yen.[98] A package of the three-day formula Jinmudan (see fig. 4.1) cost only 0.1 yen to deliver the same effect.[99] As the demand for scientific Chinese medicine rose during the 1930s, the major products of Taiwanese private manufactories were glucose and halibut liver oil.[100] The Chinese medicine drugstores continued to play an important role in Taiwanese life, although as a survival strategy, to promote sales, they eventually renamed themselves local OTC manufactories in the 1930s while keeping the same formulas from herb roborants to botanical tonics.[101] The botanical drugstores grew rapidly, especially after 1924 when the number of pharmacies started to decline. In 1942, there were 10,238 botanical drugstores of various sizes, five times the number of pharmacies (2,070).[102]

Although traditional herbal drugstores became modern botanical drugstores and survived, they still faced competition from large-scale production in Japan and doctors' legal right to dispense medicine in Taiwan. The revision of the Japanese Pharmacopoeia regulation in 1891 allowed botanical medicine to become a legal part of official prescription medicine. In the following twenty years, a growing number of botanical medicines began to show up in various medical reference books, and investment by major companies in the field, such as Takada, Shionogi, and Yamanouchi, followed.[103] Due to the small scale of local production of herbal medicines in Taiwan, most producers merely repackaged imported medicines from Japan.[104]

Even worse, the combination of prescribing and dispensing medicine, as well as the presence of some OTC drugs in private dispensaries, hurt the pharmaceutical industry. A book, Rinjyo iyaku soho zenron (Comprehensive Collection of Prescription and Dispensation for Clinical Use), provided a good case for how a dispensary clinician would sell medicines from regular OTC to prescription drugs. For a stomachache, the authors recommended treatments ranging from "take aspirin 0.5 gram with two cups of Japanese rice wine (*sake*)" to the injection of "hydrochloric morphine 0.005~0.01 gram diluted with distilled water 1 gram."[105] Treatments at the dispensary would also include prescriptions for herbal OTC drugs. A roborant tonic for adult males was made of licorice power, dried orange peel, white sugar, and red wine.[106] Advertisements for similar OTC products were often posted in major newspapers throughout the 1930s.[107] Generally speaking, as a private dispensary had a limited ability to conduct surgery, dispensing accounted for most of its major medical services. It could also provide diagnosis, physical examinations, and health education. Comparatively, pharmacies and OTC drugstores were quite limited.

In colonial Taiwan, the pharmaceutical industry shrank dramatically in the 1930s. Pharmacies in Taiwan found it difficult to survive as private dispensaries took over the dispensing of drugs and as the number of OTC and botanical drugstores grew. Chart 3.4 shows the operations of the private dispensary, pharmacy, and OTC (including botanical) drugstore. The pharmaceutical industry was clearly being squeezed from all sides.

CHART 3.4: Services provided by private dispensaries, pharmacies, and over-the-counter (OTC) drugstores.

Practice	Dispensary	Pharmacy	OTC Drugstore
Diagnosis and treatment	X		
Prescription	X		
Dispensing medicine (Western and botanical)	X	X	
Hygienic education	X	X	
Sale of OTC drugs	X	X	X
Sale of drugs for environmental and sanitary uses		X	X
Sale of packaged traditional botanical medicines		X	X

Overlap between the private dispensary and OTC drugstore services occurred in only one area, the sale of OTC drugs. However, pharmacies faced competition in all areas—with private dispensaries in the first three items and with OTC drugstores in the last three.

Takagi Tomoe's *Die hygienischen Verhaltnisse der Insel FORMOSA* (Hygienic Conditions on the Island of Formosa [Taiwan]), published in 1911, contains three interesting photographs. One shows a Japanese pharmacy in Tainan, Aiseidô, which had a front signboard carved with the word *jindan* and small notes referring to the sale of other commodities such as drugs and therapeutic equipment.[108] The other two photographs are of the Hongsheng pharmacy and a traditional herbal drugstore, Xie-feng hao, in Tainan.[109] From the context and signs in the photographs, it is impossible to tell whether the Hongsheng pharmacy sold herbal or Western medicines or both. However, the photograph of the Xie-feng hao drugstore clearly reveals that it only sold botanical and herbal materials. In that picture, besides images of patients and store helpers, the reader can see a traditional doctor who also worked at the drugstore and set his table in the shadow of the middle pillar. Compared to the hybridized sales in pharmacies and drugstores, the pictures of public hospitals in the same book—in Tainan, Taihoku (Taipei), Ako (today's Pingdong), and Taihoku Red Cross—were purely Western-style medical institutions.[110] The story behind these photographs is the inequality between medical doctors and pharmaceutical practitioners, reflecting the "medicine-preferred and pharmacy-less" bias in the design of the colonial medical system. Pharmacists and traditional practitioners were not the only medical professionals to have been sacrificed by the colonial government in Taiwan to support private practitioners of Western medicine. Moreover, colonial Taiwan also lacked institutional training for midwives and nurses, who were meant to serve as doctors' subordinates or assistants and were never seen as part of the medical profession.[111]

Discrimination in the Practice of Colonial Medicine

Acclimatization was the core principle of medical reform during the Japanese occupation of Taiwan. With regard to epidemic disease, this principle was expressed in the government's policy toward cholera and plague. The same principle guided policies addressing opium addiction and malaria, although for Japanese officials these were seen as resulting from bad habits and unsanitary behaviors that were part of the traditional Chinese heritage. Such hypotheses provided a conceptual basis for the colonizers' adoption of the German *Sozialhygiene* as a guide for their policies in Taiwan.

Before the occupation, the Japanese government had already acknowledged the seriousness of Taiwan's opium problem. In fact, like the Qing rulers in

China (1644–1895), the Meiji government saw opium addiction as a Western imperialist threat that needed to be addressed.[112] In addition, during the military actions of 1895 Japanese troops in Taiwan suffered from *fudobyô* (endemic disease), among which malaria was the major killer. The Japanese understood that malaria had been a key factor in Western colonization and carefully watched the Western malariology programs being developed in the 1900s. Therefore, the successful control of opium and endemic malaria in Taiwan would be significant for the Japanese empire in demonstrating its status as a new colonial medical power.

Opium Addiction: Profit from a Chinese Bad Habit

While German medicine remained the paradigm for Japanese medical thought, it was elaborated on and amended in colonial Taiwan's medical reforms to stress moral and social traits. Climate and topography might explain why specific diseases occurred in Taiwan, but social behavior seemed to provide a complementary explanation for other serious conditions.

Opium addiction, as a troublesome issue for the practitioners of Japanese medicine in Taiwan, had political, social, and financial aspects. Medical treatment for it was not provided in Taiwan until the mid-1930s, but the primary reason for this was not ignorance. The Meiji government had taken a restrictive stance on the matter, prohibiting opium in Japan in 1870. Death and exile were the punishments for the crimes of trading and smoking it.[113] During the 1895 treaty negotiations, Itô Hakufumi declared his confidence in the Japanese government's ability to prevent opium addiction in Taiwan.[114] However, the colonial government did not enforce the prohibition, following instead a policy of gradualism that was supported by Ishiguro Tadanori and Gotô Shinpei. Gotô's approach was rejected by Katô Naoshi, the deputy chief of the Bureau of Hygiene in Taiwan, but in 1897 the minister of home affairs, Yoshikawa Kenshô, adopted Gotô's proposal.[115] The next year Gotô took office in the colonial government and began to enforce his gradualist policy.

Gotô's proposal of 1895, "Taiwan ahenseito ni kansuru iken" (Opinions regarding the Opium Administration in Taiwan), was the blueprint for the colony's opium monopoly system. The proposal, reflecting concern about financial deficits and social unrest, argued that a monopoly system would not only reduce the number of addicts but increase government income. That is, in addition to selling opium the government would license its sale to dealers and buyers. Not only would the income gradually supplement financial shortages in the government, but over time the higher monopoly price would reduce consumption.[116] In 1897, the colonial government issued the Taiwan ahenrei (Taiwan Opium Regulation) to implement Gotô's proposal. It was amended in 1898, 1902, 1928, and 1930, but only the last amendment mentioned medical treatment for addicts; all the others were about how to increase revenues.

In the view of many medical professionals, including Gotô Shinpei, opium addiction was a major disciplinary and medical issue. Addiction, it was believed, resulted from the dark side of Chinese culture and was a leading cause of crime, insubordination, and "inefficiency" in Taiwanese society.[117] From 1900 to the 1910s, the government drew attention to "the destruction, the defiance of control, and the commission of crimes which are the consequence of the fatal habit of opium addiction."[118] However, the government criticized opium addiction as a moral crime while simultaneously asserting its need for the revenue derived from its sale.[119] In consequence, despite protests from medical officers such as Shimada Sanrô, who blamed the government for encouraging the "moral and physical poison" of opium on the one hand while punishing it on the other, the government's monopoly over the manufacture and sale of opium remained an institutionalized part of colonial life in Taiwan.[120] Between 1910 and 1930, revenue from the monopoly was so attractive that the government twice granted greater access to opium addicts and wholesale merchants.[121]

In spite of the government's concentration on the revenue derived from opium, the number of addicts did decline during the colonial period,[122] although this had no significant statistical relationship with the increased cost of the drug. Chart 3.5 shows that the number of addicts declined after 1900. However, the correlation coefficient (-0.39) suggests that this decline was not significantly related to the change in opium price. After deflating the opium price by means of a price index in the colonial period, the monopoly income from opium rose in real price as well as in nominal terms.[123] In addition, the new correlation coefficient (-0.28) still supports the previous observation. According to Chen Jinsheng's study, this means that the self-discipline movement among the Taiwanese gentry and religious groups that helped addicts after 1900 were important influences in reducing addiction.[124] However, that movement and those groups were persecuted by the government on suspicion of rebellion and conspiracy.[125]

Another explanation for the decline was coercive prohibition by sanitary policemen. In order to "isolate" the Japanese from the possibility of addiction, the government used sanitary policemen to separate addicts by ethnicity. Japanese addicts were sent back to Japan for treatment and were not permitted to buy opium in Taiwan. With Taiwanese addicts, policemen had the right to supervise their purchase of opium and determine whether their purchase charter would be renewed. The charter to purchase opium was only issued to

CHART 3.5: Income from the opium monopoly and reductions in number of addicts. (Data from Taiwansheng xingzheng zhangquang gongshu, *Taiwansheng wushiyinianlai tongjitiyao*, 1373; and Taiwan Sôtokufu senbaigyoku, *Taiwan ahenji*, 227, 513–14.)

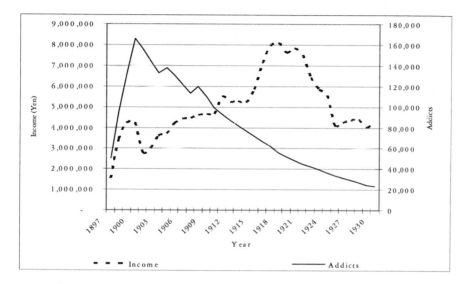

the addict and had to be renewed every two to three years. Those who could not pay the official prices and sought opium on the black market would be arrested for violation of the monopoly laws and for potentially "polluting" the Japanese community in Taiwan.[126] From this, we may deduce that the majority of "legal" addicts were wealthy Taiwanese for only these addicts could afford the rising prices of the drug. At the same time, the decline in the total number of addicts no doubt resulted from the punishment of "illegal" addicts by the sanitary police.

In 1930, the government suddenly issued new regulations providing medical treatment for addicts. There were two reasons for the change. First, with the onset of World War I, crude opium and dried opium poppy became difficult to import, and this in turn increased the cost of selling opium in Taiwan.[127] Second, international pressure forced the Japanese government to change its dual system (domestic versus colonial) of addressing opium addiction.[128] Thus, due to the shortage of raw opium and international pressure, the colonial government in Taiwan had to implement an opium policy that resembled Japan's.

Although the restrictive regulations of 1930 provided the legal basis for the medical "correction" of addiction, medical resources were in fact insufficient. Five medical institutions provided only 375 beds, which fell far short of the island's 25,527 addicts.[129] Moreover, the new regulations made opium addiction a crime: coercive measures were instituted, and the Division of Opium Policemen was established to implement the measures. The regulations also preserved ethnic segregation. The major institution addressing opium addiction was the Taihoku kôseiin (Taihoku Asylum of Correction) with 100 beds. The first Taiwanese PhD in medicine, Du Congming, was the deputy chief. On the principle that "the Taiwanese should cure Taiwanese illnesses," the government hired only Taiwanese personnel at the asylum.[130] Finally, before World War II the government's primary concern was still the income derived from the monopoly on opium. Thus, despite Du's efforts, the results of the medical treatment of addiction were not significant.

Because the *dôka seisaku* (assimilation policy) transformed to the *kominka seisaku* (Japanization policy) after the 1930s, the colonial government was asked to apply Japan's opium policy to Taiwan.[131] In doing so, the government fully supported Du's medical work and strengthened the enforcement capabilities of the opium policemen. The government also supported various social movements to eradicate addiction. In addition, the war disrupted the importation of opium materials and increased the demand for healthy manpower, thereby reducing the benefits of the opium monopoly. Both changes created a better environment for Du's work.[132] Because of Japanese politics and the war, Du's medical program came to enjoy the full support of the government, and as a result the number of addicts dropped sharply after 1940.

The Antimalaria Program

Unlike opium addiction, malaria was endemic in Taiwan. The Japanese identified the disease as an environmental problem stemming from the island's tropical climate. Therefore, malaria control was one aspect of "acclimatization" rather than "assimilation." Malarial study gained prominence in modern tropical medicine after Patrick Manson proposed his mosquito-transmission theory in 1894. For a latecomer to imperialism like Japan, attacking malaria by applying modern medicine was a way to exhibit Japan's success to the international community. In addition, for Japanese medical experts in Taiwan the antimalaria campaign was also a great opportunity to demonstrate their abilities to colleagues in Japan itself.

Before modern malariology was introduced to Taiwan, two major hypotheses existed to explain the disease, which previously had been called "unknown fever." The first was the notion of *zhangqi* from traditional Chinese medicine.[133] The second was the theory of "miasma," which was brought by early westerners, many of whom were medical missionaries.[134] The Japanese colonial authorities in 1895 were well aware of the threat to the colonizers' health posed by the many diseases on the island. In fact, many Japanese succumbed to disease when they occupied Taiwan.[135] Although malaria was endemic, the colonial government was busy dealing with other diseases, such as plague and smallpox, in the major cities and did not carry out a concerted antimalaria campaign until 1906, when a serious outbreak occurred in the camphor production areas of southern Taiwan. Although the 1906 outbreak warned the government of the prevalent thread of endemic malaria, it merely launched a small-scale campaign to deal with the problem and most preventive strategies were kept within academic circles.[136] A special meeting to map out an antimalaria strategy for the whole island was held in 1909, and a year later pilot programs were launched to experiment with Koch's method of requiring compulsory blood tests for residents and treating suspected and confirmed cases with quinine. In 1913, regulations were promulgated mandating the establishment of malarial control districts of about two thousand residents each where antimalaria stations were responsible for the enforcement of compulsory tests and treatment.[137]

Not surprisingly, the initial districts were located in areas with high concentrations of Japanese residents, natural resource development sites, and highly malarious areas. In 1932, there were 208 malaria control districts, and by the end of the decade more than three million people were undergoing routine blood examinations every year.[138] It is clear that the objective was the suppression of malaria with modern biomedical solutions, utilizing a "vertical" approach to exploit the existing centralized administrative structure where, at the *ho-kô* level, police and headmen collaborated to enforce antimalaria measures. As one historian explained, the government "avoid[ed] every possible expense in equipment and physical facilities, and [depended] on intensive use of all the administrative resources" at the government's command.[139] The coercive power of the colonial state and the hegemony of biomedical science reinforced one another to ensure the control of malaria, and the decline in malaria mortality—from 10,562 deaths in 1906 to 3,716 in 1937—testified to the success of these efforts (see table 3.4).[140]

Despite the fact that medical practitioners such as Horiuchi Takao were chiefly concerned with the practical application of quinine prophylaxis, others worried that quinine was not being taken by enough people to interrupt malaria transmission.[141] Such opinions affected the development of antimalaria policy in subsequent decades, and in 1913 the policy was reconfigured. Where quinine prophylaxis continued, it was integrated into and became barely distinct from ordinary sanitary activity. In addition, the most important function of the policy was the education it provided the public

TABLE 3.4: Blood Tests of Malaria Patients between 1910 and 1941

Year	Examination Stations	Blood Tests (A)	Positive Cases (B)	Rate (B/A) (%)
1910	no record	6,946	95	1.37
1911	12	101,064	4,311	4.27
1912	no record	218,868	2,786	2.64
1913	no record	269,999	6,366	2.36
1914	no record	286,334	6,553	2.29
1915	no record	218,361	8,389	3.84
1916	no record	354,299	11,888	3.36
1917	44	690,369	20,821	3.02
1918	58	942,605	20,073	2.13
1919	75	1,120,535	27,404	2.45
1920	68	1,032,336	20,270	1.96
1921	75	1,103,563	21,460	1.94
1922	78	1,210,432	30,278	2.00
1923	89	1,293,176	32,368	2.50
1924	117	1,636,439	47,232	2.89
1925	no record	1,732,182	42,528	2.46
1926	111	1,749,202	37,256	2.12
1927	117	1,927,826	36,523	1.89
1928	127	2,024,786	37,217	1.83
1929	132	2,188,089	38,504	1.76
1930	146	2,300,900	33,644	1.46
1931	155	2,370,553	44,329	1.88
1932	no record	2,430,740	67,265	2.77
1933	no record	2,470,950	72,092	2.92
1934	164	2,618,670	72,272	2.62
1935	no record	2,578,930	78,698	3.05
1936	186	2,771,631	83,989	3.03
1937	no record	2,811,822	85,575	3.04
1938	no record	3,214,736	106,167	3.30
1939	no record	3,459,364	116,822	3.38
1940	no record	3,595,122	98,047	2.73
1941	180	3,659,154	105,430	2.88

Sources: Taiwan Sôtokufu eiseika, *Taiwan mararia gaikyô* (Summary of Taiwanese Malaria) (Taihoku: Taiwan Sôtokufu, 1935), 8–9; Taiwansheng wenxian weiyuanhui, ed., *Taiwansheng tongzhi*, vol. 3: *Zhengshi zhi, "weisheng" pian* (Taichung: Taiwansheng wenxian weiyuanhui, 1972), 299b.

in the prevention of malaria.[142] The antimalaria program after 1913, then, was a combination of quinine prophylaxis, education, and sanitary measures.[143] Generally speaking, quinine prophylaxis was meant to improve the survival chances of Japanese settlers, and the enforcement of sanitary measures and education were ways to reform the environment. Both features endured in colonial antimalaria policy until 1945.

Endemic malaria was, in fact, the first major test of the efficacy of the colonial government.[144] The following discussion will reveal that the legacy of Japanese colonial medicine is essentially mixed and the complexity and contradictory nature of colonial medicine in Taiwan can only be understood in the detailed context of the colony, domestic Japan, and international society.

Malariology in Academic Circles. Roughly before 1910, the old miasma theory was favored in Japanese academic circles, and it appeared to be a very promising way to eliminate endemic malaria in Taiwan. In the first government report on Taiwanese sanitation in 1898, the Japanese scholar Tsuboi Jirô indicated that "humid, hot, and poisonous" air was the primary cause of malaria in Taiwan.[145] Based on Tsuboi's description, malaria in Taiwan had two obvious features: poisonous and environmental. This assertion guided the Japanese study of the disease for almost fifty years. However, the poisonous issue was technically easier to deal with than the environment issue. Japanese colonial administrators were concerned more with suppressing malaria than with understanding it, and even though they carried out entomological studies they were "largely taxonomic rather than biological or epidemiological."[146] Although malaria was classified as a local problem, Japanese scholars had to accept that it was universally transmittable once they understood the anopheles theory. In fact, by the turn of the twentieth century all of the essential knowledge needed to design an antimalaria campaign was in place.

In the 1910s, the response of Japanese malariologists to the disease was the same as that of any Western scientist. Mosquitoes replaced miasma in passing the disease. For example, Kinoshita Kashichirô was a scientist-physician and naturalist who believed that an understanding of human biology (and pathology) could be achieved only though an understanding of the biology of all living things. Collecting anopheles mosquitoes soon became a fashion in Japanese malariology as a way of identifying the target: the anopheles. As early as 1933, Morishita and Katagai had shown that 69.2 percent of malaria cases in Taiwan were transmitted by *Anopheles minimus* and 20.8 percent by *Anopheles sinensis*. They suggested that *A. minimus* was a major malarial vector in Taiwan while *A. sinensis* caused a problem only on the western plains. In 1936, Morishita listed fourteen species of anopheles found in Taiwan.[147]

Omori and Noda in 1943 discovered *A. barbumbrosus* on the east coast.[148] Within all of the anopheline species, only *A. minimus* and *A. sinensis* carried the *Plasmodium* that causes malaria.

Japanese researchers also were dedicated to finding the best treatment for malaria patients. As quinine was the most powerful medicine for malaria, twelve formulas were developed by Japanese physicians between 1926 and 1940 (see table 3.5).[149]

TABLE 3.5: Major Quinine-Based Treatments for Malaria in Colonial Taiwan

| Treatment[150] | Formula | | | Length of Treatment (days) |
| | Dosage (grams per day) | | | |
	Quinine and Others	Plasmochinum	Atebrin	
P.S. One-week method		0.04–0.06		7
P.S. Ten-day method		0.05–0.06		10
P.C. One-week method	Sulfurata 0.375–1.0	0.03–0.08		7
P.C. Ten-day method	Sulfurata 0.5–1.0	0.04–0.08		10
P.C. Two-week method	Sulfurata 0.625–0.75	0.05–0.06		14
P.Q. Five-day method	Sulfurata 0.8	0.04		5
P.Q.A.	Sulfurata 0.9	0.03		14
P.Q.B.	Sulfurata 0.9	0.04		14, 7
A			0.3	5
A.P.A.		0.03	0.3	7
Taiwan adjustment	Hydrochloride 0.8			18
Quinine I.V.	Hydrochloride 0.02–0.03 (per kilogram)			5–10

Source: Morishita Kaoru, "Taiwan chihôbyo to densen chousaiinkai ni okeru mararia chousa gaiyou," 142.

P.S. = pyrimethamine-sulfadoxine; P.C. = chloroquine-prima;

P.Q. = primaquine; P.Q.A. = type A treatment of P.Q.;

P.Q.B. = type B treatment of P.Q.; A = atebrin only;

A.P.A. = type A treatment of atebrin-primaquine; I.V. = intravenous injection.

Among these twelve treatments, the Taiwan adjustment of quinine therapy was the most common and paralleled the treatments adopted by the navy and army in Japan.[150] Postwar materials also show that the Taiwan adjustment had merged Plasmochinum and Atebrin to form a more complex treatment, lately known as the Morishita method (see chart 3.6).[151]

CHART 3.6: Treatments developed by the Central Research Institute in Taiwan

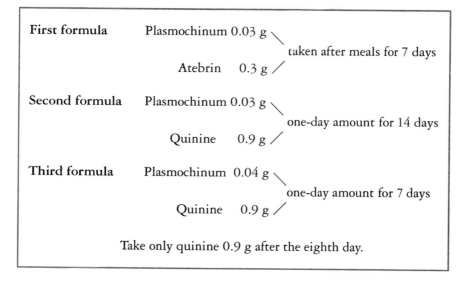

First formula   Plasmochinum 0.03 g
taken after meals for 7 days
Atebrin   0.3 g

Second formula   Plasmochinum 0.03 g
one-day amount for 14 days
Quinine   0.9 g

Third formula   Plasmochinum 0.04 g
one-day amount for 7 days
Quinine   0.9 g

Take only quinine 0.9 g after the eighth day.

In addition, like modern malariologists in the West, Japanese experts in colonial Taiwan also searched for a local replacement for imported quinine. Japanese scholars in colonial Taiwan turned to Chinese herbs: *changshan* (*Dichroa febrifuga*) and *chaihu* (*Bupleurum chinese*). Both were tested under laboratory conditions and had comparatively strong results. However, at least in 1933, neither medicine could be sufficiently and effectively produced. Additionally, the test results were questionable since each remedy was tested in fewer than twenty patients and no follow-up reports were issued following clinical observation.[152] The search for a Chinese herbal replacement for quinine seemed merely academic and had no impact on the pharmaceutical business in Japan. In 1950, a Japanese pharmacopoeia only had a very short statement on *changshan*: "a malaria antipyretic [that] contains an unknown alkaloid, and some say it has a therapeutic effect one hundred times more powerful than quinine."[153] Basically, the Japanese pharmacologists did not really expect to find a replacement for quinine, especially when importation was possible.

Pharmacological experiments on *changshan* and *chaihu* would have been seen as merely exotic.

The most exotic knowledge related to malariology in colonial Taiwan was malariotherapy.[154] Unlike their colleagues in Japan, who applied malariotherapy only to syphilis patients, Japanese physicians in colonial Taiwan saw it as a potential way to treat parasitic problems and other venereal diseases. In an article published in 1936, the author suggested malariotherapy for gonorrhea sufferers, claiming that all of his twenty-plus patients had positive responses to treatment.[155] Another article, published in 1938, suggested using malarial fever to "burn out" parasites.[156] With great confidence, Japanese malariologists not only tried to retest all the Western discoveries in Taiwan and Japan, but they also aimed to develop their own knowledge by learning modern malariology. Colonial officials hoped that success in merging malariology and modern laboratory techniques would spell victory over malaria in Taiwan.[157] This optimistic attitude soon faced a crucial challenge.

The Reality of the Antimalaria Campaign

As the "tools of empire" theory suggests, the colonial government invested a lot in antimalaria programs to increase the chances of survival for the colonizers. Antimalaria technologies developed in the academy were soon applied in Taiwan, but only in the beginning did they seem promising. Medical practitioners essentially adopted two preventive methods: the drainage or avoidance of swampy areas and quinine prophylaxis. The first method focused on residential areas such as cities and military compounds, while the second was sporadically applied at check stations in the immigrant villages.[158] Although quinine was important, the colonial government continuously complained about its cost and restricted its use.[159] Takagi once argued that as a result of malaria annual workdays lost were 150,416 for Japanese living in Taiwan and 3,365,896 for Taiwanese. Assuming a treatment fee of 0.3 yen per capita per day, the total cost would have been 2,254,893 yen a year.[160]

The limitations of the sanitation campaign and quinine usage became evident when the government applied them to a broader area. Although Governor-General Ando Teibi planned to invest a hundred million yen to solve the malaria problem in 1915, Takagi argued that eradicating malaria over the entire island would yield only half the benefit expected from the money and effort invested. He suggested suppressing malaria only in areas where public offices were located because the cost would be lower.[161] By taking such advice, during the 1920s Japanese immigrants exploiting new lands in eastern Taiwan suffered more from malaria than from other diseases.[162] The colonial government adopted quinine prophylaxis on an experimental basis from 1906 onward, but for financial reasons the experiment was only sporadically enforced among Japanese in the immigrant villages, government plantations, and major industries.[163] There is much evidence to show that the Japanese professionals pinned their faith on quinine prophylaxis for Japanese immigrants, hoping that it would prevent infection from settlement outsiders such as Taiwanese and aborigines.[164] Due to various natural disasters and epidemics, the immigration program finally encountered financial difficulties. Eventually the program became impossible to carry out satisfactorily and was ended in the 1930s.[165]

The failure to keep Japanese settlements malaria free signaled the inadequacy of Japanese malariology. All the efforts expended did not prevent the loss of life, and as a result, from around 1920 until the beginning of World War II, many settlers fled to Japan or cities in western Taiwan.[166] While government statistics showed a continuously declining trend in the malarial mortality rate, the rate of improvement varied in different regions.[167] Chart 3.7 shows the increases and decreases in malaria cases in both western and eastern Taiwan.

CHART 3.7: Regional trends in malaria morbidity rates (1917–40). (Data from Taiwan Sôtokufu eiseika, *Taiwan mararia gaikyô,* 8–9.)

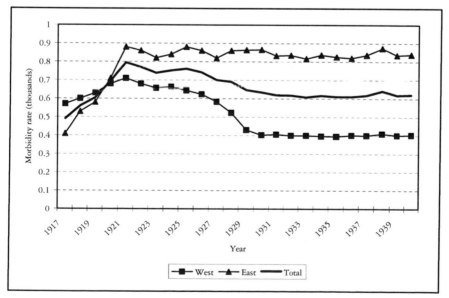

The malaria morbidity rate in western Taiwan quickly diminished after 1920 because of improved sanitation in many western cities.[168] Contrarily, as the general condition of malarial infection improved the number of cases in eastern areas surged before 1921, slightly increased after 1923, and then stayed relatively static between 1927 and 1940. While the diminishment of Japanese settlements in eastern Taiwan showed the limitations of the preventive strategy, western Taiwan had conditions more conducive to prevention and thus experienced better results.

Like other public health reforms, the antimalaria campaign started not in the countryside but in cities where better economic conditions and social organization led to better results. The growth of urbanization during the 1920s and early 1930s meant that every city had several public and private medical facilities. Compared to the average ratio of doctors to population in all of colonial Taiwan, 0.39 physicians per thousand people, the ratio of 0.62 in the three major cities—Taipei, Taichung, and Kaohsiung—was much better.[169] In addition, urban residents in western Taiwan enjoyed easy access to various kinds of medical help. Increasing numbers of pharmacies and drugstores not only sold mosquito coils and sprays but also provided medicines to relieve the suffering of malarial patients.[170] Mosquito coils and sprays were not expensive, and many over-the-counter medicines and common prescriptions such as antipyrine, aspirin, and senega were easily purchased at local pharmacies.[171] These commonly used treatments also could help *Plasmodium vivax* patients to overcome the painful cycle of relapse.[172] As a result, the chances of survival increased.[173] Besides the traditional *hokô* system and the sanitary police force, modern media also helped promote antimalaria programs in the cities. Newspapers such as *Taiwan nichinichishinpo* were powerful tools to educate people and raise the alarm about a crisis,[174] as were showings of antimalaria films.[175] Exhibitions were another popular way to promote preventive knowledge (see figure 3.3).[176]

While urbanization and higher living standards in the cities helped block malaria transmission, the agrarian countryside in western Taiwan remained under the shadow of endemic malaria. The turning point was the construction of the Great Jia'nan Irrigation System and Wushantou Dam, begun in 1929. Undertaking such a project meant that the colonial government had to invest in improving conditions for the workers. The construction resulted in more than 60 percent of the plains in western Taiwan being covered by a comprehensive antimalaria program, thus shifting the battle front to the countryside. The program not only incorporated important elements from the urban experience, but it also enhanced prevention efforts by improving infrastructure.[177]

The construction of the dam and irrigation system marked the much broader application of modern malariology. The builders were sensitive to

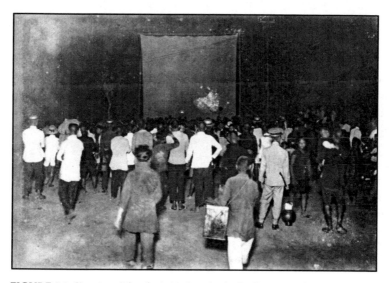

FIGURE 3.3: Showing slides about hygiene in the Da Daocheng district in Taipei. Courtesy of Chung Chin-shui.

the danger of malaria, and expert teams of malariologists, entomologists, biologists, and engineers were hired to become a permanent unit charged with figuring out how to control mosquitoes and the malaria they carried.[178] One way was draining wetlands and swamps to reduce the number of mosquito larvae, which accounted for nearly 30 percent of construction expenditures between 1929 and 1931.[179] Malaria rates did not decrease as quickly as the Japanese experts expected. In 1933, there were still about 3,021 cases of malaria annually, although better management and improved health services had reduced annual mortality to about 200 people.[180] In general, it would safe to conclude that two strategies were simultaneously applied in the Japanese antimalaria campaign: quinine prophylaxis targeted on human beings and environmental control to reduce the mosquito population.[181]

Although the strategies might be different in the cities and countryside, the means of promoting the antimalaria campaign as a whole were the same. The most influential network for preventive measures in the cities, and later in the countryside as well, was the public schools. Morishita's method of blood sampling was introduced in 1936 and soon applied in schools. Meanwhile, every school began to check students for splenomegaly as a way to identify chronic malaria.[182] Any students suspected of having the disease had to report to the local hospital, and their families underwent follow-up examinations for three to five years.[183] Preventive methods practiced during the construction mainly relied on antivector measures (mosquitoes) and quinine prophylaxis. The antivector measures were carried out in stations set up in the rural Jia'nan region. Public health officials appointed by each station taught villagers to clear bamboo bushes and water receptacles and, where possible, to install screens where the sick lay. In some cases, officials would spread larva-killing oil on large breeding sites and send squads out to destroy containers that might hold rainwater. Screens were only seen in military compounds or commercial locations because of their high cost.[184] Overall progress as a result of the preventive measures was slow but steady.[185]

The establishment of antimalaria stations in the countryside created an administrative foundation combining the *ho-kô* system, public dispensaries, a sanitary police force, and elementary schools, which grew rapidly in the mid-1920s and 1930s.[186] Stations in rural areas played a role similar to that of public hospitals in the cities, eventually shifting the focus of malariology away from the laboratory and bringing the urban prevention experience to rural Taiwan. The number of stations increased from 12 in 1911 to 185 in 1942, serving a population of 1,600 in 1910 and 6,276,695 in 1942.[187]

The success in the Jia'nan region was soon transferred to other places. A significant case reflecting the influence of the antimalaria stations was Morishita's investigation following the Great Hsinchu Earthquake. Morishita and his colleagues urged the establishment of antimalaria stations for distributing quinine following blood tests.[188] Besides the use of quinine prophylaxis, coercive blood examinations at antimalaria stations also gave researchers a tremendous opportunity to collect a sufficient number of samples. In the 1930s, three species of human malaria (*falciparum, malariae,* and *vivax*) were thus confirmed to be indigenous to Taiwan.[189] In addition to the progress in malariology during the 1930s, diagnosis and examination of *Plasmodium* also improved. According to one of Morishita's studies, his blood-screening method increased the accuracy rate to 80 percent.[190] Drawing on the increased number of cases and data collected at the stations and schools, academic experts in colonial Taiwan even developed their own quinine treatment programs in the 1930s, as noted in table 3.5.

Iijima Wataru and Wakimura Kôhei have compared differences between antimalaria policies in colonial India and Taiwan, emphasizing the political factor. The Indian colonial government, for example, made an effort to segregate colonists and local inhabitants in order to protect the former. Moreover, the authors note that the policy in Taiwan followed "Koch's method" (quinine prophylaxis), which enabled the colonial government to intervene in local society and extend its control over the Taiwanese people.[191] Their conclusion is accurate but overlooks the function of the public school system. Once the antimalaria campaign network was fully functioning, it also served the purpose of scientific research. Blood samples tested the efficacy of the Morishita method while the newer treatment was subjected to field experiments. With the rapid accumulation of data, a special unit of CIR was created at in the late 1920s to "search [for] the diagnosis and therapy of malaria patients, particularly for chronic patients, in order to provide a basis of policy making which gives priority to the treatment of patients and the eradication of carriers."[192] In this case, medicine was the tool of the colonizer for the purpose of self-approval and feedback to the empire.

As shown in a film circulated in Taiwan in 1939 to promote the antimalaria program, *Mararia no bôatsu* (The Prevention and Eradication of Malaria), during the colonial period the government strongly advocated an integrated approach to malaria control.[193] This involved the use of drugs, insecticides, and bed nets; prompt diagnosis; improved community-based systems; proper case management; improved health service systems; and proper environmental management geared toward vector control plus a continuous search for effective pharmacological prescriptions. The film highlighted three themes of the campaign: modern malariology, promising treatments, and environmental improvement. Although the film presents the themes smoothly and reasonably, the reality is that the antimalaria program was consumed with controversy. The contradictions between advanced technology and low-tech cleaning, quinine prophylaxis and environmental control, and expensive eradication and cheaper social mobilization were never resolved.

Molding the Legend of Japanese Colonial Medicine

In the 1930s, the system for reporting disease outbreaks was reliable, and laboratory and clinical medicine peacefully coexisted as a teacher (Japanese)-pupil (Taiwanese) relationship. The colonial government in Taiwan obviously had better statistics and evidence with which to persuade the Taiwanese to accept colonization as modernization, a core issue of scientific colonialism. Japanese colonialism intensified the importance of classification in the field of medicine. To know was to name; to name was to control. The colonial state soon found that "scientific" narratives of objective numbers could be a powerful tool.

While complex medical statistics and analytic models stayed mainly in academic circles, the bureaucracy in Japan and later in Taiwan used popular exhibitions to demonstrate its modernization efforts and win the cooperation of the colonized. Hygiene exhibitions are a good example. Tanaka Satoshi explores their changing meanings in the Japanese pavilion at the 1911

International Sanitary Conference in Dresden and at similar events held in Japan before 1945.[194] He suggests that they were designed to be a spectacular mass visual learning experience.[195] Such visual educational technology was even more important in colonial Taiwan. Exhibitions had been held in Japan from 1919 onward, and the governor-general in Taiwan, Den Kenjiro, soon made education beyond the classroom a priority as a way to promote assimilation.[196] The first hygiene exhibition, in 1918, was relatively shabby and only showcased the economy.[197] But by 1936 the colonial government was holding about fifty hygiene exhibitions a year with total attendance of about 150,000.[198]

Among those exhibitions, the most significant was the Keisatsu eisei tenrankai (Police Hygiene Exhibition) of December 1925 mounted by the Taihoku Prefecture Police Department. The five-day exhibition was hailed by local newspapers as unprecedented in size and scope. It vividly propagandized the colonial state's policing of public health and medical services as evidenced in the extensive record left behind. Everything was recorded, from its content (in the form of photographs of the exhibits) to its planning and intent (a textual record) and the reactions of both the Japanese and Taiwanese. Some 6,814 items were exhibited in several categories, including models, specimens, photographs, and posters. Among these publicity materials, the poster category was central.[199] Over a thousand posters hung throughout the exhibition, far outnumbering any of the other items. Police tallied the number of visitors at 308,900.[200] With a population in 1925 of 5.2 million, this means that exhibit was visited by about 2.6 percent of the people in Taiwan.[201]

The physical layout of the exhibition reflected four areas of the Japanese effort to modernize Taiwan: politics, finance, transportation, and medicine. Walking between the three buildings given over to exhibits, attendees traveled along boulevards lined with the centerpieces of Japanese colonial architecture in Taihoku, including the Taiwan Governor-General's Office (politics), the Bank of Taiwan (finance), the Taihoku train station (transportation), and the Taihoku hospital (medicine). The Eiseikan (Hall of Hygiene) was the single largest portion of the exhibition with over 2,794 items (41 percent of the total number of exhibited items). The exhibition was organized in a series of rooms devoted to sewers, city sanitation, and school and physical education hygiene followed by rooms devoted to the consumption of milk and meat, pregnancy and raising children, medicine, endemic diseases, oral hygiene, and barber hygiene. The largest section was devoted to contagious diseases.[202]

Under the comprehensive surveillance of the police force, as one poster showed, the stated goals of the Japanese colonial venture in Taiwan were to bring civilization and enlightenment to the Taiwanese through modern medicine.[203] Many exhibits compared public health conditions before and after colonial rule. One poster, captioned "Disease prevention in the thirty years of Japanese rule," graphically contrasted superstitious activities such as burning incense and dancing with shamans before the occupation with a modern vaccination administered by a doctor in a white coat in 1925.[204] The success of the colonial government in eliminating or stopping epidemics outside Taiwan was presented in an impressive way but was not entirely accurate. For example, another poster depicted a map of Taiwan with ships arriving from mainland China bringing cholera, bubonic plague, and smallpox, which in fact had been under control since 1901 when the colonial state began to systematically enforce port quarantines and vaccinations.[205] The common scenario implied that China was a major reservoir of these epidemics while simultaneously indicating that the Japanese colonial state had brought to Taiwan a scientific, secular understanding of disease prevention. However, foreigners were also responsible for bringing the diseases to Taiwan. For example, French troops brought cholera to Taiwan during the Sino-French War when they landed at Keelung in 1884.[206] And the Japanese transmitted the same germ to the whole island during their military actions after 1895.[207]

The 1925 exhibition as a whole presented the image of Japanese colonial rule in Taiwan as extending civilization along with the enlightenment of modern science. However, as discussed in previous chapters, the reality of public health improvement, disease prevention, and medical education was not always smooth going. The cowpox vaccination was successful, but its success relied heavily on the household registration system completed during the 1910s. Moreover, preventive technologies during the 1920s did not produce reliable results in the antimalaria campaign when we compare the loss of Japanese immigrant villages in eastern Taiwan with the campaign's success on the southwestern plain.

Taiwanese intellectuals at that time questioned the motives and strategies of Japanese colonial medicine in Taiwan but had little doubt about the nature of modern medicine that the colonizer had brought. The Taiwanese-run newspaper *Taiwan minpo* ran at least two articles that criticized the exhibition. In an article published on December 6, 1925, the author attacked the exhibition as intended first and foremost to improve the public's perception of the police, challenging the visual trope of presenting Japanese policemen as tall and strong while depicting the Taiwanese as children or weak. "How can one not conclude that the objective is to say that the Taiwanese lack a foundation of culture?" asked the author, pointing out the implicit discrimination.[208] Commercial interests were also promoting the image of advanced Japanese medicine. In the other article, the author focused on the statistics in one poster, noting that the number of Japanese geisha and escorts far surpassed the number of Taiwanese and Koreans engaged in these occupations but had fewer cases of sexually transmitted disease. After he learned of the overwhelming sponsorship of the exhibition by Japanese pharmaceutical companies, the author concluded that the statistics "must be incorrect" because the whole exhibition "was dominated by pharmaceutical advertisements."[209]

Both articles must be seen as not simply criticizing the colonial government's discrimination against the Taiwanese but also as a challenge to the police department's claim to be a responsible and trustworthy agent of sanitary reform. The images found most offensive were those that denied Taiwanese agency in pursuing modernity. The articles did not question the goals of the sanitary reforms—indeed, they wholeheartedly embraced them—but questioned the means by which they were being achieved. Similar reactions appeared in the 120-page official report of the exhibition. In the report, the police department stated that Taiwanese attendees resented the offensive descriptions of "evil customs" while they often praised the visual and statistical representation of progress in sanitary conditions and medical services.[210]

After the 1920s, the census data and sanitary investigations were on firmer ground. In fact, it became the fashion for central and local governments to compile numbers and conduct investigations in the 1920s and 1930s. Takekoshi Yosaburo stated in 1907, "I do not think it would be wrong to say that the degree of civilization attained by a people may be measured by the success of its sanitary administration. This is particularly true of tropical colonies."[211] That goal was set by governors-general throughout the colonial period, especially after the 1920s. For all the statistics implying the improvement of demographic and health conditions in colonial Taiwan, the same number would support the argument that Japanese colonial medicine had brought better life and health to the Taiwanese. The argument that life expectancy had been improved by modern Japanese medicine not only convinced medical professionals at that time but also led postwar researchers to shape the legend of modernity brought by Japanese colonial medicine. This historiographic tendency inspired the acceptance of the "tools of empire" theory by postwar historians in Taiwan.

In addition to reforms in the system for reporting births and deaths and the governmental census, the Department of the Police Force compiled its own census data starting in the 1920s. Various statistical books on studies of parasites, infectious diseases, and physical strength were published occasionally. Meanwhile, epidemiological investigations boomed after the 1920s when the government promoted an extensive investigation.[212] The colonial government officially initiated a series of epidemiological investigations during the mid-

1920s and early 1930s, and local governments undertook their own public health investigations.[213] Among the abundant entries in the 1925 exhibition, one-third were posters showing statistics, charts, and analyses. To the attendees, statistics was part of science and a convincing tool to prove the success of Japanese colonial medicine. Among all the statistical information, the emphasis on demographic improvements was most significant. Posters showing the infant mortality rate, improvements in life expectancy, and reductions in morbidity rates for selected diseases were there for professionals to study while the presentations impressed regular attendees.

Ruling a colony by means of scientific knowledge was a way for Japan to prove its ability to act as an imperial power in the first half of the twentieth century. The improvements in public health and medical services in colonial Taiwan were important issues amenable to "scientific" methods such as sanitary investigation and the collection of vital statistics. The meaning of gathering statistics and engaging in such investigations was, as Gyan Prakash suggests in his study of British India, that empires used colonies as a laboratory for modernity—a lifestyle set by the colonizer.[214] Institutional expansion sped up the creation of medical resources and the transfer of organizational models to Taiwan. Through the RIGG and CIR, the Sanitary Police Department provided serums and treatments against diseases. The establishment of both institutes mobilized medical scientists on behalf of colonial rule. In this institutional expansion, German *Staatsmedizin* and germ theory deserve credit for a number of major changes and medical advances. By the end of the 1930s, medical reformers were engaged in a wide range of projects in newly established laboratories, all of which were turned over to the colonial government with the coming of the war.

The change in preventive medical reform targets reveals how "politics masqueraded as science" in debates over the origin and prevention of disease. In the case of cholera and plague, the colonial government tended to identify both epidemics as threats from an unhealthy China. Opium addiction and the malaria endemic, on the other hand, were Taiwanese problems that were waiting to be cured by the Japanese. The cause and treatment of health threats were not determined by scientific criteria alone. More critical factors were beliefs about how much the colonial government should support a policy, who should take the credit or the blame, and whether Chinese heritage or the colonial environment was ultimately responsible for disease.

Despite the controversies surrounding Japanese sanitary policies, after the expansion of medical resources in the 1920s and 1930s, the Taiwanese seemed to trust modern medicine and began to willingly follow governmental regulations. In the case of the antimalaria campaign, the keynote of Japanese propaganda—that better theories would improve treatment and guarantee a healthier environment—was reflected in the background music of a 1939 film, *Malaria no bôatsu*. The film producer used a symphony for the section that addressed modern malariology, light jazz to unveil promising treatments, and, finally, a bucolic melody for the section describing improvements in the rural environment. On the whole, what the Japanese antimalaria program left the Taiwanese was a new "confidence in modern medicine"; at the same time, "grass-roots [local] experience" continued to buzz in people's ears.[215] As A-nan (a male, seventy-two years old), who was a schoolboy in the mid-1930s, stated, "In school . . . we had routine blood tests and physical examinations every semester . . . [and] at home the sanitary police were strict in upholding environmental cleanliness and clearing village surroundings. . . From newspapers, I learned a lot about malaria and . . . when I was infected I believed the doctor would give me proper medicine."[216] Academic malariology, after its application in the 1920s, eventually filtered down to popular understanding as institutional and media channels were called on to educate the colonized society. The basic principles of modern medicine, malariology in this case, became rooted in at least a generation of Taiwanese like A-nan.

Finally, in his famous book *Ecological Imperialism: The Biological Expansion of Europe*, Alfred W. Crosby concludes that human beings are biological entities before they are members of political and religious groups.[217] David Arnold criticizes Crosby's argument that colonialism was an inevitable consequence of the superiority of Western science, including medicine.[218] Instead, he asserts, medicine could be a cover-up for Western ambition in colonies. The motives for holding the 1925 Police Hygiene Exhibition in colonial Taiwan support Arnold's position. The colonial state utilized the occasion of the island-wide exhibition to circulate the colonizers' ideas about modern medicine and sanitation standards. By visiting the exhibits, the Taiwanese attendees were expected to accept the missions of "civilization" and "science" with which the Japanese legitimized their colonizing activities. Although governmental measures contributed to improvements in health, private agents of medical practice such as Taiwanese doctors, nurses, midwives, and even pharmacists should also be given some of the credit. The colonial government reduced the support to the *koi* system and left more responsibility to private practitioners, which meant the patient should pay for the treatment. *Koi* received salary from the government. Economic growth in the 1930s increased the ability of the Taiwanese to pay for their medical services. As the four themes of the 1925 exhibition showed, a combination of one-quarter politics, one-quarter medical science, and one-half economics would contribute to the improvement of indigenous health.

4

The 1930s and Beyond

From Prewar Legacy to Postwar Legend

The colonial medical service had achieved stability by the late 1920s and reached its golden age in the 1930s. Japanese medical experts and bureaucrats built systems of public health and medical services mainly on the basis of clinical rather than laboratory medicine—in contrast to Japan—and massive numbers of Taiwanese private clinicians, not doctors in government facilities, promoted the development of colonial medicine in order to achieve their goals.

The achievements of Japanese colonial medicine were manifest when researchers examined Taiwan's medical resources and demonstrated the improvement by means of demographic indices for the 1930s and early 1940s.[1] Their favorable conclusions about Japanese colonial medicine appeared in both political propaganda during the colonial period and statements by Taiwanese medical professionals in the postwar era.[2] David Arnold has pointed out that the "tools of empire" thesis neglects the role of compromise, which was essential to the provision of services when the quantity and quality of medical personnel were low.[3] Most likely for similar reasons, Taiwanese doctors were involved in the creation of medical services and were almost the only professionals accepted by the colonial government after traditional medicine declined.

Medical development in colonies did not always mean that the colonized copied the medical services of the colonial power. In one way, a new generation of Taiwanese private practitioners who accepted the values of science and civilization of Japanese colonial medicine dominated the main body of medical services in colonial Taiwan. Because of them, the colonized society was impressed with clinical medicine, a form of medicine that did not receive much attention in Japan. In another way, during the 1930s medicine in Taiwan became a model for other Japanese colonies. Japanese colonial medicine during World War II was based on Taiwan's experience rather than modeled on German *Staatsmedizin* as it had been earlier. The following discussion begins by analyzing the structure of medical manpower and the process of professionalization to illuminate the doctor-favored mechanism in Japanese colonial medicine. The close link between a growing group of

Taiwanese doctors and the expanding functions of medical services meant that Taiwanese medical practitioners were the primary contributors to and beneficiaries of Japanese colonial medicine. In addition, increasing numbers of Taiwanese doctors diversified Japanese colonial medicine in the 1930s in two directions—the growth of clinical medicine in serving local needs and the continuous expansion of laboratory medicine within academic circles.

Medicine: A State Agent in Colonial Taiwan

In most historical scholarship about Taiwan—with its origins in the writings of colonial medical officers and imperial politicians—colonial medicine's role as a "tool of empire" is the most familiar theme. Two famous slogans that the Japanese principal of the Taipei medical school used to encourage Taiwanese pupils were "*xuezuo yisheng zhiqian xianxue zuoren*" (Learn to be a human being before becoming a doctor) and "*shangyi zhiguo, zhongyi zhiren, xiayi zhibing*" (An excellent doctor can manage the state, a moderate one cures people, and a common doctor only treats illness). These slogans appeared in books, speeches, and newspaper columns.[4] It is obvious, as Takekoshi Yosaburo wrote in 1907, that the medical colonization of Taiwan meant "the responsibility of extending civilization in this island."[5] In fact, Takekoshi's words reveal one agenda of Japanese colonialism: training Taiwanese doctors to be tools of empire and agents of modern civilization. The two aspects of Japanese public health policy—science and salvation—not only influenced public health investigation but also shaped doctors' expectations of themselves and the Taiwanese image of a modern state with proper health care.

Additionally, continuous growth in Western-type medical resources was the most popular image in government propaganda, which later influenced many postwar historians. Propaganda in the 1925 Police Hygiene Exhibition portrayed the Taiwanese as beneficiaries of the colonizers' concern to improve the survival of the Japanese and to catch up with contemporary Western medicine.[6] However, politics rather than technology determined what kind of medicine would be practiced. For example, traditional practitioners worked side by side with Western doctors before 1900, but their numbers declined after the mid-1920s due to the government policy. According to the demographer Chen Shaoxin:

> In 1906, only one-tenth of all death certificates were issued by Western-trained doctors, including policemen, while the Chinese traditional physicians were responsible for the rest. . . . But by the end of 1935 the situation had been reversed: only one-tenth of death certificates were issued by Chinese traditional physicians while Western-trained doctors issued the rest.[7]

Chen's statement clearly illustrates the replacement of traditional physicians by Japanese-trained indigenous doctors. This did not happen immediately after Gotô's proposal of colonial medicine in 1902 but accelerated with the reorganization of the medical school in Taipei after 1919. The colonial government intentionally supported medical graduates by reducing the number of traditional practitioners and in the late 1920s and early 1930s issued regulations to restrict the use of herbal medicines.

As discussed previously, the number of traditional physicians decreased fairly rapidly during the colonial period, especially in the 1920s. The colonial government without doubt manipulated the licensing examination to select and support the types of medical service it preferred. The result was significant: in 1942, forty years after the only licensing examination ever given for traditional physicians in 1902, a mere ninety-seven physicians could legally practice traditional Chinese medicine.[8] Traditional physicians were replaced by doctors trained in Western medicine, who held the exclusive right to train practitioners such as nurses and midwives.[9] Chart 4.1 shows the replacement of traditional physicians by those practicing Western medicine.[10]

CHART 4.1: Proportions of major medical personnel in Taiwan, 1902–1940. (Data from *Sôtokufu eisei nenpo* [Sôtokufu Annual Report on Sanitation], 1900–1940.)

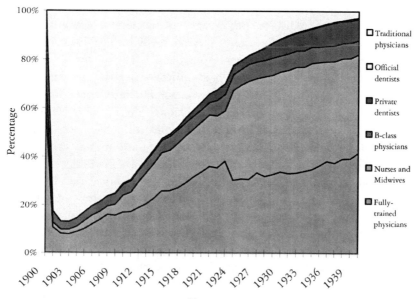

With the population growing at an average rate of 3 percent per year, at least partly due to the rapid decrease in the number of traditional physicians the growth ratio between qualified practitioners and the population in Taiwan from 1906 to 1921 became negative (see chart 4.2 and table 4.2 later in this chapter). Even with the greater numbers of medical graduates between 1922 and 1931, the ratio never exceeded 1 percent. Only in the decade prior to 1942 did it significantly improve, to 3 to 6 percent, but that still could not compensate for the loss of traditional doctors and much faster population growth.[11] In fact, the ratio between medical practitioners and population did not change dramatically and even slightly declined in the colonial period.

The change in the distribution of various medical practitioners is important to the analysis that follows. As shown in chart 4.1, increased numbers of nurses, midwives, and B-class physicians compensated for the decrease in traditional physicians between 1902 and 1924. The numbers of nurses, midwives, and B-class physicians grew much faster between 1924 and 1940, with members of those groups forming over 50 percent of the qualified medical manpower in Taiwan. Although the colonial government attributed improvements in health to formal medical education and the expanded system of public doctors (*ko i*), the numbers in chart 4.1 seem to give much credit to nurses, midwives, and B-class physicians those who seldom received formal training at the medical school.[12]

Discrimination in Japanese Colonial Medicine

The replacement of traditional physicians with doctors of Western medicine also marked the professionalization of Western medicine in Taiwan, promoting the status and social image of those who practiced it.[13] Before the establishment of the medical school and licensing examination by the government, the professional status of traditional physicians was indeterminate. According to a government investigation in 1897, traditional physicians in Taiwan were classified into six categories, none of which fit medical professional definitions in Japan after the 1870s. The standard of classification was very obscure, involving self- and ethnic identity with no indication of medical specialization such as internal medicine, surgery, or pediatrics. For instance, the classification *dojin i* meant "indigenous physician," *ryô i* referred to a doctor's "goodness," *se i* indicated family background, *jû i* revealed a Confucian background, and *ji i* meant "current medical practitioners." A total of twenty-four *yô i* (Western physicians) were listed.[14] Without disturbing the continuity of the data, Japan adopted a Western standard of classification in 1923.[15] However, the new classification of diseases caused difficulties for traditional practitioners, even the licensed ones, in the reporting of causes of the death.[16] Because of the licensing examinations and new standards of medical practice, traditional medicine no longer fit into Japanese colonial medicine after the 1920s.

The colonial government did not immediately enforce the classification of medical practitioners in Taiwan. Although the 1896 Regulation of Medical Practice in Taiwan was virtually identical to Japan's law of the same name, it was never put into practice. An amendment in Meiji 39 (1906), which classified licensed physicians in Taiwan, actually compromised the principles of the 1896 regulation by only offering medical training on the high school level. Four types of physicians with three graduated titles were qualified by the colonial government to practice medicine.[17] Obviously, the classification of legal practitioners of medicine in Taiwan copied the rules used in Japan (see chap. 2). However, the proportion of different types of the medical practitioners in Taiwan differed. After 1906, licensed physicians in colonial Taiwan were classified as follows.

A. Graduates of medical schools (*igakkô sotsugyôsei*)

B. Graduates of special schools or colleges of medicine (*igaku senmongakkô*)

C. Graduates with bachelor's degrees in medicine and medical doctors who graduated from the medical schools of imperial universities and research institutes

D. Others: graduates of qualified foreign medical schools or those engaging in the "heritage practice" of traditional medicine

Compared to the situation in colonial Taiwan, in Japan the physicians in types C and D formed the majority of medical professionals and wielded great influence in government facilities as well private practice.[18] Government statistics in Japan showed that nearly 90 percent of government institutions, including hospitals, universities, and research institutes, were the domain of type-C and type-D doctors.[19] However, type-B physicians were the most numerous. After the mid-1920s, some Taiwanese students studied medicine in Japan, but this did not increase the number of type-C physicians in Taiwan. The registration data for licensed physicians in Taiwan showed that most Taiwanese in Japan still enrolled in medical colleges (*Igaku senmongakkô*). From 1922 until 1939, according to the registration of licensed practitioners, there were eighty-seven Taiwanese doctors who had graduated from medical colleges in Japan and returned. Only four Taiwanese enrolled in the medical colleges of universities remained in Japan.[20]

Like medical colleges in Japan, medical colleges in colonial Taiwan were vocational. Even Taiwanese medical graduates from Japan were trained under the same college curriculum. For the colonial government in Taiwan, the application of clinical medicine rather than medical research in laboratories was the first priority. This state of affairs divided Japanese and Taiwanese medicine into two categories: provider and user.[21] Japanese medicine was considered to be advanced because of its emphasis on laboratory medicine. Taiwanese medicine was a user of advanced medicine and emphasized clinical treatment. Thus, laboratory medicine led Japanese medical progress while clinical medicine supported the establishment of colonial medicine in Taiwan. Naturally, then, the increase in medical practitioners in colonial Taiwan favored clinicians. Table 4.1 shows the long-term features of medical manpower in colonial Taiwan.

TABLE 4.1: Medical graduate types in Taiwan and Japan, 1910–1940.

	Type A (%)	Type B (%)	Type C (%)	Type D (%)
Taiwan	23	52	8	18
Japan	6	29	55	11

Sources: Kosesho, *Isei hyakunenshi furo,* 45–47; Taiwansheng xingzheng zhangquang gongshu, *Taiwansheng wushiyinianlai tongjitiyao,* 1249.

Note: Graduates of medical colleges (type B) formed the majority of licensed physicians in colonial Taiwan while university graduates (type C) formed the majority in Japan.[22]

Under the goals of medical education in Japan before World War II, doctors of types A and B were trained by the government to be clinicians while the imperial universities provided elite training in Western and laboratory medicine.[23] Of the medical graduates of Tokyo Imperial University between 1897 and 1901, 32.8 percent were general clinical doctors, 49.3 percent worked in hospitals, and only 17.6 percent worked in education and research. That situation changed in 1920 as the growth of government-owned medical facilities slowed and the medical graduates of imperial universities increased. In the decade of 1920s, only 2.4 percent of medical graduates were general clinical doctors, while 17.4 percent worked exclusively in education and research and 75.6 percent worked in hospitals.[24] As the Japanese government further increased the number of medical doctors after the mid-1930s, the number of type-C physicians in Japan dramatically increased, which led to the opening of many new clinics and dispensaries. Before the 1920s, type-B doctors had replaced traditional physicians in the medical services market, but their predominance vanished in the 1920s with the rapid increase in type-C doctors in Japan. More university graduates, therefore, competed with college graduates in the private medical services market. When more medical graduates began opening dispensaries in the 1930s, serious competition in private practice became common in Japan.[25] To distinguish university clinicians from college practitioners, as well to promote higher quality medical training and meet advanced research needs, practitioners with an MD title increased in the 1940s. For instance, in 1940, the Japanese government issued 13,820 doctoral degrees in twelve disciplines, with 11,891 medical doctors accounting for more than 80 percent of the total number of doctoral degree holders.[26] The role played by university graduates in clinical practice and the growth in the number of MDs imply further professionalization in Japan.

In general, in the 1930s Japan experienced the professionalization of modern medical manpower from a two-tiered (college-university) base to a three-tiered (college–university–graduate school) base.[27] However, the Taiwanese situation was different from the very beginning. Not only did the original college-university formation appear relatively late, but the colonial government kept the lower quality of vocational training in medicine on the high school–college base for nearly forty years (1897–1936).

The policy of racial discrimination before 1919 restricted medical training on the vocational level to Taiwanese.[28] Japanese were not allowed to enroll at the medical school in Taiwan. Although that policy was canceled in 1922, the new policy of "equal education" for all races in Taiwan favored students who could speak Japanese fluently, so, predictably, the majority were Japanese.[29] With the same agenda of discrimination, the colonial government retained vocational training at the Taihoku Medical College when the Taihoku Imperial University was established in 1928 and the medical school of that university was found in 1936. The dual system of medical education—the imperial university (laboratory medicine) versus the medical college (clinical medicine)—continued into the 1930s. In one way, Japanese university graduates dominated the research institutes RIGG and CIR and usually occupied higher positions in public hospitals.[30] In another way, during the fifty years of occupation the colonial government intentionally prolonged vocational training in medicine on the college level exclusively for Taiwanese pupils. Moreover, the double standard in medical education met the goals of discrimination. The medical college mainly accepted Taiwanese students while the university took equal numbers of Taiwanese and Japanese students in incoming classes of seventy.[31] But, considering the small population of Japanese in Taiwan, the ratio of Taiwanese to Japanese students enrolled in the medical school in Taihoku Imperial University was about 1 to 850 (Taiwanese) and 1 to 130 (Japanese in Taiwan).[32] The equality policy in force between 1922 and 1936 in fact reduced the quota of Taiwanese students when the total number of students in the medical college was fixed. Between 1922 and 1936, the 729 students enrolled in the medical college of Taihoku Imperial University included 423 Japanese and only 305 Taiwanese. It seems that, although most Taiwanese doctors had only vocational training in medicine, they must have been very talented as they had to pass a much more competitive entrance examination than the Japanese students did.

The pupil-teacher relationship in colonial medicine, in the long run, stunted the growth of Western medicine in colonial Taiwan. In 1928, "Nihon igaku no dokuritsu" (The Independence of Japanese Medicine), the conclusion to *Nihon igaku bunka nenbyô* (The Cultural Annals of Japanese Medicine), declared that Japanese medicine had become independent of German medicine in the early 1910s. The author emphasized that the majority of teachers in medical schools in Japan since the mid-1890s had been Japanese. Because of the policies of the Ministry of Education and the eagerness of Japanese medical scientists to catch up with the West, "Japanese physicians transferred German medicine and rapidly replaced German medical teachers to train the new generation."[33] Medical service in colonial Taiwan, however, was never intended to become independent of Japanese medicine; Japanese teachers totally controlled medical education and determined its educational goals.

Even before the 1930s, colonial Taiwan was almost like a workshop for applying advanced medical knowledge from Japan. Between 1902 and 1921, 81.87 percent of medical graduates were general clinical doctors practicing in Taiwan, 5.46 percent were B-class doctors working in official clinics, and 12.66 percent worked in hospitals.[34] That is, most of the medical graduates were general clinical doctors and Taiwanese. In fact, many Taiwanese interns were eager to open their own dispensaries because of the discrimination in training hospitals.[35] Their major concern was to apply advanced Japanese medicine in daily practice rather than improving or advancing it; that mission was supposedly carried out by university graduates.

The medical college first hired Taiwanese faculty in 1918 and employed twelve Taiwanese in 1920. However, at the peak Taiwanese teachers were only 13.5 percent of the total faculty, and the average over time was less than 2 percent. In contrast, the majority of medical students were always Taiwanese. From the beginning, the Sôtokufu medical school and college exclusively recruited Taiwanese students. The teacher-pupil relationship between Japanese and Taiwanese remained the same even after the establishment of the medical school of Taihoku Imperial University in 1936. In 1943, only eight Taiwanese instructors were hired by the university, representing only

4.9 percent of the total number of teachers. Although the medical school of Taihoku Imperial University did not exclude Japanese students, conditions did not improve until the 1940s. While Taihoku Imperial University provided more instruction in laboratory medicine and Japanese dominated the faculty, more Japanese students enrolled in the medical school of the university. The ratio of Japanese to Taiwanese students in the medical school was 0.7 to 1 in 1936, 0.9 to 1 in 1937, 0.7 to 1 in 1938, 0.96 to 1 in 1939, and only 1 to 1 in 1940.[36] Generally speaking, the hierarchical relationship between clinical and laboratory medicine in Taiwan amounted to more than the roles they played in Japan. In colonial Taiwan that relationship determined doctors' training and careers in terms of race rather than ability.

Discrimination and the hierarchical structure existed not only between Japanese experts and Taiwanese clinicians but also between Taiwanese doctors and other medical personnel. Only licensed physicians could prescribe medicine and diagnose patients. Pharmacists in Taiwan therefore lost their professional status and had to work under doctors' supervision. In addition, nurses and midwives were merely medical assistants serving directly under licensed physicians; because their training was very basic, they were prohibited from practicing without a doctor's supervision.[37] Moreover, since doctors in colonial Taiwan could train their own nurses and midwives, obedience and other "feminine qualities" became the required professional norms. That is, no questioning of their doctor-educators was allowed.[38] Thus, the prevailing teacher-pupil relationship was repeated at each dispensary and hospital where doctors trained their nurses and midwives.

Despite the growing numbers of medical personnel after the mid-1920s, the doctor was still the only legal practitioner in colonial Taiwan who had the right to diagnose, prescribe, and treat patients. As medical manpower grew, the population in colonial Taiwan also increased. But, as the increased number of Western doctors could not keep up with population growth, the policy to phase out traditional physicians had the potential to create a shortage of medical manpower.

The Significance of the Size of Professional Groups

The major change in medical manpower in colonial Taiwan was in fact the replacement of traditional physicians, not the improvement of medical resources per head. The increased number of licensed physicians, especially Western-type physicians, was not sufficient to close the gap caused by the decline in the number of traditional physicians. The shortage is obvious when we examine the ratio of physicians per population. As shown in chart 4.2, between 1906 and 1940 the decline of traditional physicians made this ratio worse.

CHART 4.2: Ratio of physicians to population in Taiwan and Japan, 1906–1940. (Data from *Koseisho gôjûnenshi* (Tokyo: Koseisho, 1988), 516–17, 572–74; Taiwansheng xingzheng zhangquang gongshu, *Taiwansheng wushiyinianlai tongjitiyao*, 44, 1249.)

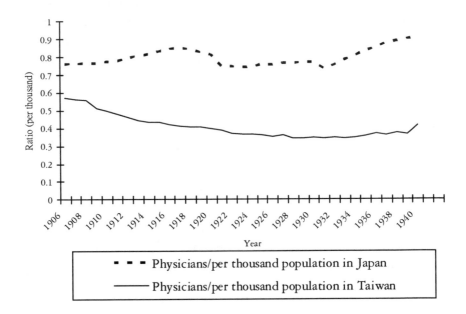

Two semilog regressions show that as the ratio in Taiwan declined the ratio of physicians in Japan generally increased—by 19 percent in thirty-four years, a rate of about 0.5 percent per year.[39] However, in the 1920s and 1930s the government in Japan still allowed the practice of traditional medicine as "alternative medicine" and continued to hold licensing examinations for its practitioners.[40] In addition, funding and medical manpower were provided for all three tiers of medical education in Japan. Formal medical education rejected traditional medicine beginning in the 1930s, and at the same time the Japanese government permitted the establishment of private medical colleges and universities.[41] The combination of these two policies eventually increased the number of physicians of western medicine and medical graduates from universities, while traditional physicians became rare. The increasing numbers of physicians caused the average income of general clinical physicians to decline. One report in a famous medical journal stated that "because of rapid growth and loosening licensing tests of medical graduates, the average income of doctors dropped one-third after the 1930s."[42] Meanwhile, the increase in medical bachelor's degree holders and medical doctors overwhelmed the market with graduates of medical schools and colleges. Declining income and economic competition among physicians became an important issue in Japanese medical magazines.[43]

From this viewpoint, however, the Japanese were better off than the Taiwanese. The ratio between physicians and population was declining in Taiwan, partly because of the rapid growth of the population (see table 4.2). Another factor was that the increase in Japanese-trained physicians was too small to balance the decline in traditional physicians. Because the ratio of doctors per thousand population was already lower in Taiwan than Japan, the sudden move to prohibit traditional medicine had a very negative effect. Looking only at the first and last years for the period 1906–40, the Taiwanese ratio declines by 27 percent, an annual rate of around 0.8 percent. This change was probably due to the establishment of two-tiered system medical education and the increase in Taiwanese medical students in Japan.

TABLE 4.2: Population-per-Doctor Ratios in Japan and Taiwan.

	Japan			Taiwan		
Year	Total Number of Doctors	Total Population	Population-per-Doctor Ratio	Total Number of Doctors	Total Population	Population-per-Doctor Ratio
1906	35,850	47,038,000	1:1,312	1,804	3,156,706	1:1,750
1910	38,055	49,184,000	1:1,292	1,649	3,039,751	1:1,843
1915	43,813	52,752,000	1:1,204	1,557	3,479,922	1:2,235
1920	45,488	55,963,053	1:1,230	1,495	3,655,308	1:2,445
1925	45,327	59,736,822	1:1,318	1,494	3,993,408	1:2,673
1930	49,681	64,450,005	1:1,297	1,626	4,592,537	1:2,824
1935	57,581	69,254,148	1:1,203	1,907	5,212,426	1:2,733
1940	65,332	71,933,000	1:1,101	2,534	5,872,084	1:2,317

Source: Liu Shiyung, "1930 niendai rizhishiqi Taiwan yixue de tezhe," 127.

The increasing population-to-doctor ratios meant that distribution of regular medical services was difficult, especially with the rapid decline of traditional medical practice. In their colonial design, the Japanese considered traditional medicine in Taiwan a legacy of Chinese superstition. Introducing scientific medicine and a public health system to Taiwan was a way in which Japan could claim its modernity and build a colony as its Western counterparts had done.[44] The introduction of public health investigation and the accumulation of data was viewed as evidence of the Japanese "enlightening" the Taiwanese through their advanced medicine science.

Japanese colonialism couched science and salvation in humanitarian terms to create a special viewpoint—the "Whiggish" interpretation of colonialism.[45] However, the connection between medical improvement and the exercise of specialist knowledge meant that the extent and nature of government power was changing as access to knowledge changed, with the result that power and the professions were open to being contested. As the numbers of Taiwanese doctors increased in colonial medical services, as well private dispensaries, replacing the ho-kô system, the elite image of modern medicine in government propaganda enhanced the influence of Taiwanese doctors. That is, in local social contexts the Taiwanese doctor was seen not as a colonial agent but as a medium of modern science and civilization.[46] It is easy to see why many Taiwanese doctors became leaders in anticolonial politics while still appreciating the science and civilization the colonizer brought to Taiwan.

As in most privatized markets, the immediate impact of the worsening ratio of population to doctors was that it kept charges for medical services relatively high. That is, an increase in the number of doctors will increase competition in a market and reduce prices and vice-versa. Although data reflecting medical service costs in colonial Taiwan are rare, several clues suggest that the average charge for medical service was high and that patients often turned to alternative remedies. For instance, in a short story in *Yangkui ji* (The Collected Works of Yangkui), the author describes a Taiwanese peasant who has to ask for help from an illegal healer because the public hospital will charge him nearly one month's income to treat his illness.[47] For those who could not afford to see legal practitioners, another alternative was to purchase over-the-counter drugs. Besides regular treatment in medical facilities such as public hospitals and private dispensaries, a popular system called *jiyaobao* (door-to-door over-the-counter drug service) provided self-treatment to rural populations (see figure 4.1).[48] In the end, especially in a privatized medical service market, level of income or economic welfare was the real factor determining an individual's health care.

Although exhibits in the 1925 exhibition attributed improvements in health to medical reforms, public health interventions, and educational campaigns undertaken by the Japanese authorities, in the privatized market of medical services before 1945 Taiwanese medical practitioners, including

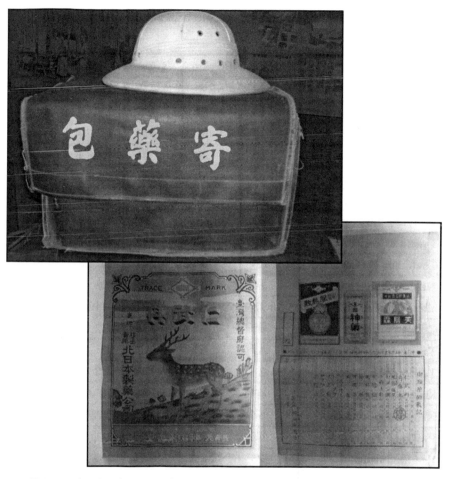

FIGURE 4.1: *Jiyaobao*: a carry box and a sample of medicine from the Taiwan yiliao shiliao wenwu zhongxin (Taiwan Center for Historical Materials in Medicine), Kaohsiung City. Courtesy of Taiwan yiliao shiliao wenwu zhongxin (Taiwan Center for Historical Materials in Medicine), Kaohsiung, Taiwan.

physicians, nurses, midwives, pharmacists, and even the OTC drug providers, deserve some of the credit. As these medical services differed, the charges for each type were determined by local economic conditions, a sign of a privatized market rather than the total control of the *Staatsmedizin* design. In the 1930s in Taiwan, the economic growth associated with urbanization compensated for the deficit in qualified practitioners by creating markets for medical services on the outskirts of major cities while the remote countryside relied on regular drugstores or *jiyaobao* services. Table 4.3 shows the ratios and distribution of qualified physicians in 1945 in Taiwan.

in mid-1930s Taiwan stimulated Japanese bioscientists to shift their epidemiological investigations to certain diseases that had been ignored in Taiwan but were prevalent in Southeast Asia. Elephantiasis, a disease caused by the parasite *Filaria,* was a good case for making such a shift. Although a British doctor named Mayer had claimed in 1886 that he observed several elephantiasis patients in Taiwan, Japanese physicians and researchers had denied the existence of local filariasis cases since 1909.[55] They also claimed that research on the disease was irrelevant to the practice of tropical medicine in the colony.[56]

Preparations for the Pacific War brought filariasis in Taiwan to the attention of Japanese researchers. To guarantee the security of the Taiwan Strait, the Japanese navy had been expanding the maintenance dock in Makung, Penghu, since 1935. A major concern during the expansion was maintaining the health of the laborers. In the course of regular health examinations, navy surgeon Tanaka Shikeo recorded 229 cases of local workers with 99 filariasis positives in blood tests and a morbidity rate of 43.3 percent. Among the infected cases, 37 patients were found to have filaria in their blood in microscope examinations. Under the microscope, Tanaka proved that the local causative agent was *Wuchereria bancrofti* and suggested that the disease was endemic throughout Penghu Isle.[57] Tanaka's report attracted the attention of a famous parasitologist, Yokogawa Sadamu, who in 1939 led an investigation team to Penghu to confirm Tanaka's observation. The team found a filarial infection rate of 8.6 percent in Penghu Isle with all cases having been caused by *W. bancrofti.*[58]

After the local cases were confirmed in Penghu, the colonial government soon began an investigation on the main island of Taiwan. Huang Dengyun investigated the Pingdong area in southern Taiwan. Among 5,267 subjects, no filarial infection was found on blood examination.[59] Since local cases of filariasis seemed to exist only in remote fishing villages, there was no motive for the government to continue its investigation.[60] Nor did launching an investigation into filariasis advance the Japanese agenda of attracting international attention. There was no incentive for the colonial government to conduct a thorough filariasis survey in poor, isolated fishing villages like those Huang studied. Yokogawa's investigation in Penghu in the 1930s was actually driven by the need for war preparations in 1939 and merely worked to secure a supply of healthy workers for the navy docks. Therefore, surveys in Taiwan were done on a limited basis and without sufficient cases.[61] In academic circles, it was assumed that filariasis did not exist because of the lack of substantial investigative evidence, a well as the lack of a practical need for its treatment.

Taiwan and the Spread of Medical Services in the Japanese Empire

From the mid-1920s and into the 1930s, colonial medicine in Taiwan differed in various ways from the original model of Japanized *Staatsmedizin*. The colonial government claimed that those differences were based on reasons related to medical education, but in fact they were based on ethnicity. While most medical care was highly privatized and generally provided by Taiwanese, Japanese medical professionals in Taiwan were university graduates and thus held higher positions at government institutes and public hospitals. The cooperation between Japanese-dominated laboratory medicine and Taiwanese-dominated clinical medicine, and the resulting improvement in public health, made Taiwan a model of Japanese colonial medicine when the empire was extended to coastal China and Southeast Asia in the late 1930s.

In the late 1930s, Taiwan was a significant model for Japanese colonial medicine in the medical circles of the empire. After the friction between Japan's National Institute of Infectious Disease and Tokyo Imperial University, their merger in 1914 caused a chain reaction that spread Western medicine from Japan to its colonies.[62] After the merger, many of Kitasato Shibasaburo's pupils left Tokyo—the center of modern medicine in Japan—to serve in various peripheral locations, including the colonies. Among the former faculty of the Institute of Infectious Disease, Takagi Tomoe, Kanai Shoji (1886–1967), and Shiga Kiyoshi (1870–1957) played key roles in introducing modern medicine to Japanese-occupied Taiwan, Manchuria, and Korea.

Takagi Tomoe's contributions to improving public health in colonial Taiwan won him the nickname Eisei Sôtoku (Governor of Hygiene).[63] As mentioned previously, because of Takagi's devotion, a process for establishing medical services and health education was established by 1910 and eventually integrated into local society. Takagi's work was not unique in the Japanese colonies; similar processes, led mainly by Kanai Shoji and Shiga Kiyoshi, were introduced in Manchuria and Korea, though much later.

Modern Medicine in Manchuria

The transfer of Gotô Shinpei to Manchuria in 1906 was a turning point in the process of disseminating modern medicine from Japan to its colonies. With full confidence based on his experience in Taiwan and using public health infrastructures developed there, Gotô soon created a reform strategy to improve public health and medical education. The Japanese government in the Guangdong Leased Territory, mainly in Dairen, established public health and quarantine systems and enacted public health regulations based on or identical to those in Taiwan. For example, the public health association, Eisei

Kumiai, was based on the Chinese native organization, Hui, following the Taiwanese model in which the public health association was based on the native *ho-kô* system.[64]

Medical education in Manchuria was established much later than in Taiwan but grew faster. The Medical College of South Manchuria was established at Hengtian by the South Manchurian Railway Company in 1911. The college played an essential role in many anti-epidemic campaigns. A former researcher at the Institute of Infectious Disease and professor at the Medical College of South Manchuria, Tsurumi Sanzo, became the chief of the Public Health Department of the South Manchurian Railway Company when the Japanese government of the Guangdong Leased Territory organized the Research Committee for Local and Infectious Disease, similar to that in colonial Taiwan.[65] Although Gotô left Manchuria in 1920 for a new position in Tokyo, the establishment of modern medical services continued. In 1922, the Medical College of South Manchuria was upgraded to the Manchurian Medical College, which housed important scientists and was a major resource for public health policies in the Manchukuo period after 1931.[66]

Because the South Manchurian Railway Company was so influential in manipulating politics in Manchuria, developing health programs within the company was much more important than expanding medical education. The establishment of the Mantetsu Eisei Kenkyujyo (Institute for Public Health of the South Manchurian Railway Company) in 1926 was essential. The chief of this institute was Kanai Shoji, who had graduated from Tokyo Imperial University and joined the Kitasato Institute, successor to the Institute of Infectious Disease, in 1918. Kanai played a role much like that of Takagi Tomoe in Taiwan. Under the influence of Kanai, scientists recruited from the Kitasato Institute formed a reliable medical service team that dealt with various public health problems in Manchuria. Because of their great similarity, the Institute for Public Health of the South Manchurian Railway Company was seen as an overseas branch of the Kitasato Institute in Japan.[67] Thus, Taiwan's experience was important for the expansion of Japanese efforts in Manchuria.

Activities in Shanghai

In the 1910s, as Takagi was initiating public health reform in Taiwan, a medical organization in Shanghai, the Hakuaikai, which was supported by the Japanese colonial government in Taiwan, established several hospitals in Fujian and Guangdong provinces, as well as in North Borneo.[68] The purpose of the Hakuaikai-affiliated hospitals was to compete with the activities of the Rockefeller Foundation in China.[69] The Shanghai Institute for Natural

Science was established in 1931, with Yokote Chiyonosuke, a professor at the Institute of Infectious Disease of Tokyo Imperial University, appointed deputy president. The original purpose of this institute was to develop cooperation between Japanese and Chinese scientists with the support of the Ministry of Foreign Affairs. The institute organized a research unit for medical science that included infectious and parasitic disease studies.[70] Institutional support and academic friendship were key issues linking the CIR in Taiwan and the Shanghai Institute.

Because of its close relationship with the colonial government in Taiwan, the Shanghai Institute became a shelter for Japanese physicians who were seen as socialists or social medicine sympathizers during the left-wing movement of the 1920s.[71] Among those physicians, Komiya Yoshitaka (1900–1976), Soda Takenume (1902–1984), and other leftist activists organized the Research Committee for Social Medicine at Tokyo Imperial University. After Komiya and Soda were arrested for "disturbing social order" in 1930, Komiya moved to Shanghai as a scientist at the Institute for Natural Science.[72] Soda worked for CIR in Taiwan, winning his professorship at Taihoku Imperial University in 1940.[73] Komiya and Soda both studied malaria and other parasitic diseases and published articles in the *Journal of the Shanghai Institute for Natural Sciences*.[74] In an article in *Toa igaku* (East Asian Medicine),[75] of which Komiya was a long-term editor, he described measures to combat the anopheles mosquito that obviously had been inspired by antimalaria strategies in colonial Taiwan.[76] In 1934, Komiya attended the Nanjing conference of the Far Eastern Association of Tropical Medicine, and Soda attended as the representative of the colonial government in Taiwan.[77]

Such relationships were significant in the Shanghai Institute's full support for the investigation and research teams sent to China by the Taiwanese government. Accepting the mission of Hakuaikai and support from the Shanghai Institute, Shimojyo Kumaichi, the chief researcher of CIR, was sent to South China to study the prevalence of infectious diseases, including malaria.[78] Shimojyo's work was not an isolated case but a sign of the cooperative network between the two colonial research institutes. In another case, Otsuru Masamitsu (1916–), a medical graduate from Taihoku Imperial University, joined the army and with support from Shanghai studied malaria in Guangzhou. After World War II, he became a leading scholar in the field of infectious and parasite studies.[79] If we compare the development of colonial medicine in Taiwan and Manchuria, the Shanghai Institute for Natural Science was like an extension of CIR in Taiwan while the Medical College of South Manchuria was like a twin of Japan's Institute of Infectious Disease.

The spread of modern medicine from Japan to the colonies offers a good case for examining George Basalla's diffusionist model of Western science proposed in 1967: "During 'phase 1' the nonscientific society or nation provides a source of European science. . . . 'phase 2' is marked by a period of colonial science, and 'phase 3' completes the process of transplantation with a struggle to achieve an independent scientific tradition (or culture)."[80] Basalla's model is correct only if we accept the story promulgated by the colonial government in Taiwan. In fact, the spread of modern medicine from Japan to its colonies was an accident caused by political friction in Japan that resulted in medical scientists pursuing their work elsewhere in the empire. The institutions in Taiwan, Manchuria, and Shanghai formed a strange relationship with Tokyo, copying institutional developments in Japan and studying assigned research topics but always in competition with each other. Basalla's model fails to take into account the political and social forces that brought about the diffusion of modern medicine, forces that were kept in balance, maintaining the status of the center in Japan, as long as the situation was peaceful. That balance was upset by Japan's preparations for the Pacific War. With the expansion of military activities during the 1940s, the relationship between the colonial subcenters and the main center in Japan broke into two major parts: *kaitaku igaku* (development medicine) in the northern Japanese empire and *nanhô igaku* (southern medicine) in the tropical zones.

From Tropical Medicine to Southern Medicine

In Taiwan, the Japanese colonial government made a great effort to establish public health programs in order to protect colonizers from infectious and parasitic diseases, which involved, in part, enforcement of regulations by sanitary policemen and the development of private and public dispensaries to control disease among the natives. The Japanese government then applied the Taiwanese model to other colonies: the Guangdong Leased Territory, Korea, and Manchuria. While the Institute of Infectious Disease and the Kitasato Institute played the role of a megacenter to spread medical professionals to colonies over time, Taiwan was the first to go through the whole process, providing a flexible model for other colonies.

As Taiwan and Manchuria jointly became subcenters of Japanese colonial medicine after the1930s, another subcenter was independently forming in Korea, which Japan had occupied since 1910. During the Lee dynasty, in the last decade of the nineteenth century, the Korean government had already established a medical school and organized the public health system.[81] Nevertheless, a similar process of providing medical education and services was launched in Japanese-ruled Korea, apparently without influence from Taiwan. In the process of colonization by Japan, medical services and education in Korea progressed farther in introducing modern medicine[82] and upgrading the old missionary medical schools.[83] The development of modern medicine in Korea took place within roughly the same time frame as that in Taiwan, progressing in parallel especially after 1915 when Kitasato's pupils began to influence the design of colonial medicine.

In colonial Korea, Shiga Kiyoshi and Kobayashi Harujiro (1884–1969), two former members of Kitasato's team, were vital in constructing public health infrastructures and medical services. Shiga, famous for discovering the dysentery virus in 1897, had served as chief of the Parasite Studies Department of the Institute of Infectious Disease since 1901. In 1920, he was became dean of Keijô Medical College (Keijô Igaku senmon gakkô, which became Keijô Imperial University in 1929 and Seoul National University in 1945), Kitasato's idea for promoting Japanese modern medicine in Korea.[84] Kobayashi Harujiro also had served at the Kitasato Institute, from 1914 until he moved to Korea and took a professorship at Keijô Medical College in 1916. He became a professor of parasitology at Keijô Imperial University and pursued research there until 1945. After carefully studying the careers of Shiga Kiyoshi and Kobayashi Harujiro in colonial Korea, Iijima Wataru characterized Korea as a laboratory of Japanese colonial medicine led by former Kitasato pupils.[85]

Despite the rapid growth of Japanese colonial medicine prior to the 1930s, Japanese experts continued to use Western-defined tropical medicine as the backbone of their colonial medical programs.[86] Before 1939, Japanese experts in tropical medicine were eager to reorganize their domestic resources for the competition with their Western counterparts. To publicize their progress in tropical medicine and present their discoveries, the government in Japan encouraged the experts to participate in major conferences of tropical medicine, especially those held in colonies.[87] The first conference of the Far Eastern Association for Tropical Medicine was held in Manila in 1910, and subsequent conferences were held in Hong Kong in 1912, Saigon in 1913, Java in 1921, Singapore in 1923, Tokyo in 1925, Calcutta in 1927, Bangkok in 1930, Nanjing in 1934, and Hanoi in 1938. The participants were mainly scientists from India and Southeast Asia, under the rule of Western countries, as well as China, Siam, and Japan.[88] Representatives from colonial Taiwan soon appeared; at the conference in Hong Kong in 1912, the Japanese representative was Hatori Jyuro (1871–1957), an entomologist engaged in malaria research for the Japanese colonial government in Taiwan.[89] When Japan hosted the conference in 1925, Prime Minister Kato Takagi addressed the participants, stating, "The success of the Suez Canal and the development of the tropical regions were due to the development of tropical medicine. The Japanese government established tropical medicine in Taiwan and the Nanyo islands [the islands of the Philippines, Malaya, and Indonesia]. As a result of this, Japanese scientists will play an important role in the field of tropical medicine."[90] In his speech, Kato stated that Japanese medical experts made great efforts to research and control tropical diseases, and their research was advanced in the colonies, especially Taiwan.[91]

However, the Japanese empire expanded after the 1930s to include various climate zones, and geographic conditions in Manchuria, Korea, and Shanghai were significantly different from those in Taiwan, so tropical medicine applied to only part of the Japanese-controlled areas. The term *kaitaku igaku* (development medicine) was invented after the establishment of the Kaitaku kagaku kenkyujyo (Institute for Development Science) in 1939 and the Kaitaku igaku kenkyujyo (Institute for Development Medicine) in 1940. The main purpose of these institutes was to conduct research on hygienic conditions and environmental survival factors relating to Japanese immigration in the frigid and temperate zones of Manchuria and Korea, respectively.[92] While the Japanese used *kaitaku igaku* to denote the application of medical science in the frigid and temperate zones, they retained a Western term, *tropical medicine,* for medicine in subtropical and tropical zones, including Taiwan and southern China. Given the Japanese desire to be independent of the Western influence of tropical medicine, the creation of the Japanese term *nanhô igaku* (southern medicine) was no accident.

As shown by the policy *Kokumin tairyuku kôjô ondo* (Campaign to improve the physical constitution of Japanese nationals), the modification of the medical administration after 1938 was a necessary step toward satisfying the requirement of conscription. The laboratory medicine developed in Taiwan soon became a model of Japanese tropical medicine.[93] The Institute of Tropical Medicine sent several malaria experts to Bangkok and established a branch there in 1939.[94] In 1940, Japanese medical researchers in Taiwan organized the Reidai igakukai (Society of Tropical Medicine), which published the journal *Tropical Medicine Japonica.* Their activities implied the similar institutionalization of tropical medicine studies in Japan, medical knowledge that would benefit the construction of the "Greater East Asia Co-Prosperity Sphere."[95]

To fulfill their mission of improving bodily strength, tropical medicine experts in Taiwan pursued research concerning the physical health of the population, epidemic prevention, and parasitism between 1938 and 1945.[96] All three subjects were major strengths of Japanese colonial medicine in Taiwan from the very beginning. At the same time, the colonial government encouraged medical students, especially those trained in clinical medicine, to serve on the battlefield in China and other parts of eastern Asia. Because of the war, the colonial government issued policies to control medical resources, including manpower and supplies. In the area of manpower, since the colonial government used membership in the Association of Taiwanese Physicians as a prerequisite for a doctor's right to practice, membership became obligatory. Meanwhile, to maintain control of medical resources, the colonial government ensured that Japanese doctors were appointed to head organizations such as the Taiwan igakukai (Taiwanese Association of Medicine).[97] Through the association, government officials and leading Japanese doctors passed many motions in support of military action.

As circumstances changed with the beginning of the Sino-Japanese War in 1937, many scientists who worked in the colonies, especially malariologists in Taiwan, were mobilized by the Japanese army and navy. As mentioned previously, Shimojyo Kumaichi was perhaps the first investigator from Taiwan to conduct a field survey of parasites in China. Morishita Kaoru, the famous malariologist in colonial Taiwan, later conducted a series of investigations on the anopheles mosquito in East and Southeast Asia.[98] In addition, Miyahara Hatsuo, a professor at Taihoku Imperial University, continued Morishita's research and stressed the importance of studying malaria on the battlefield in Southeast Asia.[99]

In 1941, the Japanese government went to war against the United States, Great Britain, and the Netherlands in Southeast Asia and New Guinea. To minimize disability and loss from disease, Japanese operations in the Pacific included measures to protect personnel from parasites and the "lethal" tropical climate. The Japanese army and navy adopted the approach of scientists in colonial Taiwan such as Koizumi Makoto and Morishita Kaoru.[100] For example, in 1941 the Japanese army established the Research Unit for Taiwan to investigate methods of disease prevention during military operations in Southeast Asia based on the experience of Taiwan. As time passed, laboratory medicine—especially as it related to tropical medicine combined with the abundant clinical experience in Taiwan—gradually formed a body of medical knowledge that the Japanese used to deal with sanitary problems and various diseases in southern China and southeastern Asia, that is, the southern part of the prosperous circle of Great Eastern Asia. Although that knowledge was essentially no different from modern tropical medicine in the West, the Japanese renamed it *nanbô igaku* (southern medicine) to indicate its main mission of health maintenance in the southern part of the Japanese empire.[101]

However, the harmony between laboratory and clinical medicine in Japanese medical circles in Taiwan soured when Japan increased its military actions in the late 1930s and established the Igakubu (Department of Medicine) at Taihoku Imperial University. Probably because their training in clinical medicine was at the vocational level and because of the academic friction in Japan between Kitasato's pupils and Todai's graduates, graduates of Taihoku Medical College had no opportunity to enroll in Tokyo Imperial University (known as Todai).[102] Nor was the Medical College allowed to merge with Taihoku Imperial University in 1936. Just as Todai graduates monopolized the positions in the Department of Medicine at the new Taihoku Imperial University after 1936, Japanese faculty at Taihoku Medical College were rejected by the university with the exception of Du Congming and Yokogawa Sadamu. A graduate from Kyoto Imperial University, Du Congming was retained because he symbolized Japanese mercy to the Taiwanese, but Yokogawa was definitely chosen because of his Todai education. The monopoly of Todai graduates caused great turbulence among the Japanese faculty at Taihoku Imperial University in 1937 and 1938—a déjà vu of the original 1910 academic feud.[103]

The concept of *nanhô igaku* implied a shift of the center of Japanese tropical medicine from Taiwan to the southern border of the Japanese empire, the occupied areas of the Philippines, Malaya, and Indonesia. To meet the military's goals and fit the geographic definition of southern medicine, Nagasaki Medical College established the Tairiku igaku kenkyukai (Research Society for Continental Medicine) to promote medical research in China proper. Furthermore, the college invited Aoki Yoshio to establish the Toa fûdobyô kenkyujyo (Institute for Endemic Disease in East Asia) at Nagasaki Medical College in 1942.[104] During the Pacific War, the institute was considered the headquarters of *nanhô igaku* while the Institute of Tropical Medicine in Taiwan functioned as a back office. By 1941, as mentioned previously, experts from Taiwan were working for the Japanese army in Southeast Asia. In fact, most of the preventive methods they applied in occupied areas had already been pioneered by scientists in colonial Taiwan.[105]

Nanhô igaku duplicated the experience of colonial medicine in Taiwan in some areas. For example, in Burma, New Guinea, and the Philippines the antimalaria program inspired by Morishita's method was adopted by the Japanese military forces in 1942. Unfortunately, bloody military operations and a continuous shortage of medical supplies undermined the antiparasite efforts.[106] Wartime circumstances were not conducive to conducting medical programs in Japanese-occupied areas of Southeast Asia.

From Legacy to Legend in Postwar Taiwanese Scholarship

Efforts to establish a new medical discipline, Japanese southern medicine, vanished with the end of the war in 1945. The prewar system of medical education and services in Japan was also demolished to meet the requirements of modernity and democracy mandated by the American General Headquarters (GHQ) and the Supreme Commander for the Allied Powers in Japan (SCAP).[107] Since southern medicine was no different in its technology and definition from Western tropical medicine, it was inevitably dropped from the medical curriculum and research topics in postwar Japan.

In Taiwan, a similar reform process was enforced starting in 1952. Efforts had been invested in importing advanced technology and copying the new health care system from the United States.[108] Due to the technology-oriented and pro-American atmosphere in postwar Taiwan, the legacy of Japanese colonial medicine was understood by many scholars to be a simple process of technological innovation. Therefore, the major concern of medical professionals in Taiwan was the replacement of old skills with new American technologies. For example, a great debate occurred in the 1960s when a younger generation of American-trained obstetrics and gynecology physicians attempted to replace the old surgical procedure radical hysterectomy—used to treat uterine cancer—which had been tried on laboratory basis in the 1940s with new radiotherapy treatment using American equipment.[109] Finally, the history of Japanese colonial medicine in Taiwan was confined to a relatively small circle of medical professionals and was intentionally neglected by Chinese nationalist historians prior to the 1980s.

Reidentification of the Colonial Legacy

Although the dream of being the center of Japanese *nanhô igaku* disappeared, the legacy of Japanese colonial medicine in Taiwan did not. With generations of Taiwanese doctors and many medical facilities having survived the war, that legacy was commonly seen as the foundation of medical modernization in training and institutions during the first two decades of postwar era. This interpretation of the Japanese contribution bypassed the unresolved debate about whether colonization was a merciful force or a brutal one.[110] Until the late 1970s, scholars of historical demography, a new discipline in postwar Taiwanese academia, first took the colonial statistics for granted and later focused on demographic improvements in colonial Taiwan.

Among the historical demographers who rediscovered the legacy of Japanese colonial medicine in Taiwan, George Barclay, the first to discuss the improved mortality rates, is frequently cited by postwar researchers, including medical historians from the 1990s on. Barclay found that the increase in life expectancy combined with the decrease in the mortality rate create the impression that health conditions probably had begun to improve by the 1930s at the latest. He argued that mortality rates in Taiwan started to decline in the first decade of Japanese rule and continued to do so through the 1906–14 period.[111] Because of the significant reduction in mortality in Taiwan starting in the 1920s, Barclay suggested that 1920 should be considered the onset of the mortality transition there.

Chen Shaoxin was the first Taiwanese scholar to notice fast growth in the colonial population and link it to the government's role in building the public health infrastructure.[112] According to his study, Taiwan had a population of around 500,000 in the 1650s and reached 2,545,731 in 1894. Since during this period there was no major improvement in public health programs, the population growth was caused more by immigration than an increasing birth rate or decreasing mortality rate. Following efforts during the colonial period to reform the medical system and public health infrastructures, Chen concludes, birth rates went up while mortality rates declined sharply. According to Chen's calculations from governmental statistics between 1906 and 1942, the total increase in birth rate in Taiwan (meaning the rate for both Taiwanese and Japanese nationals) was around 40 to 45 percent, while the death rate declined from 33 to 16 percent. This improvement increased the population growth rate from 5 percent in 1906 to 25 percent in the 1930s.[113]

Barclay's argument is further strengthened by Mohammad Mirzaee's doctoral dissertation. By modifying infant mortality rates from the original numbers, Mirzaee traced long-term trends in mortality in Taiwan between 1895 and 1975 to reveal that, with the outbreak of several contagious diseases, the rates increased during World War I.[114] Only after 1920 was there a steady and continuous decline in mortality. The overall standardized life expectancies by sex are shown in chart 4.3. Mirzaee concluded that "colonial development reduced Taiwanese mortality from a high pre-transitional level to an intermediate level by 1940. Improvements in the environment, changes in the relation between microorganism and human host (primarily as a result of increase in the resistance of the host), and therapy were regarded as immediate determinants of the reduction in mortality."[115] Chart 4.3 was generated using original statistics and Mirzaee's revisions. It shows that sexual differences in life expectancy were greatest at birth; later the differences were reduced somewhat, but females still enjoyed a higher life expectancy. Furthermore, the changing life expectancy of both sexes in Taiwan since 1906 was highly irregular during the early period of mortality transition.

CHART 4.3: Changing life expectancy at birth in colonial Taiwan, 1906–1940. (Data from Taiwan Sôtokufu, ed., *Taiwan jinkô dôtai tôke* (Taiwanese Population Dynamics Statistics) (Taihoku: Taiwan Sôtokufu, 1906, 1915, 1920, 1925, 1930, 1935.)

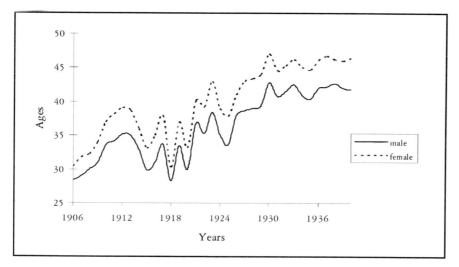

Following the impact of Western scholarship on interpreting demographic changes in colonial Taiwan, demographic improvements became essential to support the discourse of Japanese colonial modernity. More advanced analysis was eventually developed in the 1980s. For example, similar efforts by Chen Kuanzheng utilizing age-cohort analysis support the arguments of Barclay and others.[116] In the 1990s, Yang Wenshan made an extensive study of the fluctuation in life expectancy rates between the sexes, suggesting that infectious disease epidemics could have been an important factor. His results showed that changes in life expectancy before the 1940s were associated with the decline in mortality, first in infancy and then in early childhood.[117] In addition, the earlier changes represent the results of selective improvement in sanitation works in major cities and public health intervention by Japanese authorities.[118]

Making the Legacy of Japanese Colonial Medicine a Legend

With George Barclay's having attributed the demographic changes to the decline of infectious diseases through mass vaccinations and Mohammad Mirzaee's having supported Barclay's contentions, the mainstream viewpoint in contemporary historical demography seemed to favor the "tools of empire" theory. [119] More recently, John Durand attributed the same changes to other factors such as Japanese police management of hygienic affairs, the prevalence of public health education, and effective prevention and therapeutic programs.[120] These assertions were soon followed by the diligent efforts of Taiwanese historical demographers. Chen Kuanzheng identified the point of transition in mortality rates as 1920, the period during which the colonial government established a reliable reporting system and effective prevention programs.[121] In addition, Wang Demu and Chen Wenling confirmed that the decline in the mortality rate became permanent after 1920 due to government investment in the control of infectious diseases and parasiticproblems.[122] All these studies identify the 1920s as the major transition point in mortality rates and attribute that change to government actions. Although these scholars were not necessarily aware of the propaganda in the 1925 Police Hygiene Exhibition, their conclusions were accidentally similar.

These studies in historical demography not only conclude that modern medicine improved health conditions in colonial Taiwan but also identify the transition in mortality rate as unique in modern demographic history.[123] That is, after comparing the mortality transition in Taiwan and Britain (England and Wales), Mirzaee concluded that the transition in Taiwan was much faster and more extensive: Taiwan took only fifty years (1920 to 1975) to increase life expectancy by 41.5 years, while Britain needed nearly two hundred years (1786 to 1976) to increase it by 40.5 years. Because Mirzaee credits this improvement to public health policies during the colonial period, his conclusion seems to imply that Japan took advantage of being a latecomer in modern imperialism and used coercive strategies to dramatically increase the efficiency of the colonial government's actions.[124]

Almost all studies of historical demography in postwar Taiwan indicate the success of Japanese colonial medicine in providing better health conditions for the Taiwanese. The worsening ratio of doctors per population seemed to have no effect on progress in health conditions, nor did the growth of the urban economy after the mid-1920s play a role. Judging from these studies, discussion and comparative analysis of political and economic activities was absent from discourse about colonial medicalization. Nevertheless, Japanese colonial medicine in Taiwan was legendary.

Research in historical demography is important to support the modernization argument in the study of Japanese colonial medicine. However, compared to the delicate mathematical analyses of historical demography, the historian in Taiwan commonly prefers easy arithmetical calculations based on original government statistics and accepts the conclusions of historical demographers without question. For example, within the first four pages of her thesis, Li Xinfeng mentions three times the horrible public health conditions in Qing Taiwan based on government statements.[125] Another popular writer, Zhuang Yungming, in his study of the University Hospital of National Taiwan University (formerly Taihoku Imperial University), cites statistics from Japanese military resources as evidence of the "lethal" environment in Taiwan.[126] The image is strong enough to allow Chen Yungxin to arbitrarily conclude that in Taiwan "a hundred years ago, medical facilities were shabby, public health conditions horrible, and people ignorant and superstitious."[127] To such authors, the mercy and achievements of Japanese colonial medicine are demonstrated by government statistics and scientific analyses drawn from historical demography. But this unintentionally oversimplifies a conclusion: that grafting modern medicine onto existing health practices was a necessary step in colonial modernization under Japanese rule and that coercive public health policies were tolerated for their merciful benefits.[128]

Cracks in the Legend

The current mainstream historiography of Japanese colonial medicine in Taiwan accepts Alfred Crosby's viewpoint along with David Arnold's modification of it. In his famous book, Crosby asserts that human beings are biological entities before they are members of political and religious groups and that Europeans' displacement and replacement of native peoples in temperate zones was more a matter of biology than military conquest.[129] To elaborate on Crosby's argument, Arnold encourages the study of demography as providing insights into the real function and impact of colonial medicine.[130] However, as Geoffrey C. Bowker and Susan Leigh Star's *Sorting Things Out* proposes,[131] the meaning of vital statistics is usually twofold: first, classification as a ubiquitous human activity; and, second, the ramifications of classification as part of the information infrastructure and as a social practice affecting human lives.[132] These meanings of government statistics deserve much greater attention than they have received so far from researchers on Japanese colonial medicine.

At the beginning of the twenty-first century, skepticism about statistics from colonial Taiwan was rife.[133] On the individual level, Fu Dawei recalculates the infant mortality rate from government statistics in the colonial period and reveals that the data were compiled to favor licensed obstetrics and gynecology doctors and modern midwives by blaming all the dystocia cases to the traditional midwife.[134] Inspired by Chen Shaoxin's suggestion that the health transition in Taiwan occurred during the 1930s,[135] I have conducted a series of general studies to identify the time frame of the transition by checking changes in the top ten causes of death between 1906 and 1942.[136] I found that between the late 1910s and the mid-1920s the diagnosis of cause of death in colonial Taiwan was significantly improved. This improvement meant that death records were more reliable after 1925 and even more so after the 1930s. I suggest, however, that therapeutic practice did not show a comparable improvement. Therefore, the permanent change in the top ten causes of death should be attributed to better public health knowledge among the population rather than better medical technologies and medications.[137] With the raw data suggesting that the health transition occurred in the 1920s, my findings need to be confirmed by more detailed analysis.

To that end, William Siler's model of risk is employed for my decomposition analysis.[138] The model defines three essential periods (1906–15, 1915–25, and 1925–35) in the health transition before the 1940s. This analysis illustrates that the turning point in the old pattern of causes of death could only have occurred during the period 1925–35.[139] I thus suggest that the health transition began around 1925 and was completed in the 1930s.[140] My analysis also indicates that the transition period in Taiwan was not only shorter than it was in Britain but shorter than in Japan as well.[141] Based on this study, the 1925 Police Hygiene Exhibition was obviously too early to claim victory for public health programs; more credit should be given to the privatized market for medical services, a significant phenomena in the 1930s. However, with the shortage of qualified professionals and medical supplies continuing in the 1930s, the stunning speed of the health transition in colonial Taiwan remained unexplained.

Some researchers challenge the accuracy of colonial statistics. Any showing improvement in public health conditions or signs of the transition in the late 1920s are probably fraudulent because of a problem in government statistics before the mid-1920s. Wu Jiezun suggests that the unrealistically rapid drop in the mortality rate in government statistics before the mid-1920s not only created a discontinuity of classification and cast doubt on the credibility of the raw data but also exaggerated real progress.[142] Without mentioning the flaws in the census data, Kelly Olds examined data from the health and sanitation surveys conducted by the sanitation office of the colonial police force between 1921 and 1931. Olds found that adult height in late Qing Taiwan did not increase over time while the adult height of those born after the Japanese takeover increased rapidly. Data on children's height confirm that this increase continued through the 1920s. The body mass index of Taiwanese, however, did not increase in the 1920s.[143] Olds's discovery does not match the argument that the health transition took place in the 1920s or even the 1930s but suggests the possibility that health conditions had improved before the public health campaign was conducted. Although Olds's conclusion is intriguing, his data requires more thorough classification and sampling. Many of the areas from which the Japanese police collected data were considered "unhealthy," and the surveys, which included 233,911 people, were used to identify the degree of unhealthiness to enable implementation of public health measures.[144] Therefore, these surveys have a particular selection bias.

Inspired by anthropometric studies in the West, and to avoid the problem in government statistics,[145] Stephen Morgan and I compiled our own data on height from individual records.[146] Stature is the most widely used measure of nutritional status,[147] and a rise in stature in a low-income developing economy indicates widespread improvement in living standards.[148] This hypothesis is based on the observation that higher real incomes translate into more food, better quality food, and better access to public goods such as health and education, which combine to improve the nutritional status of a population.

According to our study, in which height data for the 1,864 male sample were classified into five-year periods by year of birth, the average male height increased from about 162 cm to slightly less than 165 cm between the 1880s and the first decade of the twentieth century. From around 1910 to 1945, average male height increased another 3 cm to about 168 cm.[149] Although their conclusion does not totally agree with Kelly Olds's findings, the increase in adult height occurred before 1920. These results suggest that, unlike the persistent pessimistic view that Japanese colonial policy squeezed rural incomes and constrained consumption welfare, economic development in colonial Taiwan played a more important role than medication in improving the health of the Taiwanese.[150]

However, there is little agreement about the income and welfare of the Taiwanese in the colonial period.[151] An alternative hypothesis is that changes in caloric intake could be an index with which to gauge the relationship between higher income and better health. From the conservative and pessimistic viewpoint, daily food availability was low before the 1930s; according to Samuel Ho, it averaged about 1,800 to 2,000 calories per capita.[152] However, other studies contest Ho's findings. Zhang Hanyu estimates that male adult farmers had a food intake of 3,600 calories and that farmers' incomes in the 1930s were higher than their incomes the early 1950s.[153] Samuel Ho later revised his findings.[154] There may have been positive effects from increased consumption of alternative staples such as yam and peanut, fruits and vegetables, and meat, which improved the diet mix.[155] By adjusting Ho's estimates of food energy, Yeh Shujen estimates that the adult-equivalent levels raised per capita daily food availability to 2,500 calories, which was not low, and she showed that welfare improved from 1904 to 1937, stating that "per capita consumption of the agricultural sector not only increased over the whole colonial period, but grew even faster after 1925, achieving a growth of 3.65% per annum between 1925 and 1937."[156] Generally speaking, the change of caloric intake and the sustained rise in average height indicate significant health-welfare returns to the Taiwanese from colonial economic development. In sum, prior to the completion of modern medical and public health infrastructures health conditions in Taiwan had already improved by means of higher incomes and a stabile food supply.

The adoption of Japanized *Staatsmedizin* to create colonial medicine in Taiwan occurred at the great cost of police control and racial discrimination before the 1920s. Beginning in the late 1920s, the instruments of medical service depended more on the development of clinical medicine than on social mobilization and government intervention. That is, the role of the private dispensary became more important, replacing functions formerly provided by the government. Increased numbers of physicians, nurses, and midwives compensated for the rapid decline in the numbers of traditional physicians. These Taiwanese clinicians might not have been the best medical professionals by the current Japanese definition, but they played an important role in promoting modern medicine and furthering public health reform, realizing the Japanese prediction that "Taiwanese physicians will cure their own society."[157]

As students of Japanese teachers, Taiwanese medical professionals possibly internalized the power relationship of colonization, which was reflected in the medical hierarchy in Taiwan. For example, while the 1925 Police Hygiene Exhibition treated the contributions of Taiwanese clinicians as insignificant, the clinicians themselves treated midwives and nurses as not only subordinate but anonymous. In addition, the colonial government promoted the socioeconomic status of physicians by withholding the legal right to practice medicine from nurses, midwives, and pharmacists. Numerous patients in poor economic circumstances were forced to seek help from cheaper alternatives such as low-cost midwives and questionable drugs from *jiyaobao* services. In that way, the rise of Taiwanese doctors significantly depended on colonial rules.

Beginning in 1874, Meiji Japan introduced the westernization of medicine based on the German model. The Institute of Infectious Disease was established to train the first generation of specialists in laboratory medicine. But the success of medical reform in colonial Taiwan made it a model for other Japanese-occupied areas during the 1930s. However, because of World War II the cooperation between laboratory and clinical medicine entered a new stage. After Japan's proclamation of the creation of the Greater East Asia Co-Prosperity Sphere, scientists from Taiwan developed research centers to duplicate their success on the periphery of the expanded empire. The empire promoted the Japanese-defined discipline of *nanhô igaku* (southern medicine) based on the tropical medicine model developed in European colonies.

Wartime medical policies related to military mobilization helped spur the integration of both laboratory and clinical medicine in Taiwan. Tropical medicine was officially recognized as an academic discipline after the establishment of the Society of Tropical Medicine at Taihoku Imperial University. Meanwhile, modern examination methods and new ways to deal with unsanitary conditions met Japanese needs on the battlefield after 1942. With more qualified physicians and the successful sanitary reforms, Taiwan after the mid-1930s became a center for exporting tropical medicine to other Japanese-occupied areas.

The end of the academic friction in the medical hierarchy in Japan and the success of clinical medicine in Taiwan were followed by the development of Japanese southern medicine, which can be seen as having three aspects: theory, availability, and practice. The theory of tropical medicine and associated laboratory research made Japanese medical experts confident about taking that work beyond Taiwan. They adopted preventive and curative methods already available in Taiwan in hopes of overcoming similar problems in South China and Southeast Asia. When the Japanese ambition to build a great empire in Asia was extinguished in 1945, the dream of developing southern medicine faded. The legend of Japanese colonial medicine went into hibernation within the circle of Taiwanese medical professionals.

Because of developments in postwar scholarship in Taiwan, the achievements of Japanese colonial medicine have become legendary. Indeed, a Taiwanese historian of colonial medicine might appreciate both the "tools of empire" theory and the Whiggish interpretation that colonial medicine not only ensured the survival of the colonizer but improved Taiwanese public health as part of its modernization effort.

Finally, reviewing the skeptical attitude toward colonial statistics is always fascinating. Reflecting increased skepticism, the latest anthropometric studies imply that economic development in colonial Taiwan could have been more important to improved health than medical service. The achievements of Japanese colonial medicine in Taiwan were therefore not a product or side effect of medical modernization but an unpredictable result of the privatized colonial economy and market for medical services. However, despite some authors' efforts to modify governmental statistics or generate new time-series data, these studies have had an insignificant impact on the legend of Japanese colonial medicine, which was created in the 1920s by the colonial government and revived in postwar academic circles. It will be interesting to see if developments in the twenty-first century eventually crack the legend, leading, one hopes, to the writing of a postcolonial history of medicine in Taiwan.[158]

Conclusion

This book addresses the impact of Western-influenced Japanese medicine on medical practices in Taiwan. During the colonial era (1895–1945), two related processes—the creation of medical resources and the establishment of a new medical system composed of clinical medicine, laboratory medicine, and new institutions—formed the main body of medical services in colonial Taiwan. An analysis of the procedures involved in establishing those services reveals two themes: the continuity of medical westernization in Japan since the 1870s and the role colonial medicine played in Japanese empire building between 1895 and 1945.

Regarding those themes, the globalization of Western medicine beginning in the late nineteenth century coincided with the expansion of Western colonization in East Asia. Japan soon participated in that expansion by adopting Western learning.[1] To intellectuals in Meiji Japan, Western medicine was not only a part of modern science but a necessary technique of state and later empire building. The period from the late nineteenth to the mid–twentieth century saw the triumph of modern medicine as a fully scientific discipline of proven effectiveness in curing and preventing diseases.[2] The Japanese accepted medical knowledge not only as the fruit of scientific inquiry but also as a social value and norm. Japan learned Western medicine by modeling itself after the German experience, and it developed colonial medicine in Taiwan on that basis.

Hygienic intervention and medical reform in Taiwan aimed to control epidemic diseases mainly to improve living conditions for Japanese settlers. Acclimatization of the Japanese and assimilation of the Taiwanese were the major public health policy goals, as is clear from the policies of Gotô Shinpei and the documents created by the majority of sanitation officers. Working within the framework of the German-Japanese medical tradition, they emphasized the distinctiveness of the tropical environment and the unsanitary behavior of the Taiwanese inhabitants. From the viewpoint of the Japanese colonizers, the Taiwanese people, with their "filthy" habits and "unhealthy" lifestyle, were identified as part of the sanitation problem. The "tools of empire" theory, it seems, would apply to Japanese colonial medicine in Taiwan. However, the situation involved complexities beyond what is explained by that theory.

To a supporter of the "tools of empire" theory, a common scenario in developing colonial medicine might be described as follows. The colonizing powers took advantage of technological know-how to extend their geographic and political control and maximize profits through the expansion of plantations, extractive industries, and new markets.[3] In this context, medical services were intended, first, to preserve the health of the colonizers, including colonial officials, troops, and developers; second, to limit illness among workers, who, depending on the colonial economic policy, might be either indigenous laborers or immigrants; and third, to prevent the spread of epidemics that would threaten individual health and social order. Finally, quarantine laws, vaccination procedures, hospitals, household sanitation and housing regulations, and urban settlements were oriented toward preventing infection, restricting outbreaks of disease, and treating illness.[4]

As discussed in chapters 2 and 4, the motive and sequence of building Japanese colonial medicine in Taiwan may have differed from the models proposed in Western scholarship. Medicine was indeed a tool, but it served many purposes, not only the creation and maintenance of the Japanese empire. The purposes of the colonizers were never homogeneous. To Kitasato's pupils, medicine served as a tool to restore their reputation in laboratory medicine against that of their counterparts in Japan. To bureaucrats in colonial Taiwan such as Gotô Shinpei, the success of medical and public health reform was a means of winning respect and promotion. Both groups used Taiwan as a laboratory of Japanese modern medicine for their own purposes, which differed from the purposes of medical professionals such as Todai's faculty in Japan. Interestingly, because of the friction between the medical professionals in Taiwan and Japan, medicine could be used for humanitarian purposes because it functioned as an instrument of social and political control. In addition, changes in the policy of training Taiwanese doctors that broadened their opportunities meant that the colonized medical elites used their association with "advanced modern medicine" to enhance their socioeconomic status, and they shared in colonial power by focusing on clinical medicine.

Although at first glance the development of modern medicine in colonial Taiwan might appear to conform to George Basalla's simple evolutionary model on the spread of Western science, in fact the process was not quite so simple. The term *civilization* often appeared in official propaganda as a synonym for *colonization*, consistent with Basalla's model,[5] according to which Japan's colonial actions could be interpreted as extending Western civilization, including modern medicine.[6] Basalla's model has been extensively criticized in science studies since the 1980s. This critical response was inspired in part by the more general challenge of dependency theories and world systems theory to the diffusionist models of modernization and development.[7] For instance, David Wade Chambers rejected Basalla's diffusionism and asked for more case studies of science in non-Western settings as well as more interactive models of scientific development. This study addresses that request by looking into the spread of Japanese modern medicine to its colonies. However, Chambers warned that "without a more general framework, we sink into a sea of local history."[8] That pitfall is avoided in this book by a review of contemporary studies of Taiwan's colonial medicine, which reveal—similar to the discovery by Paolo Palladino and Michael Worboys with regard to European colonialism—a significant trend of imperialism shaping "metropolitan scientific institutions and knowledge."[9]

Scenarios omitted by Basalla and included here reveal a crack in the diffusionist model and a different story of how the web of Japanese colonial medicine was constructed. The impetus for transmitting westernized medicine from Japan to the colony was not mere enthusiasm for extending knowledge and improved health practices to the imperial periphery but an academic feud in Japan. Also it was nearly twenty years before Japan thoroughly understood the medical problems in Taiwan. The fact that the Japanese had to acknowledge the growing influence of Taiwanese doctors led the colonial government to tempt its pupils, taking parts of the "tools of empire" hypothesis and creating a hybrid system that favored physicians. In addition, demographic improvements were linked to a variety of factors, including improved medical care, economic conditions, and nutritional intake; medicine was only one of many factors that prolonged human life. This view was put forth in Thomas McKeown's studies on the population of Britain. He concluded that modern medicine played only a small part in the increase in population, which he saw as largely resulting from improved nutrition and environmental reforms such as clean water supplies.[10] As noted in chapters 3 and 4, no one contribution was the sole factor in this increase, not even modern medicine.

Whether we view Japanese colonial medicine as an inevitable process of westernization or a "tool of empire," we should consider that the prevalent approach among historians in East Asia who examine it through the lens of Western theories might be flawed.[11] Andrew Cunningham and Bridie Andrews assert that "scientific medicine was a development of the native medicine of modern Western Europe, which was then made universal by exportation."[12] Japan, a non-Western empire and latecomer to colonial power, would probably share a similar motive but go through a different process in its approach to colonial medicine due to its unique historical and social heritage. In retrospect, we can see how three distinctive themes interactively frame the legend of modern medicine in Japan's colonization of Taiwan: academic conflict, polarized composition, and self-recovery of the colonial society.

This book was written as part of a new wave of scholarship on colonial medicine, science, and technology that has emerged in the past decade. Following the lead of David Arnold, Miriam Ming-cheng Lo, Warwick Anderson, and others, I reject as too simple-minded both the old diffusionist arguments, which commonly viewed colonial medicine as a boon bestowed by technologically advanced civilizations on societies considered "backward," and the more recent "tools of empire" thesis, which regards colonial medical interventions as characterized by violence—both physical and epistemological—directed against indigenous practices and beliefs.[13] Therefore, either to laud Japanese physicians and public health officials as heroes or to dismiss them reductively as handmaidens of colonialism ignores the more complicated and interesting reality of improved morbidity and mortality conditions in Taiwan under Japanese rule.

The Ripple Effect of Academic Rivalry: The Precipitating Factor in Japanese Colonial Medicine

Basalla argued that scientists coming from societies with established fields of science, such as many European countries, in effect "colonized" science in new locations. Then, given certain necessary cultural, social, and economic developments, modern science took root and prospered in formerly prescientific societies. He argued that "resistance to science on the basis of philosophical and religious beliefs must be overcome and replaced by positive encouragement of scientific research. Such resistance . . . must be eradicated when science seeks a broad base of support at home."[14] In this argument, colonial medicine was not only a tool of the empire but a route to colonial modernity. On the surface, Basalla's model may seem to explain the development of modern medical services in colonial Taiwan as "civilization" brought by Japanese imperialism. However, the spread of Western medicine from Japan to its colonies might not have been as inevitable or as smooth a process as Basalla's model implies.

In the early years of the colony, medical westernization in Japan was still in its infancy and lacked the medical manpower and funding to overcome the harsh conditions in Taiwan at that time.[15] As shown in table 1.1, Japan had 40,215 qualified doctors by the end of 1890s, of whom only 21.28 percent were trained in Western medicine, to serve its population of about forty million,[16] and Taiwan had a population 2,545,731 by 1894.[17] With the colonial government facing the threat of military resistance and financial difficulties, the overwhelmingly adverse natural conditions in Taiwan before the 1900s would hardly have been attractive to qualified Japanese doctors. Thus, Mori Ôgai's pessimism about improving Taiwan's public health conditions was understandable, and Gotô Shinpei's suggestions for improvements before his assignment in 1902 appeared at best impractical. Basically, by 1895 Japan had not yet reached the "established" stage with regard to modern Western medicine that would correspond to Basalla's model. Therefore, the establishment of colonial medicine in Taiwan was in no way inevitable.

The whole system of medical service in colonial Taiwan was in fact neither built on a surplus of medical resources in Japan nor based on purely scientific interests directed toward overcoming medical difficulties and diseases in the tropics. Rather, colonial medicine in Taiwan owed its origins to the ripple effect from an academic feud in Japan between Kitasato Kenkyujyo's team and Tokyo Imperial University (Todai). The merger of the Private Institute of Infectious Disease and Todai in the decades between 1900 and 1916 created great tension between Kitasato's pupils and Todai graduates. The first generation of Japanese laboratorists left for the colonies to avoid the tension. Although Gotô may not have been an excellent physician, he contributed much to medical services in colonial Taiwan, taking advantage of the disaffection of Kitasato's talented experts in modern Japanese medicine and recruiting them to practice in Taiwan.

Despite the emphasis placed by historians on Gotô Shinpei's desire to apply his theory of *Biologische Principien* to Japanese colonial medicine in Taiwan, more important was Takagi Tomoe's initiation of new forms of medical organization and policy goals.[18] After the serious setback of the Soma event, Gotô Shinpei, with renewed awareness of his weak educational and family background, not only restarted his political career in Taiwan but also asked Takagi Tomoe to spearhead his reform plan there.[19] Because of Takagi's reputation among the medical elite in Japan, he was in a better position than Gotô to link the medical reforms in Taiwan with the famous Kitasato team. Takagi not only largely guided the expansion of medical services between 1900 and 1920 but he also created Sôtokufu kenkyujyo (Research Institute of the Governor-General Government or RIGG) and Chûô kenkyujyo (Central Institute of Research or CIR), two Japanese-dominated centers of laboratory medicine that became the scholastic core of colonial medicine in Taiwan. Those institutes provided the opportunity for Japanese researchers to contribute to the main body of clinical medicine in the colony without losing their prestige as laboratorists. After Takagi expanded Gotô's plan, a miniature version of Japanese *Staatsmedizin* was finally implemented in Taiwan by putting more focus on clinical medicine and treating laboratory medicine as an internal activity of Japanese academics.

Thus, the academic feud in Japan marked a breakthrough in the exportation of modern medicine to the colonies. Takekoshi Yosaburô claimed to "have long believed that on their [Western nations'] shoulders alone rested the responsibility of colonizing the yet-unopened portions of the globe and extending to the inhabitants the benefits of civilization; but now we Japanese, ris[e] from the ocean in the extreme Orient as a nation to take part in this great and glorious work."[20] Although this might exaggerate Japan's status as a colonial empire in Asia at the time, by the end of 1910 one thing was certain about the spread of modern Japanese medicine: Taiwan was the first colony to benefit from the academic feud and Korea the second. The Kitasato team moved out of Japan to create a network among Japanese colonies and occupied territories that lasted until the end of World War II.

Polarization: Norms for Making Taiwan a Model of Japanese Colonial Medicine

The polarization that informed the relationship between Japan and Taiwan before 1945 was primarily one of the colonizer and the colonized. However, another polarity existed between advanced laboratory medicine in Japan and clinical medicine in Taiwan. Ironically, for nearly thirty years the polarization of medical professions veiled an academic conflict within modern Japanese medicine in Taiwan.[21] The conflict between the Kitasato team and Tokyo Imperial University remained unacknowledged as long as Taiwan focused on the infrastructure of clinical medicine. The appointment of a former army surgeon, Horiuchi Takao, to succeed Takagi as director of Taihoku Medical College, was a sign that the status quo would be maintained. Before the mid-1930s, the relatively small scale of laboratory medicine at RIGG and CIR was totally under the control of Japanese experts. Even so, as shown by the case of malariology, only such entomological activities as observation and classification were performed in Taiwan while the essential research for treatment was left to medical circles in Japan.[22] The harmony among Japanese medical professionals in Taiwan soured after the appearance of Japanese southern medicine. A conflict within the Department of Medicine at Taihoku Imperial University occurred between the elite four-year section and the vocational three-year section. The later was the former Taihoku Medical College, which merged with the new Department of Medicine at Taihoku Imperial University in 1936. As the Department of Medicine was mainly built by Todai's alumni, the faculty of the former Taihoku Medical College were not allowed to teach at Taihoku Imperial University because of their vocational training background. Only Du Congming and Yokogawa Sadamu, "Japanized" Taiwanese citizens and Todai alumni, received teaching appointments from the imperial university. In the mid-1930s, Todai graduates again took the control of the medical college, a school that had been promoted and built by many of Kitasato's pupils

Following efforts to establish Japanese southern medicine in the 1930s and 1940s, the line between clinical and laboratory medicine blurred further when Taiwan was seen as a source of scientific data and biological specimens to be used in laboratory research in Japan. Malaria treatment in colonial Taiwan demonstrates that the one-way traffic in modern medicine from Japan to Taiwan, as the Basalla model implies, could be reversed. Although the importance of clinical medicine in Taiwan increased in the 1930s, the teacher-pupil relationship between Japanese and Taiwanese, another polarized relationship in the medical profession, remained the same.[23] Part of the reason was Japanese government propaganda. As Takekoshi Yosaburô's words imply, the imperial government in Japan viewed colonization as a process of educating ignorant Taiwanese. The metaphor of educating ignorant Taiwanese particularly mirrored the development of medical education in colonial Taiwan.[24] Therefore, despite Taiwanese doctors' intentions to retain their identity with the colonized and to avoid being viewed as a "colonial agency," as Miriam Ming-cheng Lo has claimed, they barely challenged the teacher-pupil relationship and even passed it on to other professionals, nurses, midwives, and pharmacists.[25]

The pupils' acceptance of the teachers' authority in Taiwanese medical circles could have arisen from traditional Asian values rather than colonization.[26] As in the case of Japanese biologists rejecting the Nazis' racial policies in the 1930s, Ogata Norio boldly expressed his reluctance to betray a Jewish teacher by following Hitler's *Rassenhygiene* policy in Japan.[27] As pupils of Japanese teachers in the medical professions, Taiwanese doctors exhibited a similar attitude. They often criticized the ruthlessness of colonization but at the same time appreciated their Japanese teachers for bringing modern medicine, and possibly a new civilization, to Taiwan.[28] Still, since the virtue of respecting one's teacher exists in Chinese as well as Japanese culture, it is possible that Taiwanese doctors accepted their teachers' authority because of their Asian heritage.

On the other hand, the fact that Todai edged out Kitasato's team might have created sympathy for the Japanese experts among medical pupils in Taiwan. On one occasion when he was speaking about the assimilation of the alumni of Taihoku Medical College, Takagi Tomoe remarked, "the Japanese and Taiwanese should coordinate on the level of thought."[29] Using the metaphor of combining hydrogen and oxygen to make a powerful material, water, he said that assimilation would help Japan "line up with other first-class powers."[30] Takagi's expectation of integrating Taiwanese and Japanese thought via modern education was totally different from that of his Japanese colleagues, including Gotô Shinpei himself. Gotô had described colonization in Taiwan with a famous metaphor: "It is impossible to transplant a bream's eyes to a flounder. . . . They have to grow as they should for biological reasons. . . . It is the same in politics. . . . It is equally important that we should not plug civilization into a barbarian place [i.e., Taiwan]."[31]

Although Kitaoka Shinichi attempted to portray Gotô as merely a "politician with a biological mind," the metaphor of the bream and flounder was, in fact, racist,[32] bearing a notable similarity to a statement by the German racist Alfred Ploetz (1860–1940): "The reason that human beings differ from chimpanzees is biological heritage. . . . Modern education is of no use in trying to alter biological nature. . . . There is thus no way to train all kinds of dogs to be police dogs, watchdogs, or hunting dogs . . . [for] they are already determined by hereditary nature."[33] To Japanese doctors in Taiwan such as Takagi Tomoe and Horiuchi Takao, physically isolating Japanese settlers from the Taiwanese was obviously impossible. The cooperation of Taiwanese doctors was needed to reduce the immediate threat of disease, and to ensure that cooperation compromises had to be made in the partnership between Japanese teachers and Taiwanese pupils in the medical profession. The closeness of the partnership made Japanese doctors in Taiwan willing to resist the monopoly of the Todai group, which opposed Du Congming's professorship in Taihoku Imperial University.[34] Both emotional sympathy regarding Japanese oppression and the practical compromises necessitated by immediate health crises strengthened the teacher-student partnership in Taiwan. Colonial medicine served as a shield for Japanese doctors who wished to stay clear of the academic feud and create a mutually supportive group on the basis of teacher-pupil relationships in clinical medicine. Thus, medicine was a "tool of empire" that served many purposes.

Propaganda and Legacy: Weaving the Legend of Japanese Colonial Medicine

One of the flaws in the "tools of empire" theory is the belief that the imperial network became a channel for spreading disease in the colonies rather than overcoming it. Possibly inspired by William McNeil's works,[35] Sheldon Watts called cholera "the disease that imperialism kept in being for 130 years at the cost of some 25 million Indian dead."[36] To Watts, the case of cholera and other infectious diseases indicated that Western imperialism created or worsened many of the health problems in the colonies and that the disease control measures deployed directly or indirectly by Western agencies to meet those problems were, in many instances, inappropriate.[37] However, neither government propaganda nor statistical reports in colonial Taiwan support this conclusion.

It is not the astuteness of current Taiwanese historians, exemplified by John Farley's criticism of Watts's book, but the nature of scientific colonialism that allowed Japan, a latecomer to imperialism, to easily exploit scientific language and tools to legitimize its rule in Taiwan.[38] As Japan began to westernize in the 1870s, it adopted the European tradition of conducting scientific surveys. Evolved from a system of beliefs and values based on empirical documentation, this tradition aims to discover quantitative mathematical interrelationships and laws that can be represented on charts and graphs.[39] The varied objects of the 1925 Police Hygiene Exhibition —including modern visual media and over a thousand posters utilizing photographs, statistical tables, and charts— propagandized the success of Japanese colonial medicine under the aegis of the police force.[40] The value of modern science and medicine, as reflected in the exhibition, was accepted and even welcomed by Taiwanese visitors, who did not object to public health improvement through a coercive state apparatus.[41] Sadly, on major government occasions such as the exhibition the colonized Taiwanese, rather than being given opportunities to act or speak on their own behalf, were viewed as objects to be treated, talked about, and lifted up by the efforts of enlightened colonizers, those who had the necessary knowledge and capabilities.[42] To the Taiwanese viewers, the sacrifice of their autonomy was a necessary trade-off to gain the better medical services and improved public health conditions displayed in the exhibition. In that context, scientific data in colonial Taiwan contributed to the consolidation of colonial rule and the simultaneous development of modern scientific knowledge, and the Taiwanese elite could succeed with the same spirit from the onset of westernization in Japan in the 1870s. Moreover, since colonial medicine always "occupied a central place in the ideological as well as the technological processes of colonial rule,"[43] the subtle application of statistics during colonial rule functioned in the way that Eric Hobsbawm saw artifact, invention, and social engineering entering into the making of modern colonies.[44] In colonial ideology, a well-run medical service was considered a powerful and effective way to win the cooperation of colonized peoples, and reports from scientific evidence—that is, statistics—confirmed the promising role of the medical service in colonization.[45] Data and numbers from scientific investigations thus played a key role in fabricating the image of Japanese modernity in ruling the colony.[46]

The use of colonial statistics to support Japanese rule in Taiwan came to an end with the Japanese defeat in WWII in 1945. In the 1980s, scholars of historical demography opened the buried treasures of colonial statistics. Some historians also put forth the Whiggish viewpoint with regard to Japanese colonial medicine in Taiwan by citing demographers' arguments. The latest studies of Japanese colonial medicine inevitably manifest the original propaganda in the 1925 Police Exhibition by showing the complexity of the relationship between improvements in public health and the introduction of modern medicine. Analyses of data on colonial demography and epidemiology show that the government was primarily concerned with disease agents, vectors, and populations.[47] From the viewpoint of demography, it seems that Japanese rule prolonged the life expectancy of the Taiwanese by improving health conditions. The "cause-of-death" data between 1906 and 1939 indicate that the thrust of the mortality transition occurred because infectious and digestive diseases eventually lost importance in determining life expectancy for both sexes. The results also suggest that mortality patterns in colonial Taiwan followed a stage of health transition.

Despite the findings of Taiwanese researchers, some Western scholars express their appreciation of the enlightening force of modernity through colonization. For example, Soma Hewa has provided a fairly detailed account of the activities of the International Health Board in Sri Lanka from 1802 until 1948. The author states simply that the International Health Board was "necessitated by the self-interested concerns of the industrial capitalists of the United States" and was "inseparable from the capitalist pursuit of global and political domination."[48] However, this interpretation has often been criticized in Western scholarship. John Farley criticizes Soma's attempt to portray the International Health Board as attempting to spread the gospel of Western technological medicine and to set up a public health administration based on that of the United States, much of which can be criticized as inappropriate for former colonies.[49] In light of the way colonial propaganda was used to create a legend in postwar Taiwan, Farley's criticism seems to be on target.

Many contemporary Taiwanese historians believe that the rapid health transition after 1925 provides the best evidence to highlight the achievements of Japanese colonial medicine. In another way, however, the transition reflects Charles Rosenberg and Janet Golden's concern about "the way disease definitions and hypothetical etiologies can serve as tools of social control, as labels for deviance, and as a rationale for the legitimization of status relationships."[50] In colonial Taiwan, the methods of classification of diseases in government reports changed during the mid-1920s, raising concern over the discontinuity of demographic data and the reliability of statistics on health problems from the late 1930s through 1945. For instance, in the case of Spanish influenza, records of deaths during the crisis were meticulously collected in Japan,[51] but the data in colonial Taiwan were haphazard and cited different mortality rates, which confused control strategies.[52] Although data on cholera and malaria were carefully collected, the colonial government distorted the records and related statistics on the catastrophic flu, which they were unable to control. Furthermore, as the latest study of the health transition in colonial Taiwan shows, Japanese efforts to build a modern public health system there lacked the flexibility to make necessary adjustments to the original plan, creating a bottleneck and resulting in stagnation during the 1930s.

The health transition in colonial Taiwan echoes Megan Vaughan's argument that "the power of colonial medicine lay not so much in its direct effects on the bodies of its subjects . . . but in its ability to provide a 'naturalized' and pathologized account of those subjects."[53] From Vaughan's vantage point, an analysis of the epidemiological transition would also reveal the hidden notion of racial superiority in Japanese colonial medicine. While the colonial government claimed victory in improving public health conditions in Taiwan by exhibiting scientific data, the success actually depended heavily on clinical medicine and a group of Taiwanese clinicians as well as other medical care providers such as nurses, midwives, and pharmacists. If the government statistics accurately reflect the health transition in colonial Taiwan, medical reforms could not have been implemented without the advanced technologies and costly investments in laboratory medicine made by the Japanese—a field that exclusively employed Japanese professionals.

This discussion of the health transition is an attempt to question the legend of Japanese colonial medicine. With rising skepticism about government statistics in colonial period, there is a demand for new methods and data. Based on individual cases, the anthropometric analysis on physical height in chapter 4 suggests that modern Japanese medicine was an add-on factor to the improvement of health conditions in colonial Taiwan, just as clinical medicine provided services in private dispensaries and the *jiyaobao* system (door-to-door service for over-the-counter drugs) worked well in maintaining and improving Taiwanese health.

Physical stature is a sensitive indicator of the nutritional status of a population and ultimately a measure of the ability of a population to obtain the necessary food and other inputs required for human growth.[54] Economic well-being encompasses not only medicine but other factors that make for a quality lifestyle. A 2007 study by Stephen Morgan and myself implies that the increase in real income in colonial Taiwan might have alleviated population pressure if medical reform had increased population size and prolonged life expectancy. However, our study clearly shows that the surge in male physical height began in the period 1906–15, much earlier than could have been accounted for by the appearance in the 1920s of sufficient medical resources from Japan. It seems that the Taiwanese enjoyed a better chance of survival and grew taller after the colonial government stabilized the social unrest in the first decade of the 1900s. From the mid-1920s on, the economic development that accompanied modern medical services further accelerated the increase in physical height. In general, skepticism about colonial statistics and recent studies questioning the legend of Japanese colonial medicine indicate the essential impact of a privatized market for medical services and the colonial economy on the improvement of health conditions in Taiwan. Both elements were intentionally neglected by the colonial government and went unmentioned in many postwar studies.

In the context of the development of Japanese colonial medicine in Taiwan, David Arnold's assertion is greatly inspiring.

> There is indeed a sense in which all modern medicine is engaged in a colonizing process. . . . It can be seen in the increasing professionalization of medicine and the exclusion of "folk" practitioners, in the close and often symbiotic relationship between medicine and the modern state, in the far-reaching claims made by medical science for its ability to prevent, control, and even eradicate human diseases.[55]

Influenced by such hypotheses, Taiwanese scholars overvalued the advance of modern medicine, viewing it as a "magic bullet"; as a result, what is read as characteristic of colonial medicine may simply be characteristic of biomedicine generally.[56] The "magic bullet" concept obviously supports the application of Basalla's model as well as some interpretations in Taiwanese scholarship of medicine as a colonial tool in which the Japanese colonist is seen as an exacting father mercifully offering medication to ignorant Taiwanese. Many public health scholars and historians in postwar Taiwan attribute changes in health conditions in colonial Taiwan to "advanced and costly" Japanese medical reforms. This book shows that Japanese colonial medicine in Taiwan was neither as advanced nor as costly as previous scholars have implied, although it did resolve a broad array of health problems. Despite Japanese confidence in advanced laboratory-based medicine, the medical services in colonial Taiwan seem to have improved health conditions through a judicious mix of clinical medicine and better socioeconomic conditions.

In contrast to the postcolonialist view of colonial medicine presented by Shula Marks and Warwick Anderson,[57] this book implies that current interpretations of Japanese colonial medicine in Taiwan have not yet been decolonized.[58] Beyond the cliché about modern medicine advancing colonial society, the conflict in Japan between Kitasato's students and the Todai faculty, along with the traditional Asian moral value placed on the teacher-student relationship, were key factors in promoting the spread of modern medicine in the Japanese empire, which means that understanding Japanese colonial medicine is more complex than has been recognized in existing interpretations. The case study of colonial Taiwan reveals this complexity and also reflects the local diversity among the colonies in Taiwan, Korea, Manchuria, and other Japanese-occupied areas. Despite local conditions in Korea and China (multiple medical systems and nationalist resistance, respectively) that might obscure the teacher-pupil norm in Japanese medical circles, the cases of colonial Taiwan and Shanghai reveal the importance of this relationship in extending modern medicine throughout the empire. This book was not written to challenge the application of these popular models for explaining Japanese colonial medicine but to provide an alternative way to think critically along with supplemental information on important events that have been overlooked in previous studies. Generally speaking, a ripple effect from the academic rivalry in Japan followed by a relationship in developing medicine in the colonies more accurately portrays Japanese colonial medicine than do the usual Eurocentric theories.

Since the Japanese colonies served as havens for Kitasato's students after 1916, Eurocentric models are not adequate to judge the roles of these experts in the spread of Japanese modern medicine. A more accurate description of Japanese colonial medicine is that the colonies served as laboratories for experimenting with various ideas in modern medicine. In fact, the development of modern medicine within the sphere of the Japanese empire can be seen in terms of a partnership model, at least before 1940. The geography of Japan and its colonies, as well as the deficiency of its medical resources before the 1930s, postponed the expansion of the Todai group. The monopolizing of positions at the Medical School at Taihoku Imperial University in 1936 was evidence of Todai's endless thrust toward expansion. Also, because of the efforts by Kitasato's students in the colonies, the variety of Japanese colonial medicine was sustained, and many medical specialties, such as parasitology and tropical medicine, were expanded after the 1930s.

Focusing on the development of tropical medicine in European colonies, Basalla's model treats the spread of modern medicine from Japan to its colonies as a one-way route, and the "tools of empire" concept usually implies a very top-down viewpoint. Although the original impetus for that spread was a feud in Japan's academic circles, this book proposes that an unintentionally cooperative relationship between the imperial center and the peripheral colonies resulted in the development of modern medicine in East Asia. Significantly, Korea and Manchuria were not tropical colonies, and the term *tropical medicine*— used in Eurocentric models—is clearly not applicable to Japan's colonial medicine. This illustrates the important point that the study of Japanese colonial medicine cannot be limited to the conventional understanding of imperial tropical medicine and underscores the critical interaction between the metropolis and the periphery as well as the contribution of Taiwan in the development of Japanese colonial medicine.

Finally, unveiling the complexity of Japanese colonial medicine may offer a stepping-stone for a more comprehensive study of modern medicine within the sphere of the Japanese empire then and now. Thus, this book presents not a final answer to the question of how modern medicine spread from Japan to its colonies, but a fresh perspective supported by historical details that should inspire further study in a variety of areas. With this information, scholars of Asia can look beyond the Western historiographies of colonial medicine of past decades and reenvision Japan's colonial medicine within a rich contemporary argument in Western scholarship. In conclusion, far from being narrow, specialized, and technical—as the history of colonial medicine might seem—this book contains a breadth of sources in a variety of languages, and integration of the local with the general renders this a fascinating topic for contemporary scholarship.

Appendix A: Romanization of Place Names in the Wade-Giles, Pinyin, and Hepburn Systems

Readers and researchers may find it difficult to identify place names in Taiwan. While the official romanization follows the Wade-Giles system in general, the Pinyin system is more familiar in Western scholarship. In addition, the romanization system used in prewar Japanese (the Hepburn system) compounds the difficulty. Table A.1 shows all three romanizations for place names.

TABLE A.1: Taiwanese Place Names in Three Romanization Systems.

Official Romanization (Wade-Giles)	Pinyin	Prewar Japanese Romanization (Hepburn)
Taipei	Taibei	Taihoku
Yilan	Yilan	Giran
Keelung	Jilong	Kirun
Taoyuan	Taoyun	Tôen
Hsinchu	Xinju	Shinchiku
Miaoli	Maioli	Byoritsu
Taichung	Taizhong	Taichû
Changhua	Zhanghua	Syoka
Nantou	Nantou	Nantô
Yunlin	Yunlin	Unrin
Chiayi	Jiayi	Kagi
Tainan	Tainan	Tainan
Kaohsiung	Gaoxiong	Takao
Pingtong	Pingdong	Byotô
Hualien	Hualian	Karenkô
Taitung	Taidong	Taitô
Penghu	Penghu	Hôko

Appendix B: Changes to the Administrative Divisions in Taiwan Prior to 1945

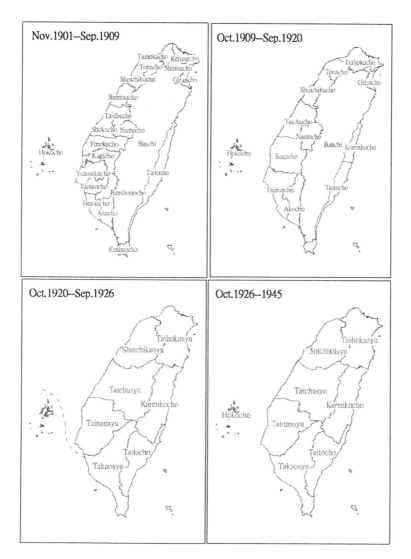

MAP B.1: Administrative boundaries were changed several times during the colonial period. Each change would effect the statistical data collected by local governments. To reduce statistical bias, I rearranged dta prior to 1940 using the 1940 administrative map. All the place names in the context match the boundary of 1940.

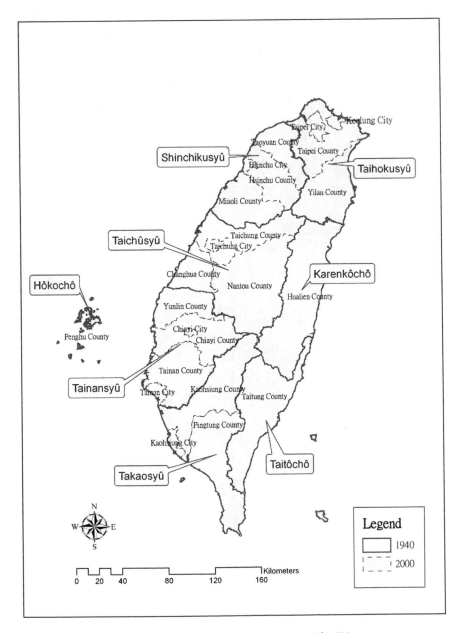

MAP B.2: Detailed map of the administrative divisions in 1940s Taiwan.

Notes

Introduction

[1] For a brief review of Taiwanese history, see Fang Hao, *Taiwan zaoqi shigang* (The Historical Outline of Early Taiwanese history) (Taipei: Taiwan xuesheng shuju, 1994).

[2] Jonathan Clements, *Pirate King: Coxinga and the Fall of the Ming Dynasty* (London: Muramasa Industries, 2004).

[3] Seiji Hishida, "Formosa: Japan's First Colony," *Political Science Quarterly* 22:2 (1907): 267.

[4] For the latest discussion of living standards in colonial Taiwan, see Stephen Morgan and Liu Shiyung, "Was Japanese Colonialism Good for the Welfare of Taiwanese?" *China Quarterly* 192 (2007): 990–1017.

[5] For more details, see Patricia E. Tsurumi, *Japanese Colonial Education in Taiwan, 1895–1945* (Cambridge: Harvard University Press, 1977); and Wu Wen-hsing et al., *Rizhi shiqi Taiwan gonggxuexiao yu guominxuexiao guoyu duben* (National Language Textbook Readers in the Taiwan Common and National Schools under Japanese Colonial Rule) (Taipei: Nantian, 2003).

[6] Seiji Hishida, "Formosa," 271.

[7] Ibid., 270–71.

[8] Ibid., 274.

[9] The concept of "model colony" appeared very early and seemed to be a main theme of Japanese colonization. See Takekoshi Yasaburo, *Japanese Rule in Formosa* (London: Longmans and Green, 1907).

[10] Cheng Jiahui, *Taiwan shishang diyida bolanhui: 1935 nian Taiwan meili show* (The Biggest Exhibition in Taiwanese History: An Appealing Exposition of Taiwan in 1935) (Taipei: Yunliu, 2004).

[11] Angela Leung, "Diseases of the Premodern Period in China," in Kenneth F. Kiple, ed., *The Cambridge World History of Human Disease* (Cambridge: Cambridge University Press, 1993), 355.

[12] Liu Ts'ui-jung and Liu Shi-yung, "Disease and Mortality in the History of Taiwan," *Taiwanshi yenjiu* (Taiwan Historical Research) 4:2 (1998): 90–132.

[13] Ibid., 92–106.

[14] Edward House, *Japanese Expedition to Formosa* (Tokyo: N.p., 1875), 53.

[15] George Mackay, *From Far Formosa: The Island, Its People, and Missions* (New York: F. H. Revell, 1896), 308–14.

[16] Chen Shaoxin, "Taiwan renkoushi de jige wenti" (Several Questions about Taiwanese Demographic History), in Chen Shaoxin, *Taiwan de renkou bianqian yu shehui bianqian* (Population and Social Changes in Taiwan) (Taipei: Lianjin, 1985), 19–21.

[17] Taiwansheng xingzheng zhangquang gongshu, ed., *Taiwansheng wushiyinianlai tongjitiyao* (A Statistical Summary of Taiwan over the Past Fifty-one Years) (Taipei: Taiwansheng xingzheng zhangquang gongshu, 1946), 1202.

[18] Chen Shaoxin, "Taiwan renkoushi de jige wenti," 101–3.

[19] Ibid., 89–91.

[20] The correlation coefficient between the aborigines and the Japanese is 0.501 while the coefficients are 0.042 for the Taiwanese and 0.005 for the Chinese.

[21] For studies of colonial medicine in British India, see David Arnold, "Medical Priorities and Practice in Nineteenth-Century British India," *South Asia Research* Vol. 5. No. 2 (1985): John Hume, "Colonialism and Sanitary Medicine: The Development of Preventive Health Policy in the Punjab, 1860 to 1900," *Modern Asian Studies* 20:4 (1986): 703 –24; and Mark Harrison, *Public Health in British India: Anglo-Indian Preventive Medicine, 1859–1914* (Cambridge: Cambridge University Press, 1994).

[22] Saurabh Dube, "Introduction," in Saurabh Dube, Ishita Banerjee Dube, and Edgardo Lander, eds., *Critical Conjunctions: Foundations of Colonialism and Formations of Modernity* (Durham: Duke University Press, 2002), 1–15.

[23] Daniel R. Headrick, *The Tools of Empire: Technology and European Imperialism in the Nineteenth Century* (Oxford: Oxford University Press, 1981).

[24] Ibid., 73.

[25] David Arnold, "Introduction," in David Arnold, ed., *Imperial Medicine and Indigenous Societies* (Manchester: Manchester University Press, 1988), 10–11.

[26] David Arnold, *Colonizing the Body: State Medicine and Epidemic Disease in Nineteenth-Century India* (Berkeley: University of California Press, 1993).

[27] For a detailed discussion, see ibid. or a review of the book, Li Shang-jen, "Review of David Arnold, *Colonizing the Body: State Medicine and Epidemic Disease in Nineteenth-Century India*," *Xinshixue* (New History) 10:4 (1999): 159–67.

[28] Philip D. Curtin, *Death by Migration: Europe's Encounter with the Tropical World in the Nineteenth Century* (Cambridge: Cambridge University Press, 1989).

[29] Nemata Blyden, "Review of David Eltis, ed., *Coerced and Free Migration: Global Perspectives (The Making of Modern Freedom.), American Historical Review* 109:1 (2004): 143.

[30] Ramon Myers and Mark Peattie, eds., *The Japanese Colonial Empire, 1895–1945* (Princeton: Princeton University Press, 1984), 4–14.

[31] Arthur Caplan, "Editorial: Misusing the Nazi Analogy," *Science* No. 22, Vol. 309, No. 5374 (2005): 535.

[32] Although the materials are often scattered, John Bowers has shown the importance of German medicine in Japan's medical westernization. See John Bower, "German Medicine," in *When the Twain Meet: The Rise of Western Medicine in Japan* (Baltimore: Johns Hopkins University Press, 1980), 58–61.

[33] Zhuang Yunmin once called this condition à la mode. See Guo Wenhua and Ye Lin, "Yixue yu renwen lishi de jiaohui: Fang Zhuang Yunmin tan Taiwan yixueshi" (The Interaction between Medicine and Humanity: An Interview with Zhuang Yunmin on Taiwan's Medical History), *Yiwang* (Hope) No. 8 (1995): 20.

[34] Ôda Toshirô, *Taiwan igaku goûnen* (The Fifty-Year History of Taiwanese Medicine), was published in 1974 and translated into Chinese by Hong Youshi (Taipei: Qianwei, 1995).

[35] Maruyama Yoshito was born in 1885 in Japan. After 1910, he held several positions in Taiwan, including researcher and teacher at the Taihoku Medical School. He taught at National Taiwan University until his repatriation in 1947. His book on public health achievements in Japanese-ruled Taiwan has had a great impact on the study of Taiwan's colonial history. See Wu Wenxing, "Maruyama Yoshito," in Xu Xueji, ed., *Taiwan lishi cidian* (Dictionary of Taiwanese History) (Taipei: Yuanliu, 2004), 75; and Ôda Toshirô, *Taiwan igaku gojûnen*, 1–11.

[36] For example, see Ôda Toshirô, "Nijin no Sawada meiyo kyôju o omou" (Thinking about Two Sawaga Professors), *Ninhon ishi shinpo*, January 8, 1983; and "Nagai Hisomu sensei no hagaki" (The Career of Master Nagai Hisomu), *Nippon ishi shinpo*, July 4, 1984.

[37] Ôda Toshirô, *Taiwan igaku gojûnen*, 62.

[38] For an account of Du's career, see Yang Yuling, *Yidai Yijen Du Congming* (A Doctor Represents a Whole Generation: Du Congming) (Taipei: Tienxia, 2002).

[39] Du Congming, *Zhongxi yixueshilüe* (A Brief History of Chinese and Western Medicine) (Kaohsiung: Kaohsiung Medical College, 1959), 486–505.

[40] As Basalla amplifies, modern science, including medicine it seems, diffused from a "Western core" and pooled on the "non-Western periphery" where the ground was ready to receive it. See George W. Basalla, "The Spread of Western Science: A Three-

Stage Model Describes the Introduction of Modern Science into Any Non-European Nation," *Science* No. 5, Vol. 156, No. 3775 (1967): 611–22.

[41] "During 'phase 1' the nonscientific society or nation provides a source for European science. . . . 'Phase 2' is marked by a period of colonial science, and 'phase 3' completes the process of transplantation with a struggle to achieve an independent scientific tradition (or culture)." Ibid., 611.

[42] Yang Yuling, *Yidai yiren Du Congming*, 156–57.

[43] Du Congming, *Zhongxi yixueshilüe*, 275.

[44] Ibid., 274.

[45] Ibid., 497.

[46] Although the terms *zhimin* (colonization) and *diguozhuyi* (imperialism) make clear Li's feelings about the Japanese, his works as a whole lack any direct argument about social reactions to or political comments on the medical reforms enacted by the Japanese. See Li Tengyue, "Zhengshizhi weishengpian" (Public Health Section of the Administration Volume), in Taiwan sheng wenxianweiyuanhui, *Taiwansheng tongzhigao* (Manuscript of the Taiwan Gazette), vol. 3 (Nantao: Taiwansheng wenxianweiyuanhui, 1953).

[47] Most of the scholars in the field of medical history in colonial Taiwan are young. Two phenomena explain this situation. First, the new wave of Taiwanese studies is the result of political liberalization after 1987, and, second, the field of medical history did not receive much attention until 2002.

[48] Xie Zhenrong, "Ribenzhiminzhuyixia Taiwanweishengzhengce zhiyanjiu" (The Study of Public Health Policy in Taiwan under Japanese Colonialism), MA thesis, Chinese Culture University, 1989.

[49] Chen Shufen, *Zhanhou zhiyi: Taiwande gonggongweisheng wenti yu jianzhi* (Postwar Epidemics: Problems and Formations of Public Health in Taiwan) (Taipei: Daoxiang, 2000), 6, n. 7.

[50] Guo Wenhua, "Taiwan yiliaoshi yanjiu de huigu: Yi xueshu mailuo weizhungxin de tantao" (A Review of Studies on Taiwan's Medical History: A Discussion Centered on the Thread of Academic Thought), *Taiwan shiliao yanjiu* (Studies of Taiwanese Historical Materials) 8 (1996): 62.

[51] Yao Rendo, "Making the Colonized Population Healthy," paper presented at the Workshop on Colonial Modernity and Body Formation, March, 22, 2003, Department of Sociology, Donghai University. For a detailed discussion, see Yao Rendo, "Governing the Colonised: Governmentality in the Japanese Colonisation of Taiwan, 1895–1945," PhD diss., University of Essex, 2002.

[52] Fan Yanqiu, "Rijuqianqi Taiwanzhi gonggongweisheng: Yi fangyi weizhongxin zhi yanjiu" (Public Health Policy during the Early Period of Japanese Occupation: A Study Focusing on Epidemic Prevention), MA thesis, National Taiwan Normal University, 1994.

[53] Fan Yanqiu, "Xinyixue zai Taiwan de shijian" (The Practice of New Medicine in Taiwan), *Xinshixue* 9:3 (1998): 49–86.

[54] Fan Yanqiu, "Redai fengtuxunhua, riben diguoyixue yu zhimindi renzhuanglun" (Tropical Acclimatization, Japanese Imperial Medicine, and Racial Discourses in the Colony), *Taiwan shehui yenjui jikan* (Radical Quarterly of Social Studies), 57 (2005): 87–132.

[55] For a case of coercive surveillance by the state for biological reasons, see Fan Yanqiu, "Rijuqianqi Taiwanzhi gonggongweisheng," 44, 83.

[56] Fan Yanqiu, "Ribendiguo fazhanxia zhimindi Taiwan de renzhuangweisheng" (Racial Hygiene in Colonial Taiwan under the Japanese Empire), PhD diss., Zhengzhi University, 2001. Fan later changed the title and published the dissertation, without major revisions, as Fan Yanqiu, *Yibing, Yixue yu Zhiming Xiandaixing: Rizhi Taiwan yixueshi* (Epidemics, Medicine, and Colonial Modernity: History of Medicine in Japan-ruled Taiwan) (Taipei: Daoxiang, 2005).

[57] If the term *Renzhung weisheng* is as Fan defines it, it would be interesting to know how the Japanese understood the German term *Rassenhygiene* and developed such different features.

[58] For one case, see Fan Yanqiu, "Ribendiguo fazhanxia zhimindi Taiwan de renzhuangweisheng," 267–69.

[59] Miriam Ming-cheng Lo, *Doctors within Borders: Profession, Ethnicity, and Modernity in Colonial Taiwan* (Berkeley: University of California Press, 2002).

[60] Ibid., 199–200.

[61] Ibid., 94.

[62] Li Shang-ren, "Yixue, diguozhuyi yu xiandaixing daodu" (Medicine, Imperialism, and Modernity: An Introduction), *Taiwan shehui yenjiu jikan* 54 (2004): 10–11, 13–14.

[63] Liu Shiyung, "Building a Strong and Healthy Empire: The Critical Period of Building Colonial Medicine in Taiwan," *Japanese Studies* 23:4 (2004): 306.

[64] Takagi Tomoe, "Reitai shokumin ni seiko noin" (On the Success of Tropical Colonization), in Nihon gôdôtsû shinsha, ed., *Taiwan taikan* (Overview of Taiwan) (Taihoku: Nihon gôdôtsû shinsha, 1932), 237–43.

[65] The concept of German *"Staatsmedizin"* had been understood by the Japanese as the process of applying medical knowledge to the building of a strong state. The Japanization of German *"Staatsmedizin"* was complex and essential to colonial medicine in Taiwan.

Chapter 1

[1] Jo Hays, *The Burdens of Disease: Epidemics and Human Response in Western History* (New Brunswick, NJ: Rutgers University Press, 1998), 182–87.

[2] Paolo Palladino and Michael Worboys take a diffusionist view, suggesting that "Western methods and knowledge were not accepted passively, but were adapted and selectively absorbed in relation to existing traditions of natural knowledge and religion and other factors." Paolo Palladino and Michael Worboys, "Science and Imperialism," *Isis* 84 (1993): 99–100.

[3] George Rosen, *A History of Public Health* (Baltimore: Johns Hopkins University Press, 1993), 223–35.

[4] By "medical reform," I mean the introduction of new ideas, methods, education, and technologies to make medical and public health services more reliable. Medical reform was an aspect of Otto von Bismarck's modernization program in Germany. A similar process in Meiji Japan would be called westernization but could also be called modernization.

[5] Claudia Huerkamp, "The History of Smallpox Vaccination in Germany: A First Step in the Medicalization of the General Public," *Journal of Contemporary History* 20 (1985): 617–35.

[6] An important collection of articles on the history and philosophy of laboratory techniques can be found in Andrew Cunningham and Perry Williams, eds., *The Laboratory Revolution in Medicine* (Cambridge: Cambridge University Press, 1992). In that book, Nicholas Jardine claims that even in 1900, when "the laboratory revolution was effectively accomplished, the roster of acknowledged practical pay-offs attributed to laboratory researches remained sparse in diagnostics and prognostics, and yet sparser in therapeutics." He also believes that laboratories were "seen to be essential years before doing anything of value for medicine." Nicholas Jardine, "Rhetorical and Aesthetic Accomplishment," in Cunningham and Williams, *The Laboratory Revolution in Medicine*, 306. Bruno Latour suggests looking for the answer in the relationship between politics and laboratory techniques. Bruno Latour, "The Costly Ghastly Kitchen," in Cunningham and Williams, *The Laboratory Revolution in Medicine*, 207, 297.

[7] Fielding Garrison, *History of Medicine* (Philadelphia: Saunders, 1960), 853–54.

[8] On state medical police, see Thomas Broman, "Rethinking Professionalization: Theory, Practice, and Professional Ideology in Eighteenth-Century German Medicine," *Journal of Modern History* 67:4 (1995): 835–72.

[9] George Rosen, "Cameralism and the Concept of Medical Police," in George Rosen, ed., *From Medical Police to Social Medicine: Essays on the History of Health Care* (New York: Science History Publications, 1974), 120–58. Cameralism was the specific form of mercantilism in Germany practiced by men usually closely connected to the bureaucracies of the German states. Cameralist science included fiscal and economic policy, legislation, administration, and public finance, and its aim was to provide methods for the efficient administration of a large population and a well-filled treasury for its noble rulers. For details, see Albion W. Small, "Some Contributions to the History of Sociology, Section 8: Approaches to Objective Economic and Political Science in Germany—Cameralism," *American Journal of Sociology* 29:2 (1923):158–65.

[10] Paul Weindling, "Medicine and Modernisation: The Social History of German Health and Medicine," *History of Science* 24 (1986): 277–301.

[11] Paul Weindling, *Health, Race, and German Politics between National Unification and Nazism, 1870–1945* (Cambridge: Cambridge University Press, 1989), 21 201.

[12] Henry Ernest Sigerist and Milton Roemer eds., *On the History of Medicine* (New York: MD Publications, 1960), 27.

[13] Han G. Schlumberger, "Rudolph Virchow, Revolutionist," *Annals of Medical History*, 3rd ser., 4 (1942): 153.

[14] Weindling, "Medicine and Modernization," 277–301.

[15] Rosen, *A History of Public Health*, 225.

[16] Stephan L. Chorover, *From Genesis to Genocide: The Meaning of Human Nature and the Power of Behavior Control* (Cambridge: MIT Press, 1979), 78.

[17] Erwin H. Ackerknecht, *Rudolf Virchow: Doctor, Statesman, and Anthropologist* (Madison: University of Wisconsin Press, 1953), 125–28.

[18] Roy Porter, *The Greatest Benefit to Mankind: A Medical History of Humanity from Antiquity to the Present* (London: Fontana, 1997), 643, 682–83.

[19] Anne Harrington, *Re-enchanted Science: Holism in German Culture from Wilhelm II to Hitler* (Princeton: Princeton University Press, 1996), 19–20.

[20] Peter E. Baldry, *The Battle against Bacteria: A History of the Development of Antibacterial Drugs for the General Reader* (Cambridge: Cambridge University Press, 1965), 48–49.

[21] For descriptions of how to identify these microorganisms, See Kenneth F. Kiple, ed., *The Cambridge World History of Human Disease* (Cambridge: Cambridge University Press, 1993), 19.

[22] Paul Weindling, "Scientific Elites and Laboratory Organization in Fin de Siècle Paris and Berlin: The Pasteur Institute and Robert Koch's Institute for Infectious Disease Compared," in Cunningham and Williams, *The Laboratory Revolution in Medicine*, 178.

[23] Sheila Faith Weiss, *Race Hygiene and National Efficiency* (Berkeley: University of California Press, 1987), 17.

[24] Andrew Cunningham and Perry Williams, "Introduction," in Cunningham and Williams, *The Laboratory Revolution in Medicine*, 10.

[25] Weindling, "Scientific Elites and Laboratory Organization," 188.

[26] Ibid.

[27] For a brief review of Grotjahn's career and his impact on German medicine, see Paul Weindling, "Soziale hygiene und eugenik: Der fall Alfred Grotjahn" (Social Hygiene and Eugenics: The Case of Alfred Grotjahn), *Das Argument: Jahrbuch fur kritische Medizin* (Argument: The Annual of Critical Medicine) (1984): 6–20; and Klemens Dieckhofer and Kaspari Christoph, "Die Tatigkeit des Sozialhygienikers und Eugenikers Alfred Grotjahn (1869–1931) als Reichstagsabgeordneter der SPD" (The Works of Social Hygienist and Eugenicist Alfred Grotjahn [1869–1913] as a Parliamentary Delegate of the SPD), *Medizinhistorische Journal* (Journal of Medical History) 21 (1986): 308–31.

[28] Dorothy Porter and Roy Porter, "What Was Social Medicine? An Historiographical Essay," *Journal of Historical Sociology* 1:1 (1988): 95, 102.

[29] George Rosen, "What Is Social Medicine? A Genetic Analysis of the Concept," *Bulletin of the History of Medicine*, 21 (1947): 674–733.

[30] For more information, see Werner Doeleke, *Alfred Ploetz, 1860–1940: Sozialdrwinist und Gesellschaftsbiologe* (Frankfurt am Main: Doeleke, 1975).

[31] Benno Müller-Hill, *Murderous Science: Elimination by Scientific Selection of Jews, Gypsies, and Others—Germany, 1933–1945* (Oxford: Oxford University Press, 1988), 10.

[32] Ibid.

[33] Weiss, *Race Hygiene, and National Efficiency*, 245.

[34] Rosen, "What Is Social Medicine?" "713. There are many studies of social hygiene in Germany and its relationship to eugenics. Also see Weindling, "Medicine and Modernization in Germany," 277–301.

[35] Harrington, *Re-enchanted Science*, 704.

[36] Roy Porter, "The Doctor and the World," *Medical Sociology News* 9 (1978): 21–28.

[37] Robert Gellately, "Medicine and Collaboration under Hitler," *Canadian Journal of History* 26:3 (1991): 479–85.

[38] Porter and Porter, "What Was Social Medicine?" 102.

[39] Weiss, *Race Hygiene, and National Efficiency*, 19.

[40] For a review of the history of health care in England and the United States, see Elizabeth Fee and Dorothy Porter, "Public Health, Preventive Medicine, and Professionalization: England and America in the Nineteenth Century," in Andrew Wear, ed., *Medicine in Society: Historical Essays* (Cambridge: Cambridge University Press, 1992), 67–83. The details of German medical development can be found in George Rosen, *A History of Public Health* (Baltimore: Johns Hopkins University Press, 1993), 137–43; and a brief review of Japan by James R. Bartholomew, *The Formation of Science in Japan: Building a Research Tradition* (New Haven: Yale University Press, 1989), 4–5, 265–66.

[41] Naimushô Eiseikyoku, ed., *Isei gojônen shi* (The Fifty-Year History of the Medical System) (Tokyo: Obunkai, 1925), 6–14. See also Bartholomew, *The Formation of Science in Japan*, 27–31.

[42] Bartholomew, *The Formation of Science in Japan*, 40.

[43] For the description of Western medicine in the Tokugawa period, see ibid., 27–31.

[44] The *bakuhan taisei* was the Japanese feudal political system in the Edo period (1603–1867). *Baku*, or "tent," is an abbreviation of *bakufu*, meaning "military government," that is, the shogunate. The *han* were the domains headed by daimyo. Vassals held inherited lands and provided military service and homage to their lords. For further reading, see James McClain, *Japan: A Modern History* (New York: Norton, 2002); and John Bowers, *When the Twain Meet: The Rise of Western Medicine in Japan* (Baltimore: Johns Hopkins University Press, 1980), 157.

[45] For a detailed discussion, see Donald Keene, *The Japanese Discovery of Europe* (Stanford: Stanford University Press, 1969), 10, 19–29, 101–3.

[46] Ibid., 126–27.

[47] A good overview of the introduction of Western medicine to Japan can be found in E. Kraas and Y. Hiki, eds., *300 Jahre deutsch-japanische Beziehungen in der Medizin* (Three Hundred Years of German-Japanese Relations in Medicine) (Tokyo: Springer-Verlag, 1992), 17–18.

[48] Masao Takenaka, *The Development of Social, Educational, and Medical Work in Japan since Meiji* (Brussels: Uitgeverij Van Keulen, 1958), 39.

[49] Bartholomew, *The Formation of Science in Japan*, 44–45.

[50] McClain, *Japan*, chap. 5, 155–82.

[51] For some cases, see Koizumi Iejiô, *Nihon kanbô iyaku hansenshi* (The History of Chinese Medicine in Taiwan) (Tokyo: Nankôdô, 1934), 142–62. In fact, the samurai constituted the majority of the Meiji scientific community. Bartholomew, *The Formation of Science in Japan*, 265.

[52] John Whitney Hall, "The Confucian Teacher in Tokugawa Japan," in David S. Nivison and Arthur R. Wright, eds., *Confucianism in Action* (Stanford: Stanford University Press, 1959), 291.

[53] On the relationship between mentors and pupils, see Bartholomew, *The Formation of Science in Japan*, 265.

[54] The number is calculated from Kurô Iseki, *Hihan enkyû hakushi jinbutu igakuhen* (Comments on and Studies of People with Doctoral Titles: The Medical Professionals) (Tokyo: Hattensha, 1925).

[55] Ibid., 16.

[56] Ann B. Jannetta and Samuel H. Preston, "Two Centuries of Mortality Change in Central Japan: The Evidence from a Temple Death Register," *Population Studies* Vol. 45. No. 3 (1991): 417–36.

[57] Naimushô Eiseikyoku, *Isei gojûnen shi*, 7–8.

[58] For a brief description of British medicine in early Meiji Japan, see Hugh Cortazzi, *Dr. Willis in Japan, 1862–1877: British Medical Pioneer* (London: Athlone, 1985).

[59] William Johnston, *The Modern Epidemic: A History of Tuberculosis in Japan* (Cambridge: Council on East Asian Studies, Harvard University, 1995), 170.

[60] Ralf Dahrendorf, *Society and Democracy in Germany* (New York: Anchor, 1969), 33.

[61] In the Japanese feudal system, The Lord of Choshu *han* occupied the region of Yamaguchi Prefecture after being defeated by Tokugawa Ieyasu in 1866. For that reason, they became the most determined enemy of the Edo shogunate and took the lead in the movement to overthrow the Tokugawa government during Meiji revolution. For details, see Albert M. Craig, *Choshu in the Meiji Restoration* (Lanham, MD: Lexington, 2000).

[62] Roger F. Hackett, *Yamagata Aritomo in the Rise of Modern Japan, 1838–1922* (Cambridge: Harvard University Press, 1972), 52–58.

[63] Ernest L. Presseisen, *Before Aggression: Europeans Prepare the Japanese Army* (Tucson: University of Arizona Press, 1965), 9.

[64] Ardath W. Burk, *The Modernizers: Overseas Students, Foreign Employees, and Meiji-Japan* (New York: Boulder, 1985), 213.

[65] For more on his career, see Erwin Baelz, *Awaken Japan: The Diary of a German Doctor, Erwin Baelz*, ed. Toku Baelz, trans. Eden Paul and Cedar Paul (New York: Viking, 1932).

[66] Sukehirô Hirakawa, "Changing Japanese Attitudes toward Western Learning: Dr. Erwin Baelz and Mori Ogai," *Contemporary Japan* 29 (1968): 138–57.

[67] Ninomi Fujiaki, "Meiji zenhanki oshui rugakusei ni tsuite" (On Overseas Students in the First Half of the Meiji Period), *Nihon ishigaku zasshi* (Japanese Journal of Medical History) 33:4 (1987): 60.

[68] Takeshi Okada, *Densenbyô kenkyûsho* (The Institute of Infectious Disease) (Tokyo: Sakai shuban senta, 1992), 1–60, 72–83.

[69] Martin Bernd, *Japan and Germany in the Modern World* (Oxford: Berghahn, 1995), 44.

[70] Kenneth B. Pyle, "Advantages of Fellowship: German Economics and Japanese Bureaucrats, 1890–1925," *Journal of Japanese Studies* 1:1 (1974): 127–64.

[71] Miora Seikô, "Gotô Shinpei shoron: Nagoya ikanjidai kara eiseikyoku made no sokubakukento" (A brief bibliography of Gotô Shinpei: From a Medical Officer in Nagoya to the Chief Deputy of the Central Bureau of Sanitation), *Ritsumeikanhôgakû* (Studies in the Law of Ritsumeikan) 3 (1980): 723–51.

[72] Sabine Fruhstuck, *Colonizing Sex: Sexology and Sex Control in Modern Japan* (Berkeley: University of California Press, 2003), 22.

[73] Dokutoru Berutsu [Erwin Baelz], "Nippon jinsho kairyôron" (On the Improvement of the Japanese Race), *Dainipon shiritsu eiseikai zasshi* (Journal of the Japanese Private Society of Hygiene) 43 (1886): 3–26.

[74] On Japanese modifications of German medicine, see Fujikawa Yu, *Nihon ikkagu shi* (Japan's Medical History) (Tokyo: Nishin, 1941), 730–33; or a brief description in Fan Yanqiu, *Yibing, Yixue yu Zhiming Xiandaixing* (Epidemics, Medicine, and Colonial Modernity) (Taipei: Daoxiang, 2005), 67.

[75] William Johnston, "Disease, Medicine, and the State: A Social History of Tuberculosis in Japan, 1850–1950," PhD diss., Harvard University, 1987, 234–52.

[76] William W. Farris, *Population, Disease, and Land in Early Japan, 645–900* (Cambridge: Harvard University Press, 1985), 52.

[77] Keishicho, ed., *Keishichoshi* (History of the Police Force) (Tokyo: Keishichoshi hensan iinkai, 1949), 10, 344.

[78] Bernd, *Japan and Germany in the Modern World*, 37, 67, n. 108.

[79] Kure Shosan, "Daiikan/ishikaku hen" (Medicine Section of the First Volume), in Kure Shosan, *Kure Shosan zanshô* (Bibliography of Kure Shosan) (Kyoto: Shibunkaku, 1982), 271–92.

[80] Johnston, "Disease, Medicine, and the State," 234–52.

[81] Takizawa Toshiyuki, "Meiji shoki ishiyosei kyôiku to eisekan" (Related Medical Affairs and Medical Officers in the Early Meiji Period), *Nihon ishigaku zasshi* 38:4 (1991): 45–64.

[82] Takeshi Okada, "Naimusho shokan densenbyô kenkyûsho" (The Institute of Infectious Disease under the Ministry of Home Affairs), *Nihon ishigaku zasshi* 35:4 (1989): 1–35.

[83] Tokyo daigaku ikagaku kenkyûjyo (Institute of Medical Science), ed., *Densenbyô kenkyûsho ikagaku kenkyûsho hyakunen no ayumi* (The One Hundred Years from the Institute of Infectious Disease to the Institute of Medical Science) (Tokyo: University of Tokyo Press, 1992), 1–20.

[84] Marius Jansen, "The Nineteenth Century," in Marius Jansen, ed., *The Cambridge History of Japan* (Cambridge: Cambridge University Press, 1989), 5:754.

[85] For the definition of a university medical graduate, see Koseisho, ed., *Iseihyakunenshi* (The Hundred-Year History of the Medical Regulations) (Tokyo: Koseishoimukyoku, 1976), 102.

[86] Literally, *senmongakkô* means "special school"; in postwar Japan these were often referred to as "colleges." My translation follows that of Herbert Passin in *Society and Education in Japan* (Tokyo: Teachers College Press, 1965), 105.

[87] Koseisho, *Iseihyakunenshi*, 45–47.

[88] Ozeki Tsuneo ed., *Meiji-shoki Tokyodaigaku igakubu sugyosei dosei ichiran* (A Statistical Summary of the Graduates of Tokyo University in the Early Meiji Period), (Tokyo: University of Tokyo Press, 1991).

[89] Japanese doctors are divided into employed hospital doctors, *kinmui*, and self-employed local doctors, *kaigyôi*.

[90] The term *social hygiene* was also used by John D. Rockefeller Jr., in 1913, as a result of his service in the Bureau of Social Hygiene in New York City. The meaning of *social hygiene* in the United States was "the study, amelioration, and prevention of those social conditions, crimes, and diseases which adversely affect the well being

of society, with special reference to prostitution and the evils associated therewith."
John Enson Harr and Peter J. Johnson. *The Rockefeller Century: Three Generations of America's Greatest Family.* (NY: Charles Scribner's Sons, 1988) pp.191. For details see *The Bureau of Social Hygiene Archives, 1911–1940,* at the Rockefeller Archive Center in New York. The application of American social hygiene in today's public health is discussed in K. K. Lo, L. Y. Chong, and Y. M. Tang, eds., *Social Hygiene Handbook* (Hong Kong: Social Hygiene Service, Department of Health, 1994).

[91] Nakano Misao, "Meiji shoki no eiseigaku" (Hygienic Studies in the Early Meiji Period), *Nihon Ishigaku zasshi* 5:1 (1954): 31–32.

[92] Izumi Hyonosuke, "Eiseigakusha Tsuboi Jirô no keireki to gyuseki" (The Career and Studies of the Hygienist Tsuboi Jirô), *Nihon ishigaku zasshi* 36:3 (1993): 3–33.

[93] Ibid., 13–16.

[94] Takizawa Toshiyuki, "Kindai Nihon ni okeru shakaieiseigaku riron" (A Brief Discussion of Social Hygiene in Modern Japan), *Nihon ishigaku zasshi* 39:1 (1995): 111.

[95] Takizawa Toshiyuki, "Kindai Nihon ni okeru shakaieiseigaku no tankai to sonotokushitsu" (Concepts behind Social Hygiene in Modern Japan),*Nihon ishigaku zasshi* 40:2 (1994): 7–9.

[96] Hoshino Tetsuo, *Kenkozoshin no tame no chishiki* (Knowledge to Improve Health) (Tokyo: Eiseibunka shisôkai, 1929), 73–74.

[97] Nakano Misao, "Meiji shoki no eiseigaku," 38–39.

[98] Kawakami Take and Agarihayashi Shigerû, *Kunisaki Tetdô* (Tokyo: Kubisoshobo, 1970), 279–87.

[99] Fujikawa Yû, "Eiseigaku ni ukeru jinruigakuno hidobi sakainoshiso" (Social Thoughts about the Evolution of Hygienic Studies), *Dai Nippon eisei shiryo zasshi* (Great Japan Journal of Hygienic Materials) 309 (1909): 6–9.

[100] Carmen Blacker, *The Japanese Enlightenment: A Study of the Writing of Fukuzawa Yukichi* (London: Cambridge University Press, 1964), 111–28.

[101] Naimusho Eiseikyoku, *Isei gojûnen shi,* 43–45, 233–42.

[102] George Fredrickson, *Racism: A Short History* (Princeton: Princeton University Press, 2002), 10.

[103] Suzuki Zenji, *Nihon no yûseigaku: Sono shisô to undôno kiseki* (Eugenics in Japan: Paths of Thought and Activities) (Tokyo: Sankyô shuppan, 1983), 155–57.

[104] Ibid., 28–30.

[105] The separation of prescribing and dispensing is common in many Western countries but was not enforced until the 1970s in Japan and the 1990s in Taiwan. For a brief discussion, see Hayase Yukitoshi, "Problems of the Separation of Prescription and Dispensing," *Yakugaku zasshi* 123:3 (2003): 121–32.

[106] Miwao Sôkô, "Iryô seido no rekishi deki haikei" (The Historical Background of Medical Service), in Kawakami On and Nakagawa Yurezô, eds., *Iryô seido* (The Medical Service System) (Tokyo: Nihon hyôlon sha, 1974), 42.

[107] Onda Shigenobu, *Obeiyakuseichushaku* (Notes on the Pharmaceutical System in Europe and America) (Tokyo: Tokyoinsatsukabushikigaisha, 1922), 1.

[108] "Regulation 41," in Koseisho, *Iseihyakunenshi*, 133–34.

[109] Koseisho, *Iseihyakunenshi*, 257.

[110] Shimada Akiseki, *Shindan shorei fuiji horei* (Cases of Diagnosis with Related Regulations) (Tokyo: Nankodo, 1916), 319.

[111] Nainmusho, ed., *Eiseikyoku Nenpo* (Annual Report of the Ministry of Home Affairs), 1913 (Tokyo: Nainmusho, 1914); Monbusho, ed., *Monbusho Nenpo* (Annual Reports of the Ministry of Education), 1913–14 (Tokyo, Monbusho 1914–15).

[112] Brian Abel-Smith, "Foreword," in Frank Honigsbaum, *The Division in British Medicine: A History of the Separation of General Practice from Hospital Care, 1911–1968* (London: Kegan Paul, 1979), xiv.

[113] K. Yamakawa, "A History of a Hundred Years of Pharmaceutical Education in Japan," *Yakushigaku zasshi* (Japanese Journal of the History of Pharmacy) 29:3 (1994): 446–51.

[114] K. Yamakawa, "Historical Sketch of Modern Pharmaceutical Science and Technology, Part 3: From the Second Half of the Nineteenth Century to World War I"), *Yakushigaku zasshi* 30:1 (1995): 1–10.

[115] Yamakawa, "A History of a Hundred Years of Pharmaceutical Education in Japan," 452–62.

[116] Yamakawa, "Historical Sketch of Modern Pharmaceutical Science and Technology," 1–10.

[117] Onda Shigenobu, *Obeiyakuseichushaku*, 40–41.

[118] H. Yamada, "The Development of the Modern Japanese Pharmaceutical Industry, Part 3: From 1886 to 1906, Coinciding with the Era between the Institution and Issue of the *Japanese Pharmacopoeia*, First Edition with Third Edition (JP I–JP III)," *Yakushigaku zasshi* 27:2 (1992): 83–89.

[119] M. C. Balfour, "Letter no. 109, M. C. Balfour to Dr. W. A. Sawyer (N.Y.), 5/21/1940," R.G. 1.1, series 609, Japan, box 3, folder 17, Rockefeller Archives.

[120] Ruth Rogaski, *Hygienic Modernity: Meanings of Health and Disease in Treaty-Port China* (Berkeley: University of California Press, 2004), 15.

[121] Nagayo Sansai, *Shôkô shishi* (Pine Fragrance Memoirs), reprint (Tokyo: Tokyo University Press, 1985), 65–66.

[122] The original context is in René Sand, *Vers la médecine* (Toward Medicine) (Paris: Bailliere, 1948), 573.

[123] Porter and Porter, "What Was Social Medicine?" 91.

[124] Sand, *Vers la médecine*, 227–311.

[125] Iguchi Jowakai, *Toshi eisei to sono kyôka* (City Hygiene and Its Education) (Tokyo: Chuô kyôka, 1936).

[126] See Teruoka Gitô ed., *Shakai eiseigaku* (The Study of Social Hygiene) (Tokyo: Iwanami shoten, 1935); and Porter and Porter, "What Was Social Medicine?" 91, 95–96.

[127] Kohinuma Bôgô, *Eisei gaku* (The Study of Hygiene) (Tokyo: Kinbara, 1937), 3–4.

[128] Porter and Porter, "What Was Social Medicine?" 95.

[129] It is worth noting that before 1945 the Japanese term *eisei* (hygiene) was much more popular than *ikagu* (medicine) in defining the application of medical knowledge to public affairs.

[130] Rosen, "What Is Social Medicine?" 702.

[131] Kohinuma Bôgô, *Eisei gaku*, 2.

[132] For the leftist movement's promotion of social medicine in Japan, see Kawakami Takeshi and S. Kanbayashi, eds., *Kunisaki Teido, teiko no igakusha* (Kunisaki Teidô as a Medical Scientist of Resistance) (Tokyo: Kieso Shobo, 1970), 122, 131, 181.

[133] Komiya Yoshitaka, "Iryo shakai ka no zengo iijyo" (The Process of Medical Socialization), in T. Kawakami and Y. Komiya, eds., *Iryo shakai ka no dohyo* (The Process of Socializing Medicine) (Tokyo: Keiso Shobo, 1969), 23–33.

[134] Iijima Wataru, *Mararia to teikoku* (Malaria and Empire) (Tokyo: University of Tokyo Press, 2005), 148–49, 165, 187–88.

[135] Quoted in Porter and Porter, "What Was Social Medicine?" 91.

[136] Miyamoto Shinobu, *Shakai Igaku* (Social Medicine) (Tokyo Mikasa, 1936).

[137] Bernd, *Japan and Germany in the Modern World*, 45.

[138] Nakano Misao, "Meiji shoki no eiseigaku," 38.

[139] Nippon minzogu eiseikai (Japanese Society of Racial Hygiene), "Kantogo," *Nihon minzoku eisei gakkaishi* (Journal of the Japanese Society of Racial Hygiene) 1:1 (1930): 1–3.

[140] Robert Proctor, *Racial Hygiene: Medicine under Nazis* (Cambridge: Harvard University Press, 1988), 29.

[141] Ibid., 25.

[142] Ibid., 55–56.

[143] Ogata Norio, *Saikin heno chôsen: Nihon no saikingakushi* (Challenges to Bacteria: The History of Bacteriology in Japan) (Tokyo: Nippon hôsô shuppan kyôka, 1940), 184.

[144] Fan Yanqiu, "Ribendiguo fazhanxia zhimindi Taiwan de renzhuangweisheng" (Racial Hygiene in Colonial Taiwan under the Japanese Empire), PhD diss., Zhengzhi University, 2001, 267–74.

[145] Mark Harrison, *Climates and Constitutions: Health, Race, Environment, and British Imperialism in India, 1600–1850* (New Delhi: Oxford University Press, 1999), 136.

[146] Although modern bacteriology seemed promising to medical professionals, traditional strategies to control diseases and improve the environment in both British and German colonies were very influential. For the example of malarial control, see Jo Hays, *The Burdens of Disease: Epidemics and Human Response in Western History*, 207–9.

[147] David Arnold, *Colonizing the Body: State Medicine and Epidemic Disease in Nineteenth-Century India* (Berkeley: University of California Press, 1993), 246.

Chapter 2

[1] Nakamura Humio, *Mori Ôgai to Meiji kokka* (Mori Ôgai and the Meiji State) (Tokyo: Sanichi shubô, 1992), 124.

[2] For a brief description of the death of Kitashirakawanomiya yoshihisa shinnô, see Cai Jintang, "Beibaichuangong nengjiu qin wang" (Kitashirakawanomiya Yoshihisa shinnô, the Consort Prince Kitashirakawanomiya Yoshihisa), in Xu Xueji, ed., *Taiwan lishi cidian* (Dictionary of Taiwanese History) (Taipei: Yuanliu, 2004), 228.

[3] Ide Kiwata, *Taiwan chisekishi* (The Achievement of Rule in Taiwan) (Taipei: Nantien, [1937] 1997), 29–30.

[4] Lu Shaoli, "Taiwan maiquelun" (The Debate on Selling Out Taiwan), in Xu Xueji, *Taiwan lishi cidian*, 1161.

[5] Seiji Hishida, "Formosa: Japan's First Colony," *Political Science Quarterly* Vol. 22, No. 2, 271.

[6] "Zhengluwan sharen shijian: Mori Ôgai yisheng zuida de beiju" (The Seirogan Killing: The Greatest Tragedy of Mori Ôgai), *Lianhe fukan* (United Daily Supplement), March 26, 2005.

[7] Takagi Tomoe was an *igakushi* (university graduate in medicine) until he passed the examination for *igakuhakushi* (doctoral graduate in medicine) in 1913. Despite the poor quality of training in Japanese medical schools (usually at the level of a vocational high school), the prewar system of medical education was mainly four years of undergraduate training at universities and three years of vocational training at colleges. To obtain a doctoral degree, the applicant had to be recommended by the faculty of the Imperial University and pass an examination administered by the Ministry of Education. For a brief description of the prewar system of medical education in Japan, see Oyamada Katsumi, *Isha wa ikanaru teido made shinyô subekika* (Trusting a Doctor's Reputation) (Tokyo: Tôatô, 1913), 86–96.

[8] For more on Takagi Tomoe's career, see Du Congming, ed., *Takagi Tomoe sensei tsuiokushi* (Collection in Remembrance of Takagi Tomoe) (Tokyo: Takagi Tomoe kinenji iinkai, 1957), 1–3.

[9] For an example, see Itô Ginchirô, *Kike Gotô Shinpei* (An Excellent Figure: Gotô Shinpei) (Taihoku: Kiyomizu shoten, 1944), 3–20. Similar portrayals of Gotô appeared in later biographies.

[10] Chang Lung-chih, "Chonggou zhiminzhe de lishi tuxiang: Houteng Xinping (Gotô Shinpei) yanjiu chuyi" (Reconstruction of the Historical Image of Colonizers: A Preliminary Discussion of Gotô Shinpei), in Cao Yunghe xiansheng pashi shouqing lunwenji pianjiweiyunhui, ed., *Cao Yunghe xiansheng pashi shouqing lunwenji* (Collection Celebrating the Eightieth Birthday of Mr. Cao Yunghe) (Taipei: Lexue, 2001), 123, n. 9.

[11] For instance, Gotô's great-grandfather, Takano Chôei (1804–50), was a famous *rangakusha* (scholar of Dutch studies) who learned Dutch medicine at the Narutaki school in Nagasaki during the late Edo period. For a brief description of Takano Chôei's career, see Satô Shuwasuke, *Takano Chôei* (Tokyo: Iwanami shoten, 1997).

[12] For a discussion of medical education in Japan before 1945, see chapter 1.

[13] Herbert Passin, *Society and Education in Japan* (Tokyo: Teachers College Press, 1965), 105.

[14] Koseisho, ed., *Iseihyakunenshi* (The Hundred-Year History of Medical Regulations) (Tokyo: Koseishoimukyoku, 1976), 45–47.

[15] Tsurumi Tasukuho, *Gotô Shinpei* (Tokyo: Kubisôshoten, 1985), 161–68, 174–95. For a brief review of the origins and interpretations of this saying and its relevance to Chinese political philosophy, see Wang Lin, "Gudai yijia renge de zhuiqiu: tan shangyi yiguo" (Pursuing a Medical Personality in the Ancient Period: On *Shangyi Yiguo*), *Henan zhongyi* (Henan Traditional Chinese Medicine) 22:6 (2002): 89.

[16] This saying is attributed to Fan Zhongyen (969–1052) of the Northern Song dynasty in China. See Ono Nishisu, "Shitamura zhangguan dui yixuexiao shengtu xunsgi," (Master Shitamura's speech to medical students) *Taiwan shinpo,* May 1917, 6.

[17] Sawada Ken, *Gotô Shinpei deh* (Biography of Gotô Shinpei) (Tokyo: Kôdansha, 1943), 40–43.

[18] Ibid., 60.

[19] Tsurumi Tasukuho, *Gotô Shinpei*, 24–97.

[20] Ibid., 247–302; Sawada Ken, *Gotô Shinpei deh*, 64.

[21] Sawada Ken, *Gotô Shinpei deh*, 63.

[22] Miyamoto Shinobu, *Mori Ôgai no igaku shisô* (The Medical Thought of Mori Ôgai) (Tokyo: Keisô shobô, 1979), 253.

[23] Gotô Shinpei, *Kokka eisei genri* (The Principles of State Hygiene) (Tokyo: Chikuma shobô, [1889] 1964).

[24] Gotô Shinpei, *Eisei seidôron* (On The Sanitation Administration) (Tokyo: Daiusha, 1890), 1–79, 90.

[25] Pappenheim was a German medical doctor and sanitary official. His book was published in Berlin in 1886. See Hino Shuitsu, "Gotô Shinpei 'kokka eisei genri' shiriron no sengen" (Gotô Shinpei's *kokka eisei genri*, a Declaration of Self-Interested Thought), *Nihon isigakushi zasshi* 34:1 (1988): 79–81.

[26] Watanabe Seikai, *Nihonjin to kindai kagaku: Seiyô heno taiô to kadai* (The Japanese and Modern Science: The Impact on the West and Its Topics) (Tokyo: Iwanami shoten, 1976), 80–88.

[27] Ibid., 105–31.

[28] Watanabe Seikai, "Asayama Jirô no seibutsugaku to fujôshiso" (Asayama Jirô's Biology and His Views on Survival), *Kagakushi kenkyû* (The Historical Study of Science) 107 (1973): 114–21.

[29] For Gotô's attitude regarding Virchow's activities, see Tsurumi Tasukuho, *Gotô Shinpei*, Vol. 1:437.

[30] Ishiguro and Nagayo did not think the sanitary police system would be necessary to improve health conditions unless an epidemic occurred. They believed its coercive power would destroy the real basis of medical westernization: the professionalization of medicine and the self-control of the people. See Ono Yoshirô, *Seiketsu no kindai: Eiseishôka kara kô kinguzzu he* (Sanitation in Modern Times: From Songs of Cleanliness to the Battle against Germs) (Tokyo: Kôdansha, 1997), 125–29.

[31] See chapter 1; and "Regulation 41," in Koseisho, *Iseihyakunenshi*, 133–34.

[32] Koseisho, *Iseihyakunenshi*, 257.

[33] Liu Shiyung, "Building a Strong and Healthy Empire: The Critical Period of Building Colonial Medicine in Taiwan," *Japanese Studies* 23:4 (2004): 302. In my opinion, at this moment Gotô was merely interested in how to "politically" colonize Taiwan. See Gotô Shinpei, *Eisei seidôron*, 95–99.

[34] Miyamoto Shinobu, *Mori Ôgai no igaku shisô*, 259.

[35] Tsurumi Tasukuho, *Gotô Shinpei*, 552.

[36] Ibid., 554–652, 751–868.

[37] Ninoshima rinji rikugun kenekijo, ed., *Ninoshima rinji rikugun kenekijo gyômu houkoku kouhen* (Business Report of the Army Quarantine Institute at Ninoshima) (Tokyo: Ninoshima rinji rikugun kenekijo, 1896), 1–5.

[38] Sawada Ken, *Gotô Shinpei deh*, 151.

[39] On Gotô's collaboration with General Kodama, see Tsurumi Tasukuho, *Gotô Shinpei*, 657–750. The resistance to Gotô's reforms at the medical school of Tokyo Imperial University is discussed on pages 855–70 of that volume and in Nagaki Daiizô, *Kitasato Shibasaburu to sono ichimon* (Kitasato Shibasaburu and His Pupils) (Tokyo: Keio University Press, 1992), 294–97.

[40] Morishita Kaoru, "Nihon ni okeru Kiseichugaku Hattatsu shi" (History of the Development of Parasite Study in Japan), in Morishita Kaoru, Y. Komiya, and H. Matsubayashi, eds., *Nihon niokeru kiseichugaku no hattastu* (The Study of Parasites in Japan) (Tokyo: Meguro Kiseichukan [Meguro Parasite Museum], 1961), 1:6–7.

[41] Iijima Wataru, *Mararia to teikoku* (Malaria and Empire) (Tokyo: University of Tokyo Press, 2005), 116–17.

[42] Iijima Wataru, *Pesuto to kindai chugoku* (Plague and Modern China) (Tokyo: Kemmbun shuppan, 2000), 33.

[43] Odaka Takeshi, *Densenbyô kenkyûjyo* (The Institute of Infectious Disease) (Tokyo: Gakkai shuppan senta, 1992), 79–80.

[44] For more on this term, see Nagaki Daiizô, *Kitasato Shibasaburu to sono ichimon*.

[45] Iijima Wataru, *Mararia to teikoku*, 118–20.

[46] Kitasato kenkyujyo (Kitasato Institute), ed., *Kitasato kenkyujyo gojunenshi* (The Fifty-Year History of the Kitasato Institute) (Tokyo: Kitasato kenkyujyo, 1966), 674–77.

[47] Kitasato kenkyujyo, ed., *Kitasato Shibasaburo den* (Biography of Kitasato Shibasaburo) (Tokyo: Kitasato kenkyujyo, 1932), 180–81.

[48] Keijo igaku senmon gakko (Keijo Medical College) ed., *Keijo igaku senmon gakko ichiran* (Handbook for Keijo Medical College) (Tokyo, Keijo University, 1931), 1–5.

[49] Tokyo daigaku ikagaku kenkyûjyo (Institute of Medical Science), ed., *Densenbyô kenkyûsho ikagaku kenkyûsho byakunen no ayumi* (The One Hundred Years from the Institute of Infectious Disease to the Institute of Medical Science). Tokyo: University of Tokyo Press, 1992, 13–15.

[50] Kitasato kenkyujyo, *Kitasato Shibasaburo den*, 175–81.

[51] Takenaka Masao, *The Development of Social, Educational, and Medical Work in Japan since Meiji* (Brussels: Uitgeverij Van Keulen, 1958), 39.

[52] Takekoshi Yosaburo, *Taiwan tôchishi* (The History of Ruling Taiwan). (Taihoku: Minsokoron sha, 1905), 466.

[53] Ibid., 468; Horiuchi Takao, "Taiwan eisei jijyô no kaiko" (The General Condition of Hygiene in Taiwan), *Taiwan shipo: Shôwa junen kan*, March issue, (1935): 42. For instance, during the bubonic plague epidemic of 1902 the Taiwanese always tried to hide the patient's body so as to keep the *quianshi* (full body) of death, as dictated by Chinese custom. see "Huanyi liangsanshi" (Several Events That Occurred during the Epidemic), *Taiwan nichinichi shinpo*, June 14, 1902.

[54] It is difficult to gauge just how serious the situation was at this time. However, several records left by army surgeons reveal that nearly 70 percent of Japanese soldiers died of various diseases rather than in battle. Rakugatsu Taisô, *Meiji nana nen seban ishi* (The Record of Conquering the Barbarians in Meiji 7 Year) (Tokyo: Nihokunibo, 1887), 42–44.

[55] "Gotô minso chôkan enzetsu hiki" (The Speech of Gotô, the Deputy Chief of Civil Affairs), in *Taiwan Sôtokufu igakkô ichiran* (Handbook of the Taiwan Sôtokufu Medical School) (Taihoku: Taiwan Sôtokufu igakkô, 1902), 1–12.

[56] It is questionable to assume that Gotô Shinpei wanted to import Western medicine to improve the health of the indigenous population. As supporters of the "tools of empire" theory have shown, Gotô's efforts to accomplish medical reform in Taiwan benefited only the colonizer. However, to guarantee the program's success a compromise had to be made between the colonizer and the colonized. For details, see chapter 3.

[57] Iijima, Wataru, *Mararia to teikoku*, 114–16.

[58] Tsuboi Jirô, "Taiwan no eisei" (Taiwan's Hygiene), *Taiwan ishi zasshi* 1:2 (1899): 1–8.

[59] Taiwan Sôtokufu keimukyoku, ed., *Taiwan Sôtokufu keisatsu enkakushi* (History of the Taiwan Sôtokufu Police Force) (Taihoku: Morikomu shoji, 1938) Vol. 1, 98–109.

[60] Li Chongsi, "Ribanshidai Taiwan jingcha zhidu zhi yenchiu" (The Police System in Taiwan during the Japanese Period), MA thesis, National Taiwan University, 1996, 72.

[61] Tong Huiwen, "Xingzhang jiankong yu yiliao quixun" (Administrative Structure and Medical Disciplines), MA thesis, Nanhua University, 2004, 83.

[62] See Fan Yanqiu, "Xinyixue zai Taiwan de shijian (1898–1906)," (The Practice of New Medicine in Taiwan, 1898–1906), *Xinshixue* (New History) 9:3 (1998): 49–86.

[63] Liu Jianhan, ed., *Rijuqianqi Taiwan beibushicheng jishi* (The Record of Administrative Works in Northern Taiwan during the Early Japanese Period) (Taipei: Taipeishi wenxian weiyuanhui, 1986), 2–3.

[64] Takagi Tomoe, "Retai shokumin ni seikô noin" (The Factors for Successful Colonization in the Tropics), in Nihon gôdôtsû shinsha, ed., *Taiwan taikan* (Overview of Taiwan) (Taihoku: Nihon gôdôtsû shinsha, 1932), 237–43; Washizu Atsuya, *Taiwan keisatsu yonjûnen shiwa* (Historical Account of the Police Force in Taiwan) (Taihoku: Washizu Atsuya, 1938), 388.

[65] The Japanese adopted the *ho-kô* system established during the Qing dynasty in Taiwan, adapting it to better address crime and epidemics. It was supported and financed by local police departments, which carried out government orders. See Suzuki Tôen, *Taiwan no ho-kô seido* (Taiwan's Ho-Kô System) (Taihoku: Taiwan Sôtokufu, 1940), 3–6.

[66] Taiwan Sôtokufu keimukyoku, *Taiwan Sôtokufu keisatsu enkakushi*, 2:746–49.

[67] "Hontônin eisei kumi ai ni tsuite" (About Hygienic Activities), *Taiwan nichinichishinpo*, 1883 (1903).

[68] Taiwansheng weixinweiyunhui (Historical Records Committee of Taiwan Provincial Government), ed., *Taiwansheng tongzhigao, zhengshi zhi, "paoan"* (The Security of Society), volium, 430.

[69] Qin Xienyu [Chin Hsien-yu], "Colonial Medical Police and the Postcolonial Medical Surveillance System in Taiwan, 1895–1950s," *Osiris* 13 (1998): 326–38.

[70] "Taiwan Sôtokufu fupo" (Report of the Taiwan Sôtokufu), no. 75, code 23 (1899) at Taiwan Historica, Nantou, Taiwan.

[71] Xu Xiqing, ed. and trans., *Taiwan zhongdufu gongwen leizhuan weisheng shiliao huibian Mingzhi 29 nian 4 yue zhi Mingzhi 29 nian 12 yue* (Sanitation Materials from the Archives of the Taiwan Sôtokufu from the Fourth Month to the Twelfth Month of Meiji 29 Year) (Nantou: Taiwansheng wenxian weiyunhui, 2000), 101–3.

[72] Ibid., 167–70.

[73] Probably because the colonial government initially overlooked the serious impact of the Spanish influenza epidemic in 1918, the police force was not assigned the mission. However, the police department's actions during the 1919 plague epidemic were tremendous due to the terrifying experience of the 1918 flu. See Yoshino Shigeru and Aida Toshirô, "Taiwan kaikyô e ken'etsu no kishi" (The Inspected Seashore on the Taiwan Strait), *Kôshû bôeki zasshi* (Public Anti-epidemic Journal) 23 (1936): 3, 5–11.

[74] Taiwan Sôtokufu minseibu, ed., *Taiwan eisei gaiiyô* (Summary of Taiwan's hygiene) (Taihoku: Taiwan Sôtokufu, 1913), 13–17.

[75] Li Xinfang, "Jidujiao yu Taiwan yiliaoweisheng de xiandaihua: Yi Zhanghua jidujiao yiyuan weizhongxin zhi tantao" (Christianity and the Modernization of Taiwanese Medicine and Public Health: A Study of the Zhanghua Christian Hospital), MA thesis, National Taiwan Normal University, 1989, 153–63.

[76] Cao Yunghe, ed., *Rijuqianqi Taiwan beipu shizhang jishi: weisheng pian* (The Record of Administrative Works in Northern Taiwan during the Early Japanese-Ruled Period: Sanitation) (Taipei: Taipeishi wenxian weiyunhui, 1986), 43–87.

[77] See Wang Junqi, "Rizhishiqi Taiwan yiliao zhi diliyenchiu" (The Geographic Study of Medical Therapy in Japanese-Ruled Taiwan), MA thesis, Chinese Culture University, 1999, 102.

[78] In the original scheme of the colonial government in Taiwan, the *kôi* was a medical assistant not a qualified practitioner. See Cao Yunghe, *Rijuqianqi Taiwan beipu shizhang jishi*, 20.

[79] Taiwan Sôtokufu minseibu, *Taiwan eisei gaiiyô*, 35–37.

[80] Tsurumi Tasukuho, *Gotô Shinpei*, 371.

[81] Xu Xiqing, ed. and trans., *Taiwan zhongdufu gongwen leizhuan weisheng shiliao huibian from Mingzhi 31 nian 1 yue zhi Mingzhi 34 nian 12 yue*, 120.

[82] "Kôi kai ni okeru Gotô enzetsu no yôshi" (The Speech of Gotô on the Kôi), *Taiwan kyôkai kaipo* 37 (1901): 25–27.

[83] This is Tong Huiwen's conclusion in "Xingzhang jiankong yu yiliao quixun," 80.

[84] "*Zheng shi zhi, weisheng bian* (volium)," *Taiwansheng tongzhigao* 3:35–36.

[85] For details, see Edward H. Forgotson and Judith Forgotson, "Innovations and Experiments in Uses of Health Manpower: A Study of Selected Programs and Problems in the United Kingdom and the Soviet Union," *Medical Care* 8:1 (1970): 11–12.

[86] Nakamura Aisuke, *Guni to gunshingaika* (Military Surgeons and Military Surgery) (Tokyo: Nippon ishu, 1944), preface and introduction.

[87] Nagasawa Kikutarô, *Hokaido ishi toran* (General Overview of Medical Affairs in Hokkaido) (Sapporo: Hokaido ishi kurabu, 1913), 1–12. Taiwanese *kôi* also charged fees for certain treatments and monitored local sanitary conditions. See Taiwan Sôtokufu minsebu, ed., *Taiwan eisei hôki* (Taiwan Sanitation Regulations) (Taihoku: Taiwan Sôtokufu minsebu, 1900), 123–31.

[88] Julius Stern, *Doitsu hinmini no jigyô* (The Business of the Doctor for the Poor in Germany) (Tokyo: Saiseikai, 1912), preface, 1–3.

[89] It might be too early to speculate on a connection between the prewar Japanese health care system and the rural hygiene program promoted by the League of Nations in the 1930s. However, Anelissa Lucas has suggested the possibility that advocacy by the League of Nations impacted Republican China and the postwar barefoot doctor system. For details, see Anelissa Lucas, *Chinese Medical Modernization: Comparative Policy Continuities* (New York: Praeger, 1982).

[90] Huang Wudong, *Huang Wudong huiyilu: Taiwan zhanglaojiaohui fazhanshi* (The Memoir of Huang Wudong: The History of the Taiwanese Presbyterian Church) (Taipei: Qianwei, 1990), 108.

[91] Russia ceded management of the South Manchuria Railroad to Japan after its defeat in the Russo-Japanese War in 1905. Japan established Mantetsu to control the management of the railroad and to function as a base for its invasion of China. See Jiang Tingfu, *Zuijinsanbainian dongbeiwaihuanshi* (The History of Foreign Invasions in Manchuria during the Past Three Hundred Years) (Taipei: Zhongyangri baoshe, 1953).

[92] Mori Ôgai was a Japanese physician, translator, novelist, and poet. He was born into a family of doctors in Tsuwano, Iwami Province. After his graduation from Tokyo Imperial University in 1884, he was sent to study for four years in Germany (in Leipzig, Dresden, Munich, and Berlin) by the Meiji government. On his return, he was appointed surgeon general of the Japanese army. For a brief biography, see Nakamura Humio, *Mori Ôgai to Meiji kokka* (Mori Ôgai and the Meiji State) (Tokyo: Sanichi shubô, 1992), 257–63.

[93] Mori Ôgai, *Ôgai zensyu* (The Collected Works of Ôgai) (Tokyo: Iwanami shoten, 1952), 33:594.

[94] Iseki Kurô, *Hihan enkyû hakushi jinbutu igakuhen* (Comments on and Studies of People with Doctoral Titles: The Medical Professionals) (Tokyo: Hattensha, 1925), 388–89.

[95] Takagi had a great reputation in the field of serum examination and application. A phenomenon involving the fixation of tetanus toxin in nervous tissue was named Wassermann-Takaki after the two researchers' discovery (Takaki is the German spelling). For more on the discovery, see A. Wassermann and T. Takaki, "Über tetanusantitoxische Eigenschaften des normalen Centralnervensystems" (Characteristics of the Central Nervous System under Tetanus Toxication), *Berliner Klinische Wochenschrift* (Berlin Clinic Weekly). 35 (1898): 5. For Takagi's contribution, see Nishida shôki, ed., *Nihon saikingakkai no 50 nen* (Fifty Years of the Japan Society of Bacteriology) (Tokyo: Nihon saikin gakkai, 1978), 427.

[96] Tsurumi Tasukuho, *Gotô Shinpei*, 361.

[97] Gotô proudly claimed that successful rule in colonial Taiwan depended heavily on various talents from the former Private Institute of Infectious Disease, among them Takagi Tomoe, who was expected to totally reform health conditions and medical services. For this reference and Takagi's early activities in Taiwan, see Nagagi Daiizô, *Kitasato Saburo to sono ichimon*, 245.

[98] "Daiichi keisatsu kikan no kôsei" (The First Duty and Mission of the Police Force), in Taiwan Sôtokufu, Keimukyoku ed., *Taiwan Sôtokufu keisatsu enkakushi*, Vol. 1, pp. 115, 122. To learn more about the establishment of the Temporary Committee of Prevention, refer to "Keisatsu honsho oku rinji hôekika" (Cooperation of the Temporary Committee on Prevention with the Police Department) and "Rinji hôe kiien kaikitai" (Establishing the Temporary Committee on Prevention), both in *Sôtokufu fupo, kunrei,* October 10, 1903.

[99] Ôda Toshirô, *Taiwan igaku gojunen* (The Fifty-Year History of Taiwanese Medicine), trans. Hong Youshi (Taipei: Qianwei, 1995), 101.

[100] Taihoku igakkô, ed., "Yamaguchi Taiwan Sôtokufu igakkôchô enzetsu" (The Speech of Yamaguchi, Dean of the Taiwan Sôtokufu Medical School), in *Sôritsu nijugo shyônen shukugakiji* (The Archive Collection of Twenty-five Years of Transformation) (Taihoku: Taihoku igakkô, 1930), 4.

[101] Ôda Toshirô, *Taiwan igaku gojunen*, 3–5, 12.

[102] For details of the career of Horiuchi Takao, see Ishigi Yoshifu, ed., *Horiuchi Takao boshi zhuidaozhi* (Collection in Memory of Dr. Horiuchi Takao), *Nanmin huazhi* (special issue), 11 (1956).

[103] The medical school changed its title to "college" after 1919. However, the education it offered remained vocational training in clinical medicine until it merged with Taihoku Imperial University in 1938. For a detailed discussion, see chapter 4.

[104] Weishengshu (Department of Health), ed , *Taiwan diqu gonggong weisheng fazhanshi* (The History of Public Health in Taiwan) (Taipei: Weishengshu, 1995), 1:104–9.

[105] Taiwansheng xingzheng zhangguan gongshu, ed., *Taiwansheng wushiyinianlai tongjitiyao* (A Statistical Summary of Taiwan over the Past Fifty-one Years) (Taipei: Taiwansheng xingzheng zhangquang gongshu, 1947), 1249–50.

[106] "Zhiyun yixu" (The Decision to Study Medicine), *Taiwan nichinichshinpo* No. 3832 (1911).

[107] Wu Yintao, *Taiwan yenyu* (Taiwanese Proverbs) (Taipei: Taiwanyinwen, 1986), 159.

[108] Yan Jinhu, *Qishi huiyi* (Memory before Seventy Years of Age) (Taipei: Longwen, 1990), 44; Zhang Yanhui "Rizhi shiqi de yishi yu Taiwan wen hua: Yi Jiang Weishui, Lai he, Wu Xinrong weili" (Doctors and Taiwanese Culture in the Japanese-Ruled Period: Case Studies of Jiang Weishui, Lai he, and Wu Xinrong), MA thesis, Taipei Medical University, 1999.

[109] For the information on training for home visits, see students' handwritten notes on internal medicine, surgery, obstetrics/gynecology, and pediatrics at the Taihoku Medical College. These notes must have been written around 1928 and currently are stored in the Institute of History and Philology, Academia Sinica, Taipei.

[110] "Fandui yishi wangzhenliao" (Objections to the Fee for Home Visits), *Taiwan minpo* No. 237 (1928), 6. Although Lin Xiantang's family was rich enough to donate a well-equipped hospital in Taizhong, his diary mentions many occasions on which he requested home visits. See Xu Shiju, ed. *Guanyun xiansheng riji* (The Diary of Lin Hsien-t'ang [Lin Xiantang]) (Taipei: Institute of Taiwanese History, 2006–7), records of March 5, 7, 14, 16, 1930, and January 7 and March 2, 1932.

[111] Oyamada Katsumi, *Isha wa ikanaru teido made shinyô subekika*, 49, 132.

[112] Stories of Taiwanese clinicians harassed by policemen are easy to find in *Taiwan minpo*. See "Shicaizuming de yisheng" (A Doctor Sees Money as His Life), *Taiwan minpo* No. 277 (1929), 6; and "Shifo weilisoqu" (If He Was Driven by Benefit), *Taiwan minpo* No. 363 (1931), 9.

[113] For examples, see "Buxiao zhi yu" (The Worst Case of Filial Piety), *Taiwan nichinichishinpo*, No. 5498, 1915; "Bupingming" (Complaining), *Taiwan minpo* No. 224 (1928), 9; and "Bupingming," *Taiwan minpo* No. 384 (1931), 9.

[114] Fan Yenchiu, *Yibing, Yixue yu zhiming xiendaixg: Rizhi Taiwan yixueshi* (Epidemics, Medicine, and Colonial Modernity) (Taipei: Daoxiang, 2005), 11.

[115] *Taiwansheng tongzhigao*, vol. 3, Zhengshi zhi, weisheng bian (volium), p. 19.

[116] Ôda Toshirô, *Taiwan igaku gojunen,* 12–23.

[117] Ôda Toshirô, "Takagi Tomoe hakase ate no shokan wo mite senjin wo shinobu"(Reading a Letter of Takagi Tomoe and Thinking about the Pioneers," *Nippon ishi shinpo* No. 2782 (1977).

[118] Xu Xiqing, *Taiwan zhongdufu gongwen leizhuan weisheng shiliao huibian*, 127, 167.

[119] An interesting and controversial topic in the history of modern medicine is the race between Alexandra Yersin and Kitasato to discover the plague bacillus in 1894 in Hong Kong. For a brief description of their competition, see Stefan Riedel, "Plague: From Natural Disease to Bioterrorism," *Baylor University Medical Center Proceedings* 12:8 (2005): 119. For Kitasato's works on the 1911 plague campaign in Manchuria, see Wu Yulin, *Memories of Wu Lienteh: The Plague Fighter* (Singapore; World Scientific Publishing, 1995), 41–45.

[120] Jennerian vaccination of cowpox was introduced to Japan in 1849. Due to its safety and high effectiveness, the *bakufu* government promoted the vaccination, which eventually came to symbolize to Japanese society the superiority of Western medicine. For the introduction of the Jennerian vaccination and Japanese trust in it in the first quarter of the twentieth century, see Itazawa Syôgokô, *Tenrento ni kansuru kenkyu* (The Study of Smallpox) (Tokyo: Tobôdô, 1925).

[121] Horiuchi Takao, "Taiwan jôgunki" (Records of Seeing Taiwan), *Minsoku Taiwan* (Taiwan Folklore) 10 (1942): 2–6.

[122] Takagi Tomoe, "Shutô no hanashi" (The Difficulty of Vaccination), *Taiwan igakukai zasshi* (Journal of the Formosan Medical Association) 66 (1908): 61.

[123] Liu Ts'ui-jung and Liu Shi-yung, "Disease and Mortality in the History of Taiwan," in Ts'ui-jung Liu, James Lee, David Sven Reher, Osamu Saito, and Wang Fang, eds., *Asian Population History* (Oxford: Oxford University Press, 2001), 260–65.

[124] Office of the Inspector General of Customs, ed., *Customs Medical Report (1876–77)* (Shanghai: Inspector General of Customs, 1886), 7, 32, 54.

[125] Zhang Jiafang, "Kangxi huangdi jieso jendoshu zhi shijin yu yunyin" (Time Frame of and Reasons Why the Kangxi Emperor Adopted Variolation), *Zhonghua yishizazhi* (Chinese Journal of Medical History) 26:1 (1996): 30–32.

[126] Kuno Yô, "Kôi hôkoku" (*Kôi* Report), in *Meiji 34 nenpo* (Annual Report of the Meiji) 34 (1901). (Taihoku: Taiwan Sôtokufu, 1902) archives of Taiwan Sôtokufu at Taiwan Historica, Nantou, Taiwan.

[127] Takekoshi Yosaburo, *Japanese Rule in Formosa* (London: Longmans, 1907), 283f. Government-General of Taiwan, *Statistical Summary of Taiwan* (Tokyo: Japan Times Press, 1912), 407.

[128] Nagano Satoru, "*Kôi* hôkoku ni getsupo" (*Kôi* Report, February), in *Meiji 34 nenpo* (1901); Imai Seishin, "*Kôi* hôkoku san getsupo" (*Kôi* Report, March), in *Meiji 34 nenpo* (1901).

[129] Saitô Hayami, "*Kôi* hôkoku san getsupo" (*Kôi* Report, March), in *Meiji 34 nenpo* (1901). (Taihoku: Taiwan Sôtokufu, 1902) archives of Taiwan Sôtokufu at Taiwan Historica, Nantou, Taiwan.

[130] David Arnold, *Colonizing the Body: State Medicine and Epidemic Disease in Nineteenth-Century India* (Berkeley: University of California Press, 1993), 135–36, 149–50.

[131] Ibid., 145.

[132] To clarify the relationship between smallpox vaccination and the death rate, the calculation was made as follows.

$X(t) = C(t) / [\text{Total Taiwanese population } (t)],$

where t = time, $C(t)$ = the number of vaccinated cases in a given year, and $X(t)$ = the ratio of total vaccinated cases in the total Taiwanese population of that year and the case mortalities shown as $D(t)$.

$D(t) = ds(t) / [\text{Total Taiwanese population } (t)],$

where t = time and $ds(t)$ = the number of deaths from smallpox in a given year.

Therefore, $D(t)$ is the ratio of total deaths from smallpox in the total Taiwanese population of that year.

[133] John Bowers, "The Odyssey of Smallpox Vaccination," *Bulletin of the History of Medicine* 55 (1981): 17–33.

[134] During the plague campaign of 1902, a problem with the reporting system had been discovered, and the government was still searching for a way to effectively reorganize the system. For one case, see "Wanli weisheng zhuangkuang" (Sanitary Conditions in Wanli), *Taiwan nichinichishinpo* (Chinese edition), May, 8, 1903. Until a complete household registration system was introduced to colonial Taiwan, the functions of surveillance and control of certain diseases, as well mass vaccinations, could not be enforced. "Yufang shuyi" (Preventing Plague), *Taiwan nichinichishinpo* (Chinese edition), January 30, 1906; Xu Xiqing, *Taiwan zhongdufu gongwen leizhuan weisheng shiliao huibian*, 126.

[135] On the reporting system, see "Baojia (*ho-kô*) jiankang diaocha" (The Investigation of Ho-Kô Functions), *Taiwan nichinichishinpo* (Chinese edition), November, 11, 1906.

[136] Zhang Shubing, "Taiwan zai rijushiqi jingcha faling yu fanzui kongzhi" (The Regulation of the Police Force and Criminal Control in Japanese-Ruled Taiwan), MA thesis, Fu-jen University, 1986, 19.

[137] "Jiazhang yizhengbaogao tingzhi" (The Enforcement of Epidemic Reporting in Jiazhang), *Taiwan nichinichishinpo* (Chinese edition), July 9, 1903.

[138] See Sanitary Sector of the Government of the Taiwan Governor-General, ed., *Sanitation Regulation in Taiwan* (Taipei: Sanitary Sector of the Government of the Taiwan Governor-General, 1900); and "Wanli weisheng zhuangkuang."

[139] Taiwan Sôtokufu, ed., *Eisei kaipo: Tennentô* (Summary Report on Sanitation: Smallpox) (Taihoku: Taiwan Sôtokufu, 1916), preface.

[140] Before 1910, complaints about unhealthy conditions in Taiwan were most likely the result of observation during the military suppression of 1895–97. Furuno Naoya, *Taiwan jindaihui mishi* (The Myth of Taiwan's Modernization) (Kaohsiung: Diyi, 1994), 62–63, 68.

[141] John Shepherd, "Smallpox and the Pattern of Mortality in Late Nineteenth-Century Taiwan," in Ts'ui-jung et al., *Asian Population History*, 283.

[142] Taiwan Sôtokufu, *Eisei kaipo: Tennentô* (1926), 6.

[143] Taiwansheng wenxian weiyunhui, *Taiwansheng tongzhigao: Zhengshizhi*, 430.

[144] Ishii Takeo, "Maruyama Yosito bokushi no jinyô de Taiwan no iryoshi hakase ate no shokan wo note" (Reading after Dr. Maruyama Yoshito's Recent Achievement regarding Taiwan's Medical and Hygienic History), *Tokyo ishi shinji* (Tokyo New Medical Magazine) 74:11 (1957): 44.

[145] Public health education in the schools was essential to the success of Japanese colonial medicine in Taiwan. Besides the success of the mass vaccinations against smallpox, the antimalaria campaigns, starting in the 1930s, benefited as well.

[146] "Shisai ni okeru shutô seiiseki" (Several Events concerning Vaccination), in *Taiwan shiryo kôhon* (A Collection of Taiwanese Historical Materials) (Taihoku: Taiwan shiryohen saniinkai, 1900), unpaginated.

[147] Chûô Eisei Kyoku (Central Bureau of Sanitation), ed., *Eisei Kyoku nenpo* (Annual Report of the Central Sanitary Bureau) (Tokyo: Central Sanitary Bureau, 1910), 50–51.

[148] Hamilton Cartwright, "Vaccination in Japan," *Lancet*, May 25, 1889, 1051–53.

[149] Lu Shaoli, "Gaoshi diaocha" (The National Census), in Xu Xueji, *Taiwan lishi cidian*, 719; Tomita Akira, "1905 nen rinji Taiwan tokô chôsa to naichjin no shisen" (1905 Temporary Household Investigation and the Viewpoint of the Japanese in Taiwan), in

Taiwanshi Kenkyubu, ed., *Taiwan no kindai to Nippon* (Taiwan's Modern Age and Japan) (Nagoya: Chôkyô daigaku, 2003), 103–5.

[150] The main themes in Tsuboi's report were interestingly similar to those of concern to European practitioners of tropical medicine. For references to European tropical medicine before the World War II, see Robert W. Steel, ed., *Geographers and the Tropics: Liverpool Essays* (London: Longmans, 1964).

[151] Horiuchi Takao, "Taiwan Weishechikuo Chihuiku" (Looking Back at Sanitation in Taiwan), *Taiwan shipo* (1935) March issue: 45–46.

[152] Taiwan Sôtokufu, ed., *Daiikai eisei chosa sho* (The First Investigation of Sanitation) (Taihoku: Taiwan Sôtokufu, 1931), 1–3.

[153] For related materials on the colonial and local governments' publications, see Nagaoka Masami, ed., *Syokuminchi shakaijigu kankei shiryoshu* (Collection of Colonization Materials) (Tokyo: Kinkendai shiryokankokai, 2000).

[154] Liu Shiyung, "Rizhishiqi Taiwandiqu de jibienjiegou gaibien" (Changes in Disease Patterns in Colonial Taiwan), *Xinshishue* 13:4 (2002): 165–208.

[155] Taiwan Sôtokufu, *Eisei chosa sho*, 1–3.

[156] "Taihoku jonai kyosei seiiketsuhô" (Issues of Public Sanitation inside Taipei City), in *Taiwan shiryo kôhon* (Taihoku: Taiwan shiryohen saniinkai, 1895), unpaginated.

[157] Taiwan igakukai, ed., *Taiwan eisei gaiyô* (Summary of Sanitation in Taiwan) (Taihoku: Taiwan igakukai, 1913).

[158] Ibid., 15.

[159] Minasaki Takena, *Igaku to eisei: Nanhô seikatsu hitsuju* (Medicine and Hygiene: The Way to Live in the South) (Tokyo: Kyoizai sha, 1937), 31–33.

[160] Ono Yoshirô, *Seiketsu no kindai*, 64.

[161] Liu Shiyung, "'Qingjie', 'weisheng' yu 'paojian': Rizhishiqi Taiwanshehui gonggongweisheng guannian zhi zhuanbian" (Sanitation, Hygiene, and Public Health: Changing Views on Public Health in Colonial Taiwan), *Taiwanshi yenju* 8:1 (2001): 6.

[162] Takagi Tomoe, "Retai shokumin ni seiko noin," 237–43.

[163] Nakahashi Tokugoro, "Shokumin seisaku to eisei" (The Success of Colonization and Hygiene), in Nihon gôdôtsû shinsha, *Taiwan taikan*, 248–51.

[164] Hino Shuitsu, "Gotô Shinpei no eisei gyôseiron no itchisei ni tsuite" (The Concepts of Gotô Shinpei's *On the Sanitation Administration*), *Nihon ishigaku zasshi* 34:3 (1988): 1–29.

[165] "Eisei kogoto" (Sanitary Mobilization), *Taiwan Sôtokufu Archives, Vol. 3., No. 54* (1896).

[166] Responding to the industrial pollution and cholera epidemics common in most cities, European governments promoted urban sanitation movements by providing clean water and building better systems to deal with waste. For a brief but clear description of the sanitation movement in European cities, see Frederick Cartwright, *A Social History of Medicine* (London: Longmans, 1977), 93–113.

[167] In table 2.1, the rate in 1905, 1.4 percent, was estimated. The rate in 1942, 16.1 percent, is an actual number; the expected rate in that year was 22.0 percent.

[168] Li Denghui, *Taiwan nongye fazhan de jingji fenxi* (An Economic Analysis of Agricultural Development in Taiwan) (Taipei: Lianjin, 1980), 2; Zhang Zhonghan, *Guangfuqian Taiwan zhi gongyehua* (Industrialization in Taiwan prior to World War II) (Taipei: Lianjin, 1980), 31.

[169] This argument was very common and even appears in the guidelines adopted by Taiwan's Ministry of Education for the editing of high school history textbooks. For a scholar's viewpoint, see Chen Qinan, "Taiwan xiandai yishi de guiji" (Tracing Taiwan's Modern Consciousness), *Xinshiji zhiku luntan* 22 (2003): 50.

[170] Zhang Yinghua, "Qingmo yilai Taiwan doshi de xingqi yu bianqian" (The Rise and Change of Cities since the Late Qing in Taiwan), in Qu Haiyuan and Zhang Yinghua, eds., *Taiwan shehui yu wenhua bianqian* (Changes in Society and Culture in Taiwan) (Taipei: Lianjin, 1986), 239.

[171] Tôgô Shi and Saitô Shinro, *Taiwan shokumin hatatsushi* (The Victorious History of Colonization in Taiwan) (Taihoku: Kôbunkan, 1916), 174–77.

[172] Taiwan suidô kenkyûkai, ed., *Taiwan suidôji* (Taiwan's Water System) (Taihoku: Taiwan suidô kenkyûkai, 1941), 619, 653, 677–82, 691, 701–4.

[173] Ibid., 641–46.

[174] Constructing and maintaining water systems took up, on average, 21.4 percent of the total budget of the Sôtokufu before 1920. After that year, local governments managed and owned their water systems. This increased the number of systems but lowered their quality. Most water systems after 1920 were "simplified" systems with low-quality purification and low quantities of water. See Zhu Zhimou, "Guojia yu gerenguanxi decongzhu" (Reconstructing the Relationship between State and Individual), MA thesis, National Normal University, 1998.

[175] See Zhu Zhimou, "Guojia yu gerenguanxi decongzhu," 94.

[176] For details on the goals and financing of building water systems in colonial Taiwan, see Zhu Zhimou, "Zhengfu yu geren guanxi de zaizu: riling shiqi de Taiwan zilaishui

shiye yu caizheng buzhu" (Reconstructing the Relationship between Government and the Individual: The Business of Supplying Water in Japanese-Ruled Taiwan), in *Caizheng yu Jindai Lishi Lunwenji* (Essays on Finance and Modern History) (Taipei: Institute of Modern History, Academia Sinica, 1999), 551–601.

[177] For instance, officials in the town of Puli asked the authorities for a subsidy in 1923. See "Pulijien shuidao bushe liyu" (Request to Establish a Water System in Puli, Taishô 12), in *Taiwan Sôtokufu Archives* 3738:001.

[178] Yanaihara Tadao, *Teikoku shokika no Taiwan* (Taiwan under Imperialism) (Tokyo: Kubisô shoten, 1988), 173–76; Du Congming, *Huiyilu* (Memoir) (Taipei: Longwen, 1989), 1:56.

[179] Taiwan Sôtokufu keimukyoku, *Taiwan Sôtokufu keisatsu enkakushi*, 2:746–49.

[180] In 1897, the colonial government added the position of police physician to local administrations. These were state agents who carried out health policies, investigations, and medical jurisprudence. See *Taiwansheng tongzhigao Vol. 3, zhenshi zhi "weisheng" bian*, 57–60.

[181] Ôta Chizuo, *Kesatsui no niiki* (The Diary of a Police Physician) (Tokyo: Shôwashoden, 1934); Weishengshu, ed., *Taiwan diqu gonggong weisheng fazhanshi* (The Development History of Public Health in Taiwan) (Taipei: Weishengshu, 1995), 48–49.

[182] Miriam Ming-cheng Lo, *Doctors within Borders: Profession, Ethnicity, and Modernity in Colonial Taiwan* (Berkeley: University of California Press, 2002), 52–54; Weishengshu, *Taiwan diqu gonggong weisheng fazhanshi*, 49.

[183] Washizu Atsuya, *Taiwan keisatsu yonj nen shiwa* (Historical Account of the Police Force in Taiwan) (Taihoku: Washizu Atsuya, 1938), 388.

[184] Taiwan Sôtokufu minsebu, ed., *Minsetsu teiyô* (Summary Report of Civil Affairs) (Taihoku: Taiwan Sôtokufu, 1898), 114–15.

[185] For example, traditional physicians and police were the main practitioners during the bubonic plague epidemic in 1896. See Taiwan Sôtokufu minsebu, comp., *Kokushibyô kaipo* (Summary Report of the Black Death) (Taihoku: Taiwan Sôtokufu, 1896); and "Taiwanjin kokushibyô chiryôsho" (Treatment of the Black Death in Taiwan), *Taiwan shipo* 68 (1896), 16.

[186] "Tahokuien ni okeru dojinishi yosetsu no jôkyô" (The Internship of Native Doctors at Taihoku Hospital), *Taiwan shinpo* 440–42 (1898), 16–21.

[187] Takekoshi Yosaburo, *Taiwan tôchishi*, 474–76.

[188] Takagi Tomoe, "Retai shokumin ni seikô noin," 237–43.

[189] Liu Shiyung, "Building a Strong and Healthy Empire," 311.

[190] David Arnold, "Medicine and Colonialism," in William F. Bynum and Roy Porter, eds., *Companion Encyclopedia of the History of Medicine* (London: Routledge, 1993), 1411.

Chapter 3

[1] Armed resistance was the main concern of the colonial government before 1900. Chen Yenhong, "Hoten Xinping (Gotô Shinpei) cai taizhimingzhengci zhi yenju," (A study of Gotô Shinpei's colonization policies in Taiwan) MA thesis, Danjiang University, 1987, 179. To suppress armed resistance, Gotô claimed to have executed 11,950 "bandits" during his stay in Taiwan (1902–6). Gotô Shinpei, *Nippon shokumin seisaku iiban* (A Case of Japanese Colonization Policy) (Tokyo: Tokushoku shinpo, 1921), 27–28.

[2] Taiwan Sôtokufu, ed., *Korera byô ryûkôji: Taishô 8, 9 nen* (The Record of Cholera Epidemics in Taishô 8 and 9 Years) (Taihoku: Taiwan Sôtokufu, 1923), 1–12.

[3] See the statistics in Taiwan Sôtokufu, ed., *Taiwan Pesuto ryûkôkji: Meiji 29 nen* (Taiwan's Record of Pestilential Epidemics in Meiji 29 Year) (Taihoku: Taiwan Sôtokufu, 1898); and Taiwan Sôtokufu, ed., *Taiwan Pesuto ryûkôkji: Meiji 31 nen* (Taiwan's Record of Pestilential Epidemics in Meiji 31 Year) (Taihoku: Taiwan Sôtokufu, 1900).

[4] Taiwan igakukai, ed., *Taiwan eisei gaiyô* (Summary of Sanitation in Taiwan) (Taihoku: Taiwan igakukai, 1913), 139.

[5] The colonial government often identified China as the origin of these diseases as indicated in various government publications. In addition, because of these accusations Taiwanese people of Han ethnicity were seen as carriers of disease and fishing harbors in Taiwan as windows that admitted "germs" from China.

[6] Tsuboi, Jirô, "Taiwan no eisei" (Taiwan's Hygiene), *Taiwan ishi zasshi* 1:2 (1899): 5.

[7] Tanaka Zenritsu, *Taiwan to nanhô shina* (Taiwan and Southern China) (Tokyo: Shin shôyôsha, 1927), 134–35.

[8] Ann Jannetta, *Epidemics and Early Modern Japan* (Princeton: Princeton University Press, 1987).

[9] Irene Taeuber, *The Population of Japan* (Princeton: Princeton University Press, 1958), 50–51.

[10] On the cholera campaign, see League of Nations Health Organization, "The Cholera Epidemic in Japan and Her Territories," League of Nations Report C.H. 18, June 1922, 20–23.

[11] Miyajima Mikinosuka, "Shibasaburo Kitasato," *Science* 74:1909 (1931): 124.

Also see Japan Office of the League of Nations, ed., "Public Health Organisation and Administration in Kwantung Province and the Territory Attached Thereto," in "Health Organisation in Japan," League of Nations Report C.H. 332, 1925, 270–80.

[12] Regarding this suggestion, see Minseibu Keisatsuka, "Hôken" (Protecting Health), in Minseibu Keisatsuka, ed., *Minsei taiyô* (Summary of Civil Affairs) (Taihoku: Taiwan Sôtokufu, 1902), 10–13; (1912), 7–8; and (1919), 12.

[13] Kono eshidan gunibu, ed., *Seitai eiseiihô* (Modern Hygienic Laws) (Tokyo: Rikugunsho, 1896), 400.

[14] Fan Yanqiu, 13. "Rijuqianqi Taiwanzhi gonggong weisheng: Yi fangyi weizhongzin zhiyanjiu," 13.

[15] Washiju Atsuya, *Taiwan keisatsu yonjûnen shiwa*, 388–89.

[16] Horiuchi Takao, "Taiwan jôgunki" (Army Service in Taiwan), *Minsoku Taiwan* (Taiwanese Folklore) 10 (1942): 2–6.

[17] Taiwan Sôtokufu, *Chûô kenkyujyo eiseibuji gyôji ikô keikka kusho* (General Report of Achievements of the Hygiene Section of the Central Institute for Research) (Taihoku: Chûô kenkyujyo eiseibu, 1930), 3.

[18] Katô Naoshi, "Taiwan no eisei" (Taiwan's Sanitation), *Taiwan kyôkaii kaipo* 46 (1910): 25.

[19] Taiwan Sôtokufu, ed., *Taiwan pesuto ryûkôkij: Meiji 32 nen,* 109–24.

[20] "Naimushô kenekigyoku jimukan Shiga Ketsu hakushi pesuto chosatsu ni okeru enzersuhikki" (Examination Report of Pestilence by Shiga Ketsu, the Administrative Officer of the Home Affairs), *Kôbun roisan, Meri* 28:10, undated; "Pesutobyô doku kenkyu hôkoku" (The Prevention and Toxic Study of Pestilential Epidemics), *Taiwan nichinichi shinpo* 159 (1898).

[21] See Horiuchi Takao, "Haiso ekikô" (Epidemics from Black Rats), *Taiwan ishi zasshi* (Taiwan Medical Affairs) 1:3 (1899): 14–22; "Sôki shindan no konnan oyobi ni byoroi" (The Pathology and Diagnosis of Plague), *Taiwan ishi zasshi* 2:2 (1900): 1–15; and "Sôki shindanhô" (The Diagnostic Method of Plague), *Taiwan igakukai zasshi* 2:7 8 (1903): 19–30.

[22] "Sôki yohôseki setauko koroe" (The Discussion of Plague Prevention), in Taiwan Sôtokufu minseibu, ed., *Taiwan pesuto ryûkôkiij: Meiji 32 nen* (Taiwan's Record of Pestilential Epidemics in Meiji 32 Year) (Taihoku: Taiwan Sôtokufu minseibu, 1900) 48–50.

[23] Taiwan Sôtokufu, *Taiwan Pesuto ryûkôkji: Meiji 29 nen ,* 126, 262–63.

[24] Taiwan Sôtokufu, ed., *Sôtokufu fu po,* August 14, 1901.

[25] "Tainan pesuto ryûkôjôkyô to yohôsekki shûseiseki hôkoku tekiyô" (Prevention and the Outbreak of Plague Epidemics), *Sôtokufu fupo,* October 5, 1901, 1–4.

[26] Rigun Gunidan (Army Surgeon Corps), ed., *Gunjin bôekigaku kyôtei* (The Teaching Principle of Military Preventive Medicine) (Tokyo: Rigun gunidan, 1930), 359–70.

[27] "Tainan pesuto ryûkôjôkyô to yohôsekki shûseiseki hôkoku tekiyô" October 5, 1901, 7.

[28] Ibid., 1–4.

[29] This is why Tsuboi believed a cleaner environment would prevent the outbreak of plague. See Tsuboi Jirô, "Taiwan no eisei," 8.

[30] Taiwan Sôtokufu, ed., *Taiwan yobôeisei gaikan* (The General Situation of Preventive Hygiene in Taiwan) (Taihoku: Taiwan Sôtokufu, 1922), 12–18.

[31] A *kasatsu i* was a sanitary policeman with official permission to practice medicine in certain areas. See Xu Xiqing, ed. and trans., *Taiwan zhongdufu gongwen leizhuan weisheng shiliao huibian Mingzhi 29 nian 4 yue zhi Mingzhi 29 nian 12 yue,* (Nantou: Taiwansheng wenxian weiyunhui, 2000) (Sanitation-related materials of Taiwan Sôtokufu Archives from Meiji 29, April–December) 35.

[32] "Pesutobyô toku kenkyu hôkoku" (About the Study of Pestilential Poison), *Taiwan nichinichi shinpo,* September 12, 1898.

[33] The number is calculated from Xu Xiqing, ed. and trans., *Taiwan zhongdufu gongwen leizhuan weisheng shiliao huibian* (Sanitation-related materials of Taiwan Sôtokufu Archives. (Nantou: Taiwansheng wenxian weiyunhui, 2000), 173–74.

[34] Takagi Tomoe, "Kanjô jûyôhachi nen no kaiko (jô)" (Rethinking the Battle against Epidemics after Eight Years [Continued]), *Taiwan jipo* (1920) March: 91.

[35] "Chûsha kaden" (Refusing Vaccination), *Taiwan nichinichi shinpo,* April 12, 1901.

[36] "Rinji bôeki" (Temporary Prevention of Epidemics), *Minsei teiyô* (1905), 139, 140–141.

[37] Paul-Louis Simond (1858–1947) was a French bacteriologist born in Beaufort-sur-Gervanne, Drôme, France. He studied medicine in Bordeaux and later joined the Pasteur Institute in Paris (1895–97) where he worked with Alexandra Yersin, who discovered the plague bacillus in 1894 in Hong Kong. Simond's subsequent work showed that plague is primarily a disease of rats spread by rat fleas, which transmit the disease to humans. In 1898, Simond suggested that the plague bacillus passed into the bloodstream of the victim through the bite of the rat flea. See Robert Forest and Orest Ranun, eds., and Elborg Forster and Patricia Ranun, trans., *Biology of Man*

in History: Selections from the Annals, Economics, Societies, Civilisation (Baltimore: John Hopkins University Press, 1975), 115–17.

[38] "Chûô koso eisei hikitei no ken" (Central Public Hygiene), *Kôbun roisan, tsuika* 2 *kan* 16 (undated).

[39] "Rinji bôeki," *Kôbun roisan, tsuika* 2 *kan* no. 16, 140–41, 152–53. Also see "Bôeki kumiaiki yakuhyôjon" (Actions and Drugs for Prevention), *Taiwan nichinichi shinpo* 2971, March 30 (1908).

[40] Fan Yanqiu, "Shuyi yu Taiwan zhi gonggong weisheng" (Plague and Taiwan's Public Health), *Guoli zhongyang tushuguan Taiwan fenguan guankan* (Journal of the Taiwan Branch of National Central Library) 1:3 (1995): 76–79.

[41] "Pesuto mondai" (The Pest Problem), *Taiwan nichinichi shinpo* 1201, May 6 (1902).

[42] "Bengi yohô" (Immunization Prevention), *Taiwan nichinichi shinpo* 1166, March 25 (1902).

[43] Taiwan Sôtokufu, *Taiwan eisei gaiyô,* 112–48. See also Kuraoka Hikosuke, *Taiwan ni okeru pesuto no ryûkôbyôgaku kenkyu* (An Epidemiological Study of Taiwan's Pests) (Taihoku: Taiwan igakukai, 1920), 20–24.

[44] Zheng Zhiming, "Ererba qiansi yujianan diqu de chuanranbing fangzhi" (The Prevention of Infectious Diseases in the Yunjianan Region on the Eve of the 228 Incident), *Taiwan wenhua* (Taiwan culture) 56 (2004): 101–2, 119–20.

[45] Henry Ernest Sigerist and Milton Roemer, eds., *On the Sociology of Medicine* (New York: MD Publications, 1960), 121–23.

[46] For a brief description of the Shiritsu Densenbyô Kenkyujyo, see Tokyo daigaku ikagaku kenkyûjyo (Institute of Medical Science), ed., *Densenbyô kenkyûsho ikagaku kenkyûsho hyakunen no ayumi* (The One Hundred Years from the Institute of Infectious Disease to the Institute of Medical Science) (Tokyo: University of Tokyo Press, 1992), 3–4.

[47] Odaka Takeshi, *Densenbyô kenkyujyo,* (The Insititue of Infectious Disease) (Tokyo: Gakkai shuppan senta, 1992) 83, 87–88.

[48] Ibid., 97–158.

[49] Ôda Toshirô, *Taiwan igaku gojûnen* (The Fifty-year History of Taiwanese Medicine). Trans. Hong Youshi (Taipei: Quianwei, 1995), 101.

[50] "Taiwan Sôtokufu kenkyujyo kansei, March 27, Meiji 42," in *Taiwan shiryo kôhon;* "Chûô kenkyujyo no shinkansei ni tsuite," *Taiwan jipo,* September issue (1921): 8–12.

[51] Taiwan Sôtokufu Chûô kenkyujyo, ed., *Taiwan Sôtokufu Chûô kenkyujyo eiseibu nenpo* (Annual Report of the Central Research Institute of Taiwan Sôtokufu) (Taihoku: Taiwan Sôtokufu Chûô kenkyujyo, 1922), 10.

[52] Laboratory medicine, not clinical application, was the most significant feature of Japanese medicine under the influence of the Densenbyô Kenkyujyo. See Odaka Takeshi, *Densenbyô kenkyujyo*, 258–59.

[53] Ôda Toshiro, *Taiwan igaku gôjûnen*, 101–4.

[54] See summaries of annual reports in *Taiwan Sôtokufu Chûô kenkyujyo eiseibu gyôseiki* (General Report of the Hygiene Section of the Central Research Institute of Taiwan Sôtokufu) (Taihoku: Taiwan Sôtokufu Chûô kenkyujyo eiseibu, 1922, 1942).

[55] Horiuchi Takao, "Soeki sôki shindanhô" (A New Method for Diagnosing Plague), *Taiwan igakukai zasshi* 2:7 (1903): 19–21.

[56] Sugimoto Mahito, *Mandan: Taiwan no zaisei* (Fullness: The Finance of Taiwan) (Tahoku: Matsuda sha, 1929), 56.

[57] "Tôkyoku no eisei sekei" (The Hygienic Design of the Bureau of Statistics)," *Taiwan minpo* September, 1, 1925.

[58] Liu, Shiyung. "1930 niandaiqian RijushiqiTaiwanyixuedi tezhi" (The Characteristics of Medicine in 1930s Japanese-Ruled Taiwan), *Taiwanshi yanjiu* 4:1 (1998): 97–147.

[59] This is a common complaint about colonial medicine. See Radhika Ramasubban, *Public Health and Medical Research in India: Their Origins and Development under the Impact of British Colonial Policy* (Stockholm: SAREC, 1982), 39.

[60] Ozeki Tsuneo, "Meiji-shoki Tokyodaigaku Igakubu Ssugyosei Dosei Ichiran" (A Statistical Summary of the Graduates of Tokyo University in the Early Meiji Period), (Tokyo: Tokyo University Press, 1991).

[61] Monbusho (Ministry of Education), comp., *Monbusho Nenpo* (Annual Report of the Ministry of Education), 1902.

[62] For Takagi's opinion, see Takaki Tomoe (Takaki Tomoeda in German), *Die hygienischen Verhältnisse der Insel Formosa* (Hygienic Conditions on the Island of Formosa) (Dresden: Druck von C. C. Meinhold and Sohne, Kgl. Hofbuchdruckerei, 1911), 45–58; and Yamaguchi's suggestion in "Yamaguchi Taiwan Sôtokufu igakkôchô ehzetsu," *Soritsu nijugo shunen kinen shoku gakiji* (The Archive Collection of Twenty-five Years of Transformation) (Taihoku: Taihoku igakkô, 1930), 1–6.

[63] *Taiwansheng tongzhigao,* zhengshi zhi, "weisheng," (Part), 333–39.

[64] It was very common for many countries to try to organize low-cost medical practitioners and provide a substantial level of medical care at the beginning of medical

reform. For example, in China the Rockefeller Foundation helped Peking Union Medical College train many "rural medical helpers" in the 1920s. This effort could have been one source of the "barefoot doctor" system that developed in China in the 1960s. However, there is no evidence that the *genji i* system (where doctors were prohibited to practice medicine in areas where medical resources were rare) in colonial Taiwan had any influence on developments in pre-war China. However the system is succeeded by Republican China in Taiwan when states expanded low-cost medical care.

[65] "Sôtokufu furei dai 54 ko: Sôtokufu Igakkô kisoku Meiji 32" (The Sôtokufu Code 54: About the Establishment of Sôtokufu Igakkô in Meiji 32), in Taiwan kyôikukai, ed., *Taiwan kyôiku engakuji* (The Development of Taiwanese Education) (Taihoku: Taiwan kyôikukai, 1939), 919–23.

[66] Wu Wenxing, "Rijushiqi Taiwan de gaodengjiaoyu" (Higher Education in Japanese-Occupied Taiwan), *Zhungguo lishi xuehui shixue huigan* (Journal of the Chinese History Association) 25 (1991): 166–69.

[67] Sôtokufu igakkô, "Yamaguchi Taiwan Sôtokufu igakkôchô enzetsu," in Taihoku igakkô, ed., *Sôritsu nijugo shyônen shuku gakiji*; *Taiwan kyôiku engakuji*, 927–36.

[68] Sôtokufu igakkô, ed., *Sôtokufu igaku senmongakkô ichiran* (An Overview of Sôtokufu Medical College) (Taihoku: Sôtokufu igakkô, 1933), 36.

[69] *Taiwan kyôiku engakuji*, 927–36.

[70] Taiwansheng xingzheng zhangquang gongshu ed., (The Office of the Chief Executive in Taiwan Province) *Taiwansheng wushiyinianlai tongji tiyao* (A Statistical Summary of Taiwan over the Past Fifty-One Years) (Taipei: Taiwansheng xingzheng zhangquang gongshu, 1947).

[71] *Taiwansheng tongzhigao*, zhengshi zhi, "weisheng," part, 33b–40a.

[72] For the original regulation and numbers as they changed over time, see Sôtokufu kesatsukan oyobi shigokukan ranshûjo, ed., *Taiwan eisei gyôseihô yôron* (The Principle of Regulations for Taiwan's Sanitary Administration) (Tahoku: Sôtokufu kesatsukan oyobi shigokukan ranshûjo, 1928), 120–36.

[73] Sôtokufu igakkô, ed., "Fuki: Takagi igakkôchô hôkoku" (Appendix: Takagi, the Dean of the Medical School), in *Sôtokufu igakkô ichiran* (Tahoku: Sôtokufu igakkô, 1905), 5.

[74] For one case, Han Shiquan's career in a Tainan hospital, see Zhuang Yungming, *Han Shiquan ishi de shengming gushi* (The Life Story of Dr. Han Shiquan) (Taipei: Yunliu, 2005), 102–3.

[75] "Takagi igakkôchô no hôkoku," *Igakkô hakken* 2040 (1905): 1–6; *Taiwan nichinichi shinpo* 2148, 2152, and 2154 (1905).

[76] Shuhei Ikai, "Becoming Hospital Owners: The Evolution of Doctors' Career Paths in Japan from the 1870s to the 1930s," paper presented at the History of Medicine Seminar, Wellcome Institute, London, January 1, 2005, 6.

[77] Taiwansheng xingzheng zhangquang gongshu, ed., *Taiwansheng wushiyinianlai tongjitiyao* (A Statistical Summary of Taiwan over the Past Fifty-one Years) (Taipei: Taiwansheng xingzheng zhangquang gongshu, 1947), 1249–50.

[78] Zhang Henghao, ed., *Yangkui ji* (The Collected Works of Yangkui) (Taipei: Qianwei, 1991), 85–96.

[79] Liu Shiyung, "Building a Strong and Healthy Empire: The Critical Period of Building Colonial Medicine in Taiwan," *Japanese Studies* 23:4 (2004): 305.

[80] Amano Ikuo, *Kyôseii senmon gakkô ron* (On the Special College in the Old Education System) (Tokyo: Tamagawa University Press, 1993), 25–27.

[81] *Taiwansheng tongzhigao*, zhengshi zhi, "weisheng," part, 445–52.

[82] Miriam Ming-cheng Lo, *Doctors within Borders: Profession, Ethnicity, and Modernity in Colonial Taiwan* (Berkeley: University of California Press, 2002), 199–200.

[83] "Kankô ritsuiin no kaizô" (Reforms on Health Care), *Taiwan minpo*, May 9, 1926; Mita Sadamaru, "Taiwan ni okeru nettai igaku no shimei" (Characteristics of Taiwan's Tropical Medicine), in Chugai maiji shinbunsha, ed., *Yakushin Taiwan taikkan* (Overview of Leap-Forward Taiwan) (Tokyo: Chugai maiji shinbunsha, 1941), ii–iii.

[84] Taiwan Sôtokufu, ed., *Taishô 9 nen Taiwan tôkei yôran* (Statistical Summary of Taiwan in Taishô 9 Year) (Taihoku: Taiwan Sôtokufu, 1916), 463.

[85] *Taiwansheng tongzhi*, 3:35–36.

[86] Shimada Akiseki, *Shindan shorei fuiji horei* (Cases of Diagnosis with Related Regulations) (Tokyo: Nankodo, 1916), 319–37.

[87] Japanese doctors are classified as employed hospital doctors, called *kinmui*, and self-employed local doctors, called *kaigyôi*. For the numbers of doctors in the two categories, see Kosesho (Ministry of Health), comp., *Ishi, shikaishi, yakuzaishi chôsa* (The Investigations of Doctors, Dentists, and Pharmacists) (Tokyo: Kosesho), from 1953 to 1996.

[88] Shimada Akiseki, *Shindan shorei fuiji horei*, 319.

[89] For background, see the discussion in chapter 2; "Regulation 41," in Koseisho, ed., *Iseihyakunenshi* (The Hundred-Year History of Medical Regulations) (Tokyo: Koseishoimukyoku, 1976), 133–34; and Shimada Akiseki, *Shindan shorei fuiji horei*, 319.

[90] Fan Zuoxun, ed., *Taiwan yaoxue shi* (History of Taiwan Pharmaceuticals) (Taipei: Zhenshi yaoxue jijinhuei, 1991), 16–18.

[91] Taiwain Sôtokufu, ed., *Taiwan Sôtokufu minseijihu seiseki taiyô* (Summary of Works of Civil Affairs in Taiwan) (Taihoku: Taiwain Sôtokufu, 1897), 105–6.

[92] Taiwansheng xingzheng zhangquang gongshu, *Taiwansheng wushiyinianlai tongjitiyao*, 1249.

[93] Fan Zuoxun, *Taiwan yaoxue shi*, 11, 16.

[94] *Taiwan sheng wushiyi nien lai tongji tiyao* (A Statistical Summary of Taiwan over the Past Fifty-One Years) (Taipei: Taiwansheng xingzheng zhangquang gongshu, 1947), table 529.

[95] Fan Zuoxun, *Taiwan yaoxue shi*, 16.

[96] Shimizu Tôtarô, *Nippon yakugakushi* (History of Japanese Pharmaceuticals) (Tokyo: Nanzandô, 1971), 270–71, 419–20.

[97] Fan Zuoxun, *Taiwan yaoxue shi*, 195.

[98] Shionogi shôden, ed., *Yakumei benran* (A List of Medicines) (Tokyo: Shionogi shôden, 1938), 2, 11.

[99] The price was printed on the back of the package. See figure 4.1.

[100] Fan Zuoxun, *Taiwan yaoxue shi*, 196–97.

[101] Zhu Delan, "Rizhishiqi Taiwan de zhongyaocai maoyi" (The Trade in Chinese Pharmaceuticals in Japanese-Ruled Taiwan), in *Taiwan shangye chuantong luanwenji* (A Collection on Taiwan's Commercial Tradition) (Taipei: Institute of Taiwan History, Academia Sinica, 1999), 233–68.

[102] *Taiwan sheng wushiyi nienlai tongji tiya*, (A Statistical Summary of Taiwan over the Past Fifty-One Years) (Taipei: Taiwansheng xingzheng zhangquang gongshu, 1947), table 529.

[103] For details on the development of scientific Chinese medicine in Japan, see Fujimoto Hajime, ed., *Yakkyoku kampo: Sono reimei kara* (Chinese Medicine in Pharmacies: From the Beginning) (Tokyo: Nippon yakkyoku kyoreikai, 1997).

[104] Fan Zuoxun, *Taiwan yaoxue shi*, 195.

[105] Nippon yakgaku kyokai, ed., *Rinjyo iyaku soho zenron* (A Collection on Clinical Prescriptions) (Tokyo: Meishinto, 1938), 1–3.

[106] Ibid., 202.

[107] For one example, see an advertisement for "*kaien akaiishu*," by Siseito, in *Nichinichi shinpo*, January 23, 1933.

[108] *Jindan* was the most successful and popular OTC drug made from traditional materials such as sandalwood powder, licorice root, menthol, and cinnamon. For more information about its creation in 1895 and subsequent history, visit the online historical museum of Morishita jindan at http://www.jintan.co.jp/museum/index.html.

[109] Adopting the German system, Japanese medical instructors had a clear classification system for the pharmaceutical business. Takagi calls pharmacies (*yaakyoku* in Japanese) *Apotheker,* while drugstores (*yakuden* in Japanese) are called *Drogistenladen*. See Takagi Tomoe, *Die hygienischen Verhältnisse der Insel Formosa*, 64–68. The three photographs are on pages 64, 66, and 67. The German translation is Takagi's.

[110] Ibid., 46, 49, 52, 55.

[111] The development of obstetrics and gynecology in colonial Taiwan also reveals the inequality between doctors and other medical professionals. The subordination of midwives and nurses in a male-centered system of medical care was significant. See Fu Dawei, *Yaxiya de xinshengti* (The Asian New Body) (Taipei: Socio, 2005), 123–24, 160–61, 166.

[112] Kinebuchi Yoshifusa, *Taiwan shakai jigyôshi* (History of the Social Welfare Business in Taiwan) (Taihoku: Tokuyûkai, 1940), 881–83.

[113] Taiwan Sôtokufu minseibu, ed., *Taiwan ahen seido yôshi* (The Materials of Taiwan's Opium System) (Taihoku: Taiwan nichnichshinpo sha, 1898), 23; Taiwan Sôtokufu senbaigyoku, ed., *Taiwan ahenji* (Opium in Taiwan) (Taihoku: Taiwan nichnichshinp sha, 1927), 21–23.

[114] Wu Zhuoliu, "Taiwanlianqiao" (Taiwanese Forsythia), *Taiwan xinwenxue* (Taiwanese New Literature) 1 (1986): 56.

[115] Hong Minling, ed., *Riju chuqi zhi yapian zhengce* (Opium Policy in the Early Japanese-Occupied Period) (Taichung: Historical Research Commission of Taiwan Province, 1978), Vol 1, 239–43.

[116] Tsurumi Tasukuho, *Gotô Shinpei* (Tokyo: Kubisôshoten, 1985), 2:261–63.

[117] Taguchi Tsuitatsu, "Ôkokumin no dôryô" (The Poisonous Tumor of Our Nationals), *Tokyo keisai zasshi* (Tokyo Journal of Economy) 790 (1895): 372.

[118] Hong Minling, *Riju chuqi zhi yapian zhengce*, Vol. 1, 13–16.

[119] Huang Zhaotong, *Taiwan zongdufu* (The Taiwanese Government of the Governor-General), trans. Huang Yinzhe (Tapei: Qinwei, 2002), 85; Ryo Meishu, *Taiwan tôji to ahen mondaii* (The Rule of Taiwan and Opium Problems) (Tokyo: Yamakawasha, 1983), 105–18.

[120] Chen Jinsheng, "Rijushiqi Taiwanyapian jianjinzhengce zhiyanjiu (1895–1930)"

(The Gradualist Policy of Opium Prohibition in Japanese-Occupied Taiwan," MA thesis, National Taiwan University, 1988, 65–95.

[121] Taiwan Sôtokufu eiseika, ed., *Taiwan ni okeru ahenseido no kenkyu* (Studies of Taiwan's Opium System) (Taihoku: Sôtokufu, 1932), 10.

[122] Taiwan Sôtokufu senbaigyoku, *Taiwan ahenji*, 405–6.

[123] I took the price index from Toshiyuki Mizoguchi's calculation of Taiwan's gross domestic product before 1945. For details, see Toshiyuki Mizoguchi, "Revising Long-Term National Accounts Statistics of Taiwan, 1912–1990: A Comparison of Estimates of Production Accounts to Expenditure Accounts," in Hitotsubashi University, ed., *The Long-Term Economic Statistics of Taiwan, 1905–1995: An International Workshop* (Tokyo: Hitotsubashi University Press, 1999), 1–41.

[124] Chen Jinsheng, "Rijushiqi Taiwanyapian jianjinzhengce zhiyanjiu," 95–142.

[125] Wang Shiqing, "Rijuchuqi Taiwan zhi jiangbihui yu jieyan yundong" (The Jiangbi Society and the Quit Opium Movement in Early Japanese-Occupied Taiwan), *Taiwan wenxin* (Taiwanese Historical Materials) 37:4 (1986): 111–52.

[126] Ryo Meishu, *Taiwan tôji to ahen mondaii* (The Rule of Taiwan and Opium Problems) (Tokyo: Yamakawasha, 1983), 74–95; Taiwan Sôtokufu senbaigyoku, *Taiwan ahenji*, 279–81.

[127] Xu Jienlin, *Taiwan Shiji* (The Great History of Taiwan) (Taipei: Wenyintong, 2001), 4:8.

[128] Ryo Meishu, *Taiwan tôji to ahen mondaii,* 117–88.

[129] Taiwan Sôtokufu Eiseika, *Taiwan ni okeru ahenseido no kenkyu,* 59–60.

[130] Ryo Meishu, *Taiwan tôji to ahen mondaii,* 207–18.

[131] The assimilation policy in Taiwan was subject to several transformations and debates in the colonial period. See Cai Jintang, "Huangminhua (kominka) yundongqian Taiwan shehuijiaohua yundong de zhankai" (Beginning of the Movement of Social Discipline on the Eve of the Kominka Movement), in Danjian University, ed., *Taiwanshi guoji xueshu yentaohui: Shehui, jingji yu kentuo* (The International Conference on Taiwanese History: Society, Economy, and Exploitation) (Taipei: Danjian University Press, 1995), 378–83. After 1931, a much more restrictive strategy, *kominka* (Japanization), was adopted to assimilate Taiwanese and incorporate the laws formerly applied in Japan. See Yanaihara Tadao, *Shokuminchi oyobi shokuminseisaku* (The Colony and the Colonial Administration) (Tokyo: Iwanami shoten, 1933), 310.

[132] Du Congming, *Du Congming huiyilu* (Memoir of Du Congming) (Taipei: Du Congming jiangxuejin guanliweiyuanhui, 1973), 111, 573–75; Taiwan Sôtokufu, ed.,

Taiwan tôji gaiyô (Summary of Rule in Taiwan), in Hara shobô, comp., *Meiji hyakunenshi* (The Hundred-Year History of the Meiji Era) (Tokyo: Hara shobô, 1973), 79–80.

[133] Liu Ts'ui-jung and Liu Shi-yung, "Disease and Mortality in the History of Taiwan," *Taiwanshi yenjiu* 4:2 (1998): 90–132.

[134] George Mackay, *From Far Formosa: The Island, Its People, and Missions* (New York: F. H. Revell, 1896), 308–14.

[135] George W. Barclay, *Colonial Development and Population in Taiwan* (Princeton: Princeton University Press, 1954), 136.

[136] Without realizing the unique development of Japanese malariology in colonial Taiwan, scholar Fan Yanqiu accidentally exposed these features by chronologically arranging related materials. See Fan Yanqiu, "Yixue yu zhimin kuozhang: Yi rizhi shiqi Taiwan nueji yenjiu weili," *Xin shixue* (New History) 7:3 (1996), 133–73.

[137] Fan Yanqiu, "Nueji fangesho" (Malaria Prevention Station)," in Xu Xueji, ed., *Taiwan lishi cidian* (Dictionary of Taiwanese History) (Taipei: Yuanliu, 2004), 1032.

[138] Taiwan sheng wenxian weiyuanhui ed., *Taiwansheng tongzhigao*, 198–200; Weishengshu, *Taiwan diqu gonggong weisheng fazhan shi* (The History of Public Health in Taiwan) (Taipei: Weishengshu, 1995), 216–17.

[139] Barclay, *Colonial Development and Population in Taiwan*, 136. See also Ts'ui-jung Liu and Liu Shiyung, "Disease and Mortality in the History of Taiwan," in Ts'ui-jung Liu et al., eds., *Asian Population History* (Oxford: Oxford University Press, 2001), 262.

[140] *Taiwansheng tongzhigao*, 183–84.

[141] Horiuchi Takao, "Bankin Taiwan ni okeru eiseijôtai gakuten no genin to sono kyûkyûsaku" (The Latest Developments and Research on Hygiene in Taiwan), *Taiwan jipo* (March 1921): 53–61.

[142] "Code 5, Mararia bôatsukisei" (The Prevention and Strategy of Malaria), *Sôtokufu fupo* 192 (April 10, 1913).

[143] Morishita Kaoru, *Mararia no bôekigaku to yobô: Taiwan ni okeru Nihon tôji jitai no kiroku to kenkyu* (The Prevention and Precaution of Malaria: Records and Research in Taiwan under Japanese Rule) (Tokyo: Nippon itaikikuya, 1976), 125–29.

[144] Liu Ts'ui-jung and Liu Shiyung, "Disease and Mortality in the History of Taiwan," in Ts'ui-jung Liu et al., *Asian Population History*, 249–55; Mohammad Mirzall, "Trends and Determinants of Mortality in Taiwan, 1895–1975," PhD diss., University of Pennsylvania, 1979, 174.

[145] Tsuboi Jirô, "Taiwan no eisei," *Taiwan ishi zasshi* 1:2 (1899): 1–8.

[146] Ts'ui-jung Liu and Liu Shiyung, "Disease and Mortality in the History of Taiwan," 262.

[147] N. Omori, *Kotosho no Anafuelesu ni tsuite* (On the Anopheline Mosquitoes of Kotosho), *Taiwan igakukai zasshi* 36:393 (1937): 2800–2801.

[148] N. Omori and H. Noda, "On an Anopheline Mosquito, *Anopheles arbumbrosus*, Newly Found in Taiwan," *Studia medica Tropicalis* (Formosa) 1 (1943): 83–89.

[149] Morishita Kaoru, "Taiwan chihôbyo to densen chousaiinkai ni okeru mararia chousa gaiyo" (Summary of the Malaria Investigation in the Survey of Taiwan's Endemic Diseases and Infectious Routes), *Taiwan igakukai zasshi* 34:362 (1935): 142.

[150] Kobayashi Hiroshi ed., *Hikone shi no mararia taisaku* (The Elimination of Malaria in Hikone City) (Hikone City: Hikone shi eiseika, 1951), 152–53.

[151] Hata Chôsan, Kuriyagawa shô, and Takeishi Hirodan, *Gentai iyakuhin no jisai* (Progress in Modern Medical Treatment) (Tokyo: Nansandô, 1950), 197, 230–31.

[152] Ôda Taifumi, Morishita Kaoru, and Nabika Hiroshi, "Mararia chiryo kansuru kenkyu 3" (Studies to Treat Malaria 3), *Taiwan igakukai zasshi* 30:310–21 (1933): 99–109; Morishita Kaoru and Nabika Hiroshi, "Mararia chiryo kansuru kenkyu 5" (Studies to Treat Malaria 5), *Taiwan igakukai zasshi* 30:310–21 (1933): 741–46.

[153] Hata Chôsan, Kuriyagawa shô, and Takeishi Hirodan, *Gentai iyakuhin no jisai*, 225.

[154] In 1915, a Viennese physician, Julius Wagner von Jauregg, came up with the idea of "burning" *Treponema pallidum* out of the central nervous system. Charles Dennie, *A History of Syphilis* (Springfield, IL: Charles C Thomas, 1962), 113, 118.

[155] Senbon Nobuo, "Rinshitsu no hanetsu ryohô ni tsuite" (About the Temporary Method of Treatment), *Taiwan igakukai zasshi* 35 (1936): 1143–45.

[156] Ishioka Heizou, "Mararia to chonai kiseichu" (Malaria and Intestinal Parasites), *Taiwan igakukai zasshi* 37 (1939): 678–84.

[157] Morishita Kaoru, *Maraia no bôekigaku to yobô*, 130.

[158] "Mararia netsu yobôhô taii" (On the Prevention of Malaria), *Taiwan shinpo*, April 1, 1897; "Mararia yobôhô ni tsuite" (About the Preventive Method for Malaria)," *Taiwan shinpo*, October 10, 1898.

[159] Miyahara Daisuke, *Mararia no chiryô* (Malaria Treatment) (Taihoku: Taiwan Sôtokufu, 1939), 9–10, 18. Miyahara's book did not reveal how much the colonial government paid for imported quinine. However, according to the continuous records of the annual reports of the Central Bureau of Sanitation, Japan continued to import quinine and the amount always topped the figures for other imported medicines.

Therefore, the amount of quinine available in colonial Taiwan depended largely on the government budget.

[160] Taiwan Sôtokufu keimukyoku eiseika, ed., *Mararia bôatsu si* (The Prevention of Malaria) (Taihoku: Taiwan Sôtokufu keimukyoku eiseika, 1932), 18.

[161] Takagi Tomoe, "Kanjyô 18 nen kaiko" (Review of an Eighteen-Year Political Career), *Taiwan jihô* (Taiwan Times) *January, February, and March 1920*.

[162] Taiwan Sôtokufu eiseika, ed., *Mararia) bôatsuj* (Preventing Malaria) (Taihoku: Taiwan Sôtokufu, 1931), 14–16.

[163] See "Mararia hokumetsu" (Malaria Prevention), *Taiwan nichinichi shinpo*, 2945–48 (Fenruary 29, 1908).

[164] Kanazawa Gintsurô, "Taiwan ni okeru shokumin jigyô no tenhô" (On Colonization in Taiwan), *Taiwan jipo* (May, 1933) 8–15, (June, 1933) 20–30, (July, 1933) 5–14.

[165] Zhang Shubing, *Taiwan de riban nongye yimin, 1909–1945* (Japanese Agricultural Immigrants in Taiwan, 1909–1945) (Taipei: Goushiguang, 2001), 107–11.

[166] Lin Zhengjung, "The Japanese Experience in Taiwan: The Immigrant Village during the Japanese Period," http://www.twhistory.org.tw/20010730.htm.

[167] For collective data on colonial Taiwan, see Weishengshu, *Malaria Eradication in Taiwan* (Taipei: Executive Yuan, 1991), 11; and Taiwansheng xingzheng zhangquang gongshu, *Taiwansheng wushiyinianlai tongjitiyao*, 326–27.

[168] Wu-Dar Huang, Ja-Haur Tsay, and Naito Akira, "The Evolution of Building Legislation in Colonial Taiwan: Case Studies in Taipei City," *Jienzhu Xuebao* (Journal of Architecture) 23 (winter 1997): 37.

[169] Taiwansheng xingzheng zhangquang gongshu, *Taiwansheng wushiyinianlai tongjitiyao*, 1249.

[170] See, for example, an advertisement posted by Shinogi seiyaku kabushikikaisha in Shimizu Hideo, *Jiyô eiseikowa* (Stories of Hygiene and Pharmacy) (Tokyo: Tomikura shoten, 1925), back page.

[171] A box (twelve rolls) of mosquito coils cost 0.3 yen in 1932. Compared to the monthly salary of an elementary school teacher (roughly 40 yen), the price was not exorbitant. For prices, see Dainibon seiyaku kabushikikaisha, *Shiyaku yôran* (Handout of New Medicine) (Osaka: Dainibon seiyaku kabushikikaisha, 1932), 33. For teachers' salaries, see Wu wenxing, *Rijushihqi Taiwan shihfanjiaoyu zhi yanjiu* (Normal Education in the Japanese-Occupied Period) (Taipei: National Taiwan University, 1983), 168–76.

[172] *Plasmodium vivax* is the most common of the four species of malarial parasites that affect humans.

[173] Nakamura Yuzuru, Imai Yô, and Akashi Mataka, "Kaitô" (Reply), *Taiwan igakukai zasshi* 197 (1919): 483–91.

[174] "Shakoku" (Editorial), *Taiwan nichinichi shinpo*, November, 5, 1919.

[175] "Kôku" (Public Announcement), *Taiwan nichinichi shinpo*, August 5, 1939.

[176] Zhuang Yungming, "Taiwan geyao," http:/library.taiwanschoolnet.org/cyberfair2004/a67560/m2023.htm.

[177] The transportation network in western Taiwan grew rapidly between the 1909 and 1924. Although passenger coaches were rare, freight cars carried medical supplies and promptly delivered experts to afflicted sites. Jiaotongbu (Transportation Bureau), ed., *Taiwansheng jiaotong jianshe* (The Development of Transportation in Taiwan) (Taizhung: Taiwanshengzhegfu, 1987); Morishita Kaoru, Sugida Nobusuke, and Hitougawa Hachigorou, "Shinchikushôshita shisaichihô ni botsuhatsu seru ryukosei mararia ni tsuite," *Taiwan igakukai zasshi* 36 (1937): 1156.

[178] Morishita Kaoru, Nabika Hiroshi, Matsûra Ho, and Tanigawa Kuniyasushi, "Wusandôni okeru mararia ryukô kyûsono bôatsuni All Quinization no kôkoni tsuite" (The All-Quinization Treatment in Addressing the Malaria Problem at Wusantou), *Taiwan igakukai zasshi* 30:310–21 (1933): 713.

[179] Ibid., 715–20.

[180] Morishita Kaoru and Nabika Hiroshi, "Mararia chiryo kansuru kenkyu 4" (Studies on the Treatment of Malaria 4), *Taiwan igakukai zasshi* 30:310–21 (1933): 735–36.

[181] The strategies were called "hito ni taisuru hôhô" (the method for human beings) and "ka ni taisuru hôhô" (the method for mosquitoes). See Tsukiyama Kiichi, "Mararia yobôhô" (Preventive Methods on Malaria), *Taiwan igakukai zasshi* 29 (1905): 89–101. Ku Ya Wen has discussed these policies and carefully examined the results. See Ku Ya Wen, "Taiwan ni okeru mararia ryûkô oyobi bôatsutaisaku no sui" (A Historical View of Malaria and Its Countermeasures in Taiwan), PhD diss., Yokohama National University, 2005.

[182] J. L. Zeigler, "Editorial: Tropical Splenomegaly Syndrome," *Lancet* 15:1 (1976): 1058–59.

[183] C. T. Chen, , Y. T. Wu, and, H. C. Hsieh, "Differences in Detectability of Minor Splenomegaly through Variation in the Recumbent Position of the Patient," *Taiwan yixuehui zhazhi* 53:9 (1954): 561–67.

[184] Weishengshu, *Malaria Eradication in Taiwan*, 14–15.

[185] Hitougawa Hachigorou, "Tainanshôshita niokeru 'mararia bôatsusagyô no jisai to sono seiseki" (The Preventive Works and Progress of Malaria in Tainan County), *Taiwan igakukai zasshi* 34 (1935): 56–76.

[186] Wang Zhiting, *Taiwan jiaoyushihliao shinbian* (The New Edition of Historical Materials on Education in Taiwan) (Taipei: Shangwu, 1978), 46.

[187] Morishita Kaoru, *Maraia no bôekigaku to yobô*, 18.

[188] Morishita Kuro, Sugida Nobusuke, and Hitougawa Hachigorou, "Shinchikushôshita shisaichihô ni botsuhatsu seru ryukosei mararia nit suite," 1151–66, 1666–1746.

[189] K. Morishita and T. Katagai, "Examination of the Blood Meals of Formosan Anophelines by Precipitin Tests," *Journal of Zoology* 45 (1933): 137–39.

[190] Morishita Kaoru, "Mararia Daisôshindan niokeru ketsueki atsusôhô no kôko sono jishihô kyûkoreni iru genchûshubetsu no yôten nitsuite," (The accumulation rate of erythrocyte as an index for clinical diagnosis of malaria) *Taiwan igakukai zasshi* 274–85 (1931): 1169–1208.

[191] Iijima Wataru and Wakimura Kôhei, "Eisei to teikoku-nichiei shokuminchi shugi no hikakusiteki kôsah e mukete" (Hygiene and Empire: A Comparative History of Japanese and British Colonialism), *Nihonshi kenkyû* (Journal of Japanese History) 462 (2001): 3–25; Iijima Wataru and Wakimura Kôhei, "Kindai ajia niokeru teikoku shugi to iryo, kôshu eisei" (Imperialism, Medicine, and Public Health in Modern Asia), in Miichi Masatosi, Saito Osamu, Wakimura Kôhei, and Iijima Wataru, eds., *Kaihotsu teikoku iryô* (Development, Disease, and Imperial Medicine) (Tokyo: Tokyo University Press, 2001), 75–94; Wakimura Kôhei, "Shokuminchi tôchi to kôshu eise: Indo to Taiwan" (Colonial Rule and Public Health: India and Taiwan), in Wakimura Kôhei, *Kikin ekibyô shokuminchi to tôchi* (Famine, Disease, and Colonial Rule) (Nagoya: Nagoya University Press, 2002), 216–44.

[192] "Mararia kihonteki kenky" (An Essential Research Unit on Malaria), *Taiwan jipo*, April, 1926; Taiwan Sôtokufu Chûôkenkyûjyo Eiseikabu, ed., *Taiwan Sôtokufu chûôkenkyûjyo eiseikabu nenpô (Annual Report of the Taiwan* Sôtokufu) 1 (1930): 60–62.

[193] Ôda Toshiro and Morishita Kaoru, *Mararia no bôatsu* (The Prevention and Eradication of Malaria) (Taihoku: Taiwan Sôtokofu, 1939).

[194] For the exhibition in Dresden, Takagi Tomoe wrote *Die hygienischen Verhältnisse der Insel Formosa,* describing sanitary conditions and related medical reforms in colonial Taiwan. The book made the application of Tanaka's interpretation to the exhibition in Taiwan more acceptable.

[195] Tanaka Satoshi, *Eisei tenrankai no yokubô* (The Meaning of Hygiene Exhibitions) (Tokyo: Seikyûsha, 1994).

[196] Tsurumi Tasukuho, *Gotô Shinpei*, 2:93.

[197] Taichûchô, ed., *Taichûchô kyoiku eisei tenrankai shashinchô* (A Photo Album of the Taichû Education Hygiene Exhibition) (Taihoku: Arita shashinkan, 1918).

[198] Weishengshu, *Taiwan diqu gonggong weisheng fazhanshi*, 230.

[199] Although some advice was received from Japan, the posters were mainly designed in Taiwan. Taihokushû keimubu, ed., *Taihoku keisatsu eisei tenrankai kiroku* (A Record of the Taihoku Prefecture Police Hygiene Exhibition) (Taihoku: Taiwan nichinichi simposha, 1926), 2–3.

[200] Ibid., 25–30.

[201] Taiwansheng xingzheng zhangquang gongshu, *Taiwansheng wushiyinianlai tongjitiyao*, tables 56.

[202] For the arrangement of the Hall of Hygiene and the exhibition as a whole, see the map in Taihoku shû keimubu, *Taihoku keisatsu eisei tenrankai kiroku*, first page.

[203] See, for example, the image of a policeman as a thousand-handed bodhisattva in Taihokushû keimubu, ed., *Taihoku keisatsu eisei tenrankai shashinchô* (A Photo Album of the Taihoku Prefecture Police Hygiene Exhibition) (Taihoku: Taiwan nichinichi simposha, 1926), 44.

[204] Ibid., 40.

[205] Ibid., 73.

[206] Zhuang Yungming, *Taiwan yiliaoshi* (The History of Medicine and Therapy in Taiwan) (Taipei, Yunliu, 1998), 28–29.

[207] Taiwan Sôtokufu ed., *Korera byô ryûkôji: Taishô 8, 9 nen.*

[208] "Ping jingcha weisheng zhanlanhui de jiazhi" (A Critique of the Value of the Police Hygiene Exhibition), *Taiwan minpo*, December 6, 1925.

[209] "Jingcha weisheng zhanlanhui: Gaodeng guan zhuanyong fengci, weisheng guan guanggao maiyao" (The Police Hygiene Exhibition: the High Police Hall Uses Caricatures, the Ads in the Hygiene Hall Sell Drugs), *Taiwan minpo*, December 6, 1925.

[210] Taihokushû keimubu, *Taihoku keisatsu eisei tenrankai kiroku*, 113–17.

[211] Takekoshi Yosaburo, *Japanese Rule in Formosa*, trans. George Braithwaite (London: Longmans, 1907), 27.

[212] Taiwan Sôtokufu, ed., *Dai ichi kai eisei chôsa houkoku* (The First Public Health Investigation) (Taihoku: Taiwan Sôtokufu, 1931), 1–3.

[213] For details, see Liu Shiyung, "Public Health Investigation and Statistics in Colonial Taiwan," in *Introduction: The Archives of Social Affairs in Colonies—Taiwan* (Tokyo: Modern Information Publishers, 2001), 1–21.

[214] Gyan Prakash, *Another Reason: Science and the Imagination of Modern India* (Princeton: Princeton University Press, 1999).

[215] The Kuomintang government that took over in Taiwan after World War II also realized that an "impressive sequence of directors had both administrative and technical talent, and shared field-oriented skills and capabilities with personal at all staff levels, many of whom had developed innovative methods of overcoming many obstacles quiet commonly found in a truly 'grass-roots' campaign." Weishengshu, *Malaria Eradication in Taiwan*, 271.

[216] A-nan is a pseudonym for a man interviewed by Liu Shiyung in Baiho, Tainan County, on July 27, 2002. A-nan was born in 1929 and became a member of the local DDT spraying team in 1956.

[217] Alfred W. Crosby Jr., *Ecological Imperialism: The Biological Expansion of Europe, 900–1900* (Cambridge: Cambridge University Press, 1986).

[218] David Arnold, *The Problem of Nature: Environment, Culture, and European Expansion* (London: Blackwell, 1996), 90–91.

Chapter 4

[1] This viewpoint of colonial modernization of medicine in the Japan-ruled period was welcomed by scholars and was very prevalent in Taiwan. For a case, see Jingdian zhazhi, ed., *Cirri yenyen: Taiwan, 1895–1945* (The Sun Was Burning: Taiwan, 1895–1945) (Taipei: Jingdian zhazhi, 2005), 120–29.

[2] Besides her book *Doctors within Borders: Profession, Ethnicity and Modernity in Colonial Taiwan*, Miriam Ming-cheng Lo discusses the *kominka*, which was a movement to form Taiwan's medical profession and transform, or Japanize, Taiwanese identity in the 1930s. "Between Ethnicity and Modernity: Taiwanese Medical Students and Doctors under Japan's *Kominka* Campaign, 1937–1945," *positions* 10:2 (2002): 285–332.

[3] David Arnold, "Crisis and Contradiction in India's Public Health," in Dorothy Porter, ed., *The History of Public Health and the Modern State* (Amsterdam: Rodopi, 1996), 345.

[4] Most famously, the colonial doctors Gotô Shinpei and Takagi Tomoe encouraged their medical students using these two slogans. In the 1990s, physician-historians such as Chen Yungxin used them in their works to recall the social responsibility of doctors. See Chen Yungxin and Chen Chongquang, comp., "Cong renwen fangmian

tantao gujin yixue liul" (Using the Viewpoint of Humanity to Study Medical Ethics in the Past and Present), *Newsletter of Mackey Memorial Hospital* 1:5 (1991): 29–32.

[5] Takekoshi Yosaburo, *Japanese Rule in Formosa*, trans. George Braithwaite (London: Longmans, 1907), 289.

[6] Malariology in colonial Taiwan offers a good case for examining this effort. See chapter 3.

[7] Chen Shaoxin, *Taiwan de renkou bianqian yu shehui bianqian* (Population and Social Change in Taiwan) (Taipei: Lianjing, 1985), 125.

[8] Taiwansheng xingzheng zhangquang gongshu, ed., *Taiwansheng wushiyinianlai tongjitiyao* (A Statistical Summary of Taiwan over the Past Fifty-one Years) (Taipei: Taiwansheng xingzheng zhangquang gongshu, 1947), 1250.

[9] For the numbers over time, see the table in ibid., 1249–50. It is worth noting that, in this table, the colonial government did not distinguish between hospitals and clinics. The Japanese word *byôin* could mean "hospital," "ward," or "clinic" in English. Also Taiwanese medical schools did not offer instruction in dentistry. Most dentists studied and earned their licenses in Japan.

[10] A graph, as in chart 4.1, is the best way to show changes in the distribution of various medical practitioners during the colonial period. For instance, out of a total of 5,045 medical practitioners in 1940, 41.82 percent were fully trained, Western-type physicians. The figures are 40.53 percent for nurses and midwives, 8.78 percent for private dentists, 5.77 percent for B-class physicians (including *ko i*), 2.64 percent for traditional physicians, and 0.46 percent for official dentists. We can see that the number of private dentists grew rapidly from none in 1910 to 8.78 percent of all medical practitioners in 1940, leaping from last place into the top three. These data are drawn from Taiwan sôtokufu eiseika ed., (Taiwan Sôtokufu Sanitation Sections) (Taihoku: Taiwan Sôtokufu eiseika, 1941), *Sôtokufu eisei nenpo 1941*.

[11] Liu Shiyung, "1930 niendai rizhishiqi Taiwan yixue de tezhe" (The Characteristics of Taiwanese Medicine in the 1930s Japanese-Ruled Period), *Taiwanshi yenjiu* (Taiwanese Historical Research) 4:1 (1999): 126–29.

[12] "Ko i no kaizô (About ko i)," *Taiwan minpo* 104 (May 9, 1926).

[13] Nagaki Daisô, *Kitasato Shibasaburo to sono ichimon* (Kitasato Shibasaburu and His Pupils) (Tokyo: Keio University Press, 1992), 247.

[14] Taiwain Sôtokufu, ed., *Taiwan Sôtokufu minseijibu seiseki taiyô* (Summary of Works of Civil Affairs in Taiwan) (Taihoku: Taiwain Sôtokufu, 1897), 105–6.

[15] Tôkeikyoku, ed., "Kaidai" (Introduction), in *Nippon jinkôtôkeishôsei* (A Collection of Japan's Demographic Statistics) (Tokyo: Harashobô, 1994), 1:3.

[16] The new standards of classification of illness caused various changes in the classification of disease and required new medical expertise. For example, in government reports some ambiguous causes of death were replaced with diseases as these were defined in Western medicine after 1930. See Taiwansheng xingzheng zhangquang gongshu, *Taiwansheng wushiyinianlai tongjitiyao*, tables 487–1 and 487–2.

[17] Naimushô eiseikyoku, ed., *Isei gôjûnenshi* (The Fifty-year History of Isei), 59 (Tokyo: Naimushô eiseikyoku, 1925).

[18] See chapter 3 for a discussion of these four types.

[19] The numbers are estimated from Kosesho, ed., *Isei hyakunenshi furo* (The Hundred-Year History of Isei), (Tokyo: Koseshoimukyoku, 1976) appendix, 45–47, and table 4.1.

[20] Nippon ijishinôsha, ed., "Taiwan," in *Nippon ijirenkan* (Annual Account of Registered Doctors in Japan) (Tokyo: Nippon ijishinôsha, 1939), 1–39.

[21] Takagi Tomoe once said that Taiwan was a place to apply and advance the research on tropical medicine conducted in Japan. See Itadeo Ichitarô, "Sofu Takagi Tomoe o haru" (About the Master Teacher Takagi Tomoe), in Du Congming, ed., *Takagi Tomoe sensei tsuiokushi* (Collection in Remembrance of Takagi Tomoe) (Tokyo: Takagi Tomoe kinenji iinkai, 1957), 9.

[22] Similar information has already been given in charts 3.2 and 3.3. However, table 4.1 gives a quicker comparison between professional groups in the two areas. Because the Sôtokufu medical school (vocational high school level) lasted for twenty-one years (1897–1918), Taiwan had many type-A doctors, which is the major difference between the majority of medical professionals in Taiwan and Japan, namely, 75 percent types A and B in Taiwan and 84 percent types B and C in Japan.

[23] See chapter 3 and the discussion of Gôto's career in chapter 2.

[24] Kosesho, ed, *Isei hyakunenshi furo*, 124.

[25] For a detailed discussion of the commercialization of medical practice in 1930s Japan, see Morôka Son and Shimakage Chikai, *Idôgakushinron* (The New Argument of Medical Ethnicity) (Tokyo: Taito, 1937).

[26] Nakano Misao, *Kôkoku ishi dainenbyô* (Great Japan's Annals of Medical Affairs) (Tokyo: Nankôdô, 1942), 314.

[27] Because of the second reform in medical education, the medical colleges became medical universities in 1928. However, Taihoku Medical College in Taiwan, the only exception, retained its old status until it merged with the Medical School of Taihoku Imperial University as an affiliated department in 1936. See Lin Jichong, ed., *Taida yiyun bainianshi (I) Rizhishiqi (1897–1945)* (The Hundred-Year History of the Medical School of National Taiwan University: The Japanese-Occupied Period, 1897–1945)

(Taipei: National Taiwan University Medical College, 1997), 93. For the transition and educational function of the college in prewar Japan, see Han Min, *Gendai Nihon no senmon gakkô: Kôto shokugyô kyôiku no igi to kadai* (The Special College in Modern Japan: The Beginning of Vocational Education), (Tokyo: Tamagaku daigaku shuppanbu, 1996).

[28] Zheng Zhimin, "Zhimin yangban huo tairen yingxiong: Shirun Du Congming yu rizhishiqi Taiwan de yixue jiaoyu" (A Colonist's Sample or a Taiwanese Hero: The Studies of Du Congming and Medical Education in the Japanese-Ruled Period), *Taiwan tushuguan guanli jikan* (Taiwanese Journal of Library Management) 1:1 (2005): 102.

[29] Yanaihara Tadao, *Rihan diguozhuyi xia zhi Taiwan* (Taiwan under Imperialism), trans. Zhou Xienwei (Taipei: Haixia xueshu, [1988] 1999), 176.

[30] See *Sôtokufu Taihoku byôin nenpo* (Annual Report of the Sôtokufu Taihoku Hospital), (Taihoku: Taihoku byôin) vols. 3–40, 1900–1937.

[31] Lin Jichong, *Taida yiyun bainianshi (I) Rizhishiqi*, 93.

[32] These ratios were provided Dr. Hu Shuiwan during an interview conducted on May 19, 2006. Hu was in the last class to graduate from Taihoku Medical College in 1937; in 1938, the school merged with Taihoku Imperial University as the Department of Vocational Training in Medicine.

[33] Fujii Namiku ,ed., *Nihon igaku bunka nenbyô* (The Cultural Annals of Japanese Medicine) (Tokyo: Nishin shôin, 1928), 199.

[34] Taiwan Sôtokufu igakusenmon gakkô, ed., *Sôtokufu igaku senmon gakkô ichiran* (Overview of the Sôtokufu Medical College) (Taihoku: Taiwan Sôtokufu igaku seimon gakkô, 1922), 162.

[35] Zhuang Yungming, *Han Shiquan yishi de shengmingushi* (The Life of Dr. Han Shiquan) (Taipei: Yunliu, 2005), 102–3; Lai Ho, "A-si," in Lin Ruiming, ed., *Lai Ho quanji: Xiaoshuojuan* (The Collected Works of Lai Ho: The Novels) (Taipei: Qianwei, 2000), 266–67.

[36] Nakano Misao, *Kôkoku ishi dainenbyô*, 1214, 1218.

[37] "Taiwan isei menkyo kisoku" (Studying to Be a Taiwanese Doctor), in Taiwan eipôsha, ed., *Taiwan eisei nenkan* (Taiwanese Annals of Hygiene) (Taihoku: Taiwan eipôsha, 1932), 179.

[38] Ishikawa Nobuo, *Kameikangogaku* (The Simplified Textbook of Nursing) (Tokyo: Nanzandô, 1939), 2–3.

[39] To study the growth rates of the two trends, the semilog regressions are calculated as follows.

Semilog regression: $\ln Y(t) = a + bt$, where $\ln$ = natural logarithm, t = time, and Y = physicians per thousand population.

The regression coefficient b will give the average annual percentage change in Y, resulting in:

Japan: $\ln Y_J = -0.2667 + 0.0022t$

Taiwan: $\ln Y_T = -0.6879 - 0.0124t$

[40] Kosesho ed., *Isei hyakunenshi furo*, 136–38.

[41] Amano Ikuo, *Kyôsei seimon gakkô ron* (On the Special College in the Old Educational System) (Tokyo: Tamagawa University Press, 1993), 229–39.

[42] "Saikin no ikai" (The Latest Medical Cycle), *Ikai shipo* 1782 (1935): 10–11.

[43] See, for example, "Fukaina iyakubunri" (About the Relationship between Therapy and Pharmacy), *Ikai shipo* 1687 (1925): 8.

[44] Yamaguchi Hidetaka, "The Founding of Taiwan Governor-General Medical College and Its Hope in the Future," trans. by L. C. Han, *Taiwan Historical Materials Studies* 8 (1996): 52.

[45] In the medical realm, Whiggish interpretation rested on a pair of assumptions. First, past actions that do not conform to present concepts of normality must be pathological. Second, past ideologies that fail to match present scientific constructions of reality are sure indicators of ignorance, malice, or both. For details, see Herbert Butterfield, *The Whig Interpretation of History* (Harmondsworth, Middlesex: Pelican, 1973).

[46] Although they are merely a collection of various documents (memoirs, yearbooks, and so on), the narratives in *Taida yiyun hainianshi (I) Rizhishiqi* clearly reveal such Whiggish features. For a general description of those sources, See Lin Jichong, *Taida yiyun hainianshi (I) Rizhishiqi,* preface, i–iii.

[47] Zhang Henghao, ed., *Yangkui ji* (The Collected Works of Yangkui) (Taipei: Qianwei, 1991), 85–96.

[48] For a brief description of this system, see Fan Tianji, "Jiyaobao: Banshijiqian de jijiuxiang" (Jiyaobao: The First-Aid Box a Half Century Ago), *Mingshenghao*, October 13, 2001.

[49] Yang Wenshan, "Trends in Life Expectancy and Cause-Specific Death in Colonial Taiwan, 1906–1935." In *Proceedings of the Conference on Asian Population History.* Taipei: Academia Sinica, 1996, 5.

[50] Although the policy of Taihoku Imperial University was nondiscrimination, according to Wu Mincha the university accepted no more than 20 percent Taiwanese

students each year. Wu Mincha, *Taiwan jindaishi yenchiu* (the Study of Modern Taiwanese History) (Taipei: Daoxiang, 1991), 171–72.

[51] Xu Ruiyun, "Taiwan quangfuqian de yixue jiaoyu ji wode huiyi" (Medical Education in Taiwan before World War II and My Memories of It), in Lin Jichong, *Taida yiyun baimianshi (I) Rizhishiqi,* 66.

[52] Tsukahara Togô, ed., *Toajia no kagaku to teikokushogi* (Articles on Science and Technology in East Asia) (Tokyo: Kôseisha, 2006), 210–14.

[53] Kôseishô, *Kôse shô gojunenshi* (The Fifty Years of the Ministry of Health and Welfare) (Tokyo: Kôsheishô, 1988), 339–43.

[54] National Archives of Japan, Digital Archive System, Call No. 01-2A-012-00, "Reitai igaku kekyushô kansei" (About the Institute of Tropical Medicine), document in the archives of the Diet Library, Tokyo, Japan.

[55] "Sanjunenmae ni okeru Taiwan no eiseijôkyô" (Sanitary Conditions in Taiwan Thirty Years Ago), *Taiwan igakukai zasshi* 10:107 (1911): 785.

[56] Fan Pingzhen, "A Review of Filariasis Study Focusing on Eradication in Quemoy," *Parasitology of National Yang-min Medical College,* special issue (1982): 136–38.

[57] Tanaka Shikeo, "Taiwanjin ni okeru Mikrofilaria nokensaku kiranabini rinsôdeki kansatsu" (The Temporary Investigation and Examination Results for *Microfilaria* in Taiwanese Cases), *Taiwan igakkukai zasshi* 389 (1937): 1815–25.

[58] Yokogawa Sada, Kobayashi Hidekazu, Kmoto Yushika, Osaka Kiyoshi, Io Mandoku, and Yokogawa Mulejyo, "Penhu Jima ni okeru bankerofuto shisoshô no ikigaku no chôsa" (The Epidemiological Investigation of *Bancrofti* at Penhu Isles), *Taiwan igakukai zasshi* 38:415 (1939): 1452–65.

[59] Huang Dengyun, "Taiwan Peingtong te wandanshô to ryukrusyo ni okeru bankerofuto shisoshô no ikigaku no chôsa" (The Epidemiological Investigation of *Bancrofti* at Wendan and Liuqiu of Peington, Taiwan), *Acta Japonia Medicina Tropicalis* 1:2–3 (1939): 411–35.

[60] Fan Pingzhen cited investigations between 1958 and 1962 that found filariasis cases in southwestern coastal Taiwan. His studies suggest that endemic filariasis in that area is caused by a single parasite, *Wuchereria Bancrofti.* The average infection rate is 1.5 percent, much lower than in Penghu Isle. See Y. T. Wu and C. T. Chen, "Filariasis Endemic Areas in Taiwan Proper, Part 1: Incidence of Bancroftian Microfilarial Infection among the Native People of Southern Taiwan," *Taiwan igakkukai zasshi* 59 (1960): 262, 1163; and Y. T. Wu, P. T. Tseng, and C. T. Chen, "Recent Advances in the Study of Filariasis and Its Control in Taiwan," *Gonggongweiseng* (Public Health) 1 (1963): 1.

[61] Fan Pingzhen, "A Review of Filariasis Study" 137.

[62] Tokyo daigaku ikagaku kenkyûjyo (Institute of Medical Science), ed., *Densenbyô kenkyûsho ikagaku kenkyûsho byakunen no ayumi* (The One Hundred Years from the Institute of Infectious Disease to the Institute of Medical Science) (Tokyo: University of Tokyo, 1992), 13–15.

[63] Iijima Wataru, *Mararia to teikoku* (Malaria and Empire) (Tokyo: University of Tokyo Press, 2005), 36–37.

[64] Iijima Wataru, *Pesuto to kindai Chugoku* (Plague and Modern China) (Tokyo: Kemmbun shuppan, 2000), 113–14, 180–84.

[65] Ibid., 176–86.

[66] Iijima Wataru,, *Mararia to teikoku*, 168–71. Manchukuo was the Japanese name for Manchuria.

[67] Odaka Takeshi, *Densenbyo kenkyujyo* (The Institute of Infectious Disease) (Tokyo: Gakkai shuppan senta, 1992), 369.

[68] Taiwan Sôtokufu, ed., *Nanshi Nanyo no Iryoshisetsu* (The Medical Institutions of South China and Southeast Asia) (Taihoku: Taiwan Sôtokufu, 1936).

[69] Iijima, *Mararia to teikoku*, 122–23.

[70] Kato Shigeo, "Shanhai shizen kagaku kenkyujyo no setsuritsu kouso" (The Establishment Plan for the Shanghai Institute for Natural Science), *Nenpo kagaku gijutsu,shakai* (Japanese Journal of Science, Technology, and Society) 6 (1997): 1–34.

[71] For the leftist movement's promotion of social medicine in Japan, see T. Kawakami and S. Kanbayashi, eds., *Kunisaki Teido, teiko no igakusha* (Kunisaki Teido as a Medical Scientist of Resistance) (Tokyo: Kieso Shobo, 1970), 122, 131, 181.

[72] Komiya Yoshitaka, "Iryo shakai ka no zengo iijyo" (The Process of Medical Socialization), in T. Kawakami and Y. Komiya, eds., *Iryo shakai ka no dohyo* (The Process of Socializing Medicine) (Tokyo: Keiso Shobo, 1969), 23–33.

[73] Iijima, *Mararia to teikoku*, 148–49, 165, 187–88.

[74] Y. Yamane, "Shanhai shizen kagaku kenkyujyo iho somokuji" (Catalogue of Academic Articles in the *Journal of the Shanghai Institute for Natural Science*), in *Tokyo joshi daigaku kiyo ronshu* (Essays and Studies: Science Reports of Tokyo Women's Christian University) 30:1 (1979), 22–38.

[75] The journal was published by the Shanghai Union Medical Association. See *Toa igaku* (East Asian Medicine) 1 (1940): 2, 11, 139.

[76] Komiya Yoshitaka, "Mararia boatsu no ichijuyo shudan toshiteno anoferesu

bokumetsu ni tsuite" (On the Anti-anopheles Method of Malaria Control), *Toa igaku* 1 (1940): 188.

[77] Iijima, *Mararia to teikoku*, 165.

[78] Shimojyo Kumaichi, "Nanshi kanton chihou ni okeru mararia chosa hokoku" (Report on Malaria in Guangdong, South China), *Tokyo iji shinshi* (Tokyo Medical Journal) 3177 (1940): 116–38.

[79] Iijima, *Mararia to teikoku*, 212–13.

[80] George Basalla, "The Spread of Western Science," *Science* 156 (1967): 611.

[81] These medical schools were mainly supported by Christian missionaries. T. Umakoshi, *Kankoku kindai daigaku no seiritsu to tenkai* (The Formation and Development of the Modern University System in Korea) (Nagoya: University of Nagoya Press, 1995), 65–66.

[82] Keijo igaku senmon gakkô (Keijo Medical College), *Keijo igaku senmon gakkô ichiran* (Handbook for Keijo Medical College) (Keijo: Keijo igaku senmon gakkô, 1931), 5.

[83] Umakoshi, *Kankoku kindai daigaku no seiritsu to tenkai*, 65–66.

[84] Kitasato kenkyujyo (Kitasato Institute), *Kitasato kenkyujyo gojunenshi* (The Fifty-Year History of the Kitasato Institute) (Tokyo: Kitasato kenkyujyo, 1966), 676–81.

[85] Iijima, *Mararia to teikoku*, 136–38.

[86] For the process through which *tropical medicine* became a synonym for *colonial medicine* in the nineteenth and twentieth centuries in Western medicine, see two important books: Roy Macleod and Milton Lewis, eds., *Disease, Medicine, and Empire* (London: Routledge, 1988); and David Arnold, ed., *Warm Climates and Western Medicine: The Emergence of Tropical Medicine, 1500–1900* (Amsterdam: Rodopi, 1996).

[87] For example, although the League of Nations launched a campaign of international relief for victims of the plague epidemic in Manchuria in 1910–11, the Japanese claimed the credit for preventive action by providing their own epidemiological statistics at conferences in 1910 in Manila and 1912 in Hong Kong. Hiroshi Nishiura, "Epidemiology of a Primary Pneumonic Plague in Kantoshu, Manchuria, from 1910 to 1911: Statistical Analysis of Individual Records Collected by the Japanese Empire," *International Journal of Epidemiology* 35:4 (2006): 1059–65.

[88] Iijima, *Pesuto to kindai Chugoku*, 267–68.

[89] Far Eastern Association of Tropical Medicine, ed., *Transactions of the Biennial Congress Held at Hong Kong* (Hong Kong: Far Eastern Association of Tropical Medicine, 1912), v.

[90] *Tokyo mainichi shinbun*, October 18, 1925.

[91] Ibid.

[92] Iijima, *Mararia to teikoku*, 171–80.

[93] Shimojyo Kumaichi, "Nanhôseikatsuken to wa ga retaiigaku kenkyûjyo" (The Southern Life Cycle and the Study of Tropical Medicine), *Taiwan jipo* 24:1 (1942): 66–70.

[94] For details, see Miyahara Hatsuo, "Taikoku no mararia chyôsa owarite" (About the Empire and the Malaria Survey), *Taiwan no ikai* (Taiwan's Medical Circle) 2:6 (1943): 330–33.

[95] Setoguchi Akihisa, "Igaku, kiseichôgaku, konchôgaku: Nippon niokeru retaibyôkenkyu no tenkai" (Medicine, Epidemiology, and Public Health: The Beginning of Tropical Medicine in Japan), *Kagakutetsugaku kagakushi kenkyu* 1 (2006): 134.

[96] Liu Shi-yung, "Zhanqian riwen yixue quanxi shumu" (Medical Books in the Prewar Period), research report submitted to the Japan-Taiwan Exchange Center, Taipei, 1998.

[97] *Taiwan no ikai* 1:1 (1942): 23.

[98] Yokogawa Sadamu and Morishita Kaoru, "Minamitaiheiyô no kokukoku no jûyôna kiseichôbyo" (Important Parasites in Various Countries in the South Pacific Ocean) and "Shinatairiku no kiseichôbyo no gaikyô," both in *Saishin jintaikiseichôgakuteiyô* (The Latest Study of Human Parasitology) (Tokyo: Tobôdô, 1943), 16–18, 50–52.

[99] Miyahara Hatsuo, "Mararia no chiryo" (A Treatment for Malaria), *Kyudai iho* (Kyushu University Medical Journal) 12:6 (1938): 1.

[100] Iijima, *Mararia to teikoku*, 208–9.

[101] Hiroshige Tôru, *Kagaku no shakaishi* (The Social History of Science) (Tokyo: Chûô koronsha, 1973), 200–203.

[102] Although Zheng Zhimin blamed the situation on the long-term friction between Tokyo Imperial University and other schools, the explanation might be more complicated than that. See Zheng Zhimin, "Zhimin yangban huo tairen yingxiong," 107–9.

[103] To protest the unfair promotion of colleagues from Todai, Japanese faculties at the affiliated Medical College of Taihoku Imperial University resigned en masse in 1937. See Lin Jichong, *Taida yiyun hainianshi (I) Rizhishiqi*, 47, 53.

[104] Reidai igaku kenkyujyo (Institute of Tropical Medicine), ed., *Nekken gojunen no ayumi* (The Fifty-Year History of the Institute of Tropical Medicine) (Nagasaki: Reidai igaku kenkyujyo, 1993), 16–18.

[105] Iijima, *Mararia to teikoku*, 208–9.

[106] Ibid., 208–17.

[107] S. E. Moolton, "Measures Taken for Reform of Medical Education in Japan," *Nippon ishi shinpo*, February 27, 1946.

[108] Wang Jinmao, "Taiwan weisheng xingzheng" (The Hygienic Administration in Taiwan), in *Taiwan yiyao weisheng zonglan* (A General Overview of Hygiene in Taiwan) (Taipei: Yiyaoixinwenshe, 1972), 17.

[109] Fu Dawei, *Yaxiya de xinshengti* (The Asian New Body) (Taipei: Socio, 2005), 197–207.

[110] For the details of this debate and its impact on historiography in Taiwan, see Chang Lung-chih, "Zhiminxindaixing yu Taiwan jindaishi yenjiu: Bentu shixueshi yu fangfalun chuyi" (Colonial Modernity and the Modern History of Taiwan: A Preliminary Discussion of Local Historiography and Methodology), in Wakabayashi Masahiro and Wu Mizha, eds., *Kuajie de Taiwanshi yenjiu: Yu dongyashi de jiacuo* (The Taiwan Study on the Crossing Zone: Interacting with the History of East Asia) (Taipei: Bozhongzhe, 2004), 133–60.

[111] George W. Barclay, *Colonial Development and Population in Taiwan* (Princeton: Princeton University Press, 1954), 145–46.

[112] Chen Shaoxin, "Taiwan renkoushi de jigewenti," in Chen Shaoxin, *Taiwandi renkou bianqian yu shehui bianqian* 18.

[113] Ibid., 96–97.

[114] Mohammad Mirzaee, "Trends and Determinants of Mortality in Taiwan, 1895–1975," PhD diss., University of Pennsylvania, 1979, 191–94.

[115] Ibid., 205.

[116] Chen Kuanzheng and Yeh Tienfeng, "Rijushidai yilai Taiwan diqu renko nianling zucheng zhi bianqian" (Changes in Age Cohorts of the Taiwanese Population since the Japanese-Occupied Period), *Taiwandaxue renkoxuekan* (National Taiwan University Journal of Demography) 6 (1982): 99–114.

[117] Ibid., 105.

[118] Yang Wenshan, "Trends in Life Expectancyand Cause-Specific Death in Colonial Taiwan, 1906–1935," in *Proceedings of the Conference on Asian Population History* (Taipei: Academia Sinica, 1996), 4–5.

[119] Barclay, *Colonial Development and Population in Taiwan*, 133–73.

[120] John D. Durand, "Comments on S. H. Preston's Paper: Causes and Consequences of Mortality Declines in Less Developed Countries during the Twentieth Century," in Richard A. Easterlin, ed., *Population and Economic Change in Developing Countries*

(Chicago: University of Chicago Press, 1980), 341–47.

[121] Chen Kuanzhang, "Rinkozhuanxing de xingshidontai" (The Dynamic Form of Demographic Transition), *Rikoxuekan* (Journal of Population Studies) 8 (1985): 1–23.

[122] Wang Demu and Chen Wenling, "Rizhishidai yilai Taiwandiqu zhi siwanglu bianqian" (Changes in Mortality Rates in Taiwan since the Japanese-Ruled Period), in *Ershi shiji de Taiwan renko bianqian yentaohui lunwenji* (Proceedings of the Symposium on Demographic Transition in Twentieth-Century Taiwan) (Taizhong: Zhonggong renko xuehui, 1986), 57–78.

[123] Chen Shaoxin, *Taiwan renko de bianqian yu shehui bianqian*, 20–21.

[124] Mirzaee, "Trends and Determinants of Mortality in Taiwan," 205.

[125] Li Xinfeng, "Jidujiao yu Taiwan yiliao weisheng de xiandaihua: Yi Zhanghua jidujiao yiyuan weizhongxin zhi tantao" (Christianity and the Modernization of Taiwanese Medicine and Public Health: A Study of the Zhanghua Christian Hospital), MA thesis, National Taiwan Normal University, 1989, 19–23.

[126] Zhuang Yungming, *Taiwan yiliaoshi: Yi Taida yiyun wei zhuzhou* (The History of Medicine and Therapy in Taiwan) (Taipei: Yunliu, 1998), 12.

[127] Chen Yungxin, *Taiwan yiliao fazhanshi* (The Development History of Medicine and Therapy in Taiwan) (Taipei: Yuedan, 1997), 44–45.

[128] For one example of such an attitude, see Xu Xiqin's words on plague control: "The colonial government adopted necessary activities because the plague epidemic indiscriminately harmed the population in Taiwan." Xu Xiqin, ed. and trans., *Taiwan zongdufu gongwen leizhuan weisheng shiliao huibian* (Nantou: Taiwansheng wenxian weiyunhui, 2000), 179.

[129] See Alfred Crosby, *Ecological Imperialism: The Biological Expansion of Europe, 900–1900* (Cambridge: Cambridge University Press, 1993).

[130] David Arnold, "Medicine and Colonialism," in William Bynum and Roy Porter, eds., *Companion Encyclopedia of the History of Medicine* (London: Routledge, 1993), 2:1394.

[131] Geoffrey C. Bowker and Susan Leigh Star, *Sorting Things Out: Classification and Its Consequences* (Cambridge: MIT Press, 2000).

[132] Henry Lowood, Review of Geoffrey C. Bowker and Susan Leigh Star, *Sorting Things Out: Classification and Its Consequences, Technology and Culture* 42:2 (2001): 392–93.

[133] It is interesting to note that skepticism about colonial statistics is, again, arising among young graduate students at the master's degree level. For examples, see the discussion of tuberculosis statistics in Wu Jieru, "Feilao yu feijiehe: Rizhisiqi consumption yu tuberculosis zha Taiwan de jiaohui" (Consumption and Pulmonary

Tuberculosis: The Interaction between Consumption and Tuberculosis in Japanese-Occupied Taiwan), MA thesis, Taipei Medical University, 2006, 63–64; Cai Chenghao, "Bingdu, tingke, chucao: Xibanyaliukan qinxixia de Taiwan (1918–1920)" (Virus, Suspending Class, and Hunting Head: Taiwan under the Invasion of Spanish Flu (1918–1920), in *Proceedings of the Conference of Medical Humanity* (Taipei: Taipei Medical University, 2004), 28; and Wu Jiezun, "Rizhishidai yilai Taiwandiqu jibing zhuanxing mushi zhi tantao" (The Transition Model of Disease Patterns since Japanese Rule in Taiwan), in *Proceedings of the Annual Meeting of the Taiwan Association of Demography* (Taipei: Taiwan Association of Demography, 2006), 11–12.

[134] Fu Dawei, *Yaxiya de xinshengti*, 94–96, 99.

[135] Chen Shaoxin examined the mortality trend and concluded that the health transition took place during the 1930s in Taiwan. However, Chen did not study the trend from the viewpoint of epidemiology. See Chen Shaoxin, *Taiwan de renkou bianqian yu shehui bianqian,* 140.

[136] Liu Shiyung, "Differential Mortality in Colonial Taiwan (1895–1945)," *Annales Démographie Historique* 1 (2004): 231.

[137] Liu Shiyung, "Rizhishiqi Taiwandiqu de jibienjiego yenbian" (Changing Disease Patterns in Colonial Taiwan), *Xinshixue* 13:4 (2002): 203.

[138] William Siler, "A Competing-Risk Model for Animal Mortality," *Ecology* 60 (1979): 750–57.

[139] See the figure in Liu Shiyung, "Differential Mortality in Colonial Taiwan," 238.

[140] Ibid., 245–46.

[141] In Japan, Saito Osamu's study of the Tokugawa to Meiji periods suggests that the level of infant mortality was not very high after the late Tokugawa. See Saito Osamu, "Infant Mortality in Pre-transition Japan: Levels and Trends," in Alain Bideau, Bertrand Desjardins, and Hector Perez Brignoli, eds., *Infant and Child Mortality in the Past* (Oxford: Clarendon, 1997), 135–53.

[142] Wu Jiezun, "Rizhishidai yilai Taiwandiqu jibing zhuanxing mushi zhi tantao," 11–12.

[143] Kelly Olds, "The Biological Standard of Living in Taiwan under Japanese Occupation," *Economics and Human Biology* 1:2 (2003): 187–206.

[144] Liu Shiyung, "Public Health Investigation and Statistics in Colonial Taiwan," in *Introduction: The Archives of Social Affairs in Colonies—Taiwan* (Tokyo: Modern Information Publishers, 2001), 1–21.

[145] Western scholars have already contributed a lot to such study. See Richard Fogel et al., eds., "Secular Changes in American and British Stature and Nutrition," *Journal of Interdisciplinary History* 14:2 (1983): 445–81; and John Komlos, ed., *Stature, Living Standards, and Economic Development: Essays in Anthropometric History* (Chicago: University of Chicago Press, 1994).

[146] The primary data are the health examination records from individual personnel files of Taiwan provincial government employees measured in the 1950s and 1960s. These records are not officially open, and I thank the archive and its staff for their support in locating suitable records and allowing our research assistant to collect the relevant personal data. These are held at the provincial archive, Nantou. Height and other individual data were collected for 2,878 subjects. There were 2,783 males born between 1899 and 1945 and 95 females born between 1921 and 1945. Later we discovered that we had a male subsample whose occupations and education differed markedly. They were unskilled farm laborers with only elementary education, most born in Chiayi or nearby areas in South Taiwan in 1928, and their file indicated that the record was related to the military .

[147] James M. Tanner, "Introduction: Growth in Height as a Mirror of the Standard of Living," in Komlos, *Stature, Living Standards, and Economic Development,* 1–6.

[148] Richard H. Steckel, "Stature and the Standard of Living," *Journal of Economic Literature* 33 (1995): 1903–40.

[149] In that article, Stephen Morgan and Liu Shiyung, "Was Japanese Colonialism Good for the Welfare of Taiwanese?" *China Quarterly* No. 192 (2007):990–1017, figures 4 and 5 and table 6 reveal that the height of male Taiwanese increased continuously after 1900.

[150] For instance, Samuel Ho claims that colonial Taiwan was "an agricultural appendage of Japan" in an unfair sugar-rice exchange relationship. See Samuel P. S. Ho, *Economic Development of Taiwan, 1860–1970* (New Haven: Yale University Press, 1978), 29. Christopher Howe, in a recent review of Taiwan's economic development, wrote that income data are "too aggregated" to estimate the effects of colonialism on individual welfare, but the Taiwanese rice and sugar farmers were "controlled in their income and choices" by "Japanese monopolistic power in the processing and commercial sectors." See Christopher Howe, "Taiwan in the Twentieth Century: Model or Victim? Development Problems in a Small Asian Economy," in Richard Louis Edmonds and Steven M. Goldstein, eds., *Taiwan in the Twentieth Century: A Retrospective View*, China Quarterly Special Issues, new ser., no. 1 (Cambridge: Cambridge University Press, 2001), 43–45.

[151] For instance, Samuel Ho argued that rural income and consumption rose slowly until the 1930s and thereafter declined. He reasoned that Japanese control of the rice

and sugar markets depressed prices for farmers and monopolistic taxes on consumer goods further reduced income. Yujiro Hayami and Verno Ruttan make a similar argument. See Samuel P. S. Ho, "Agricultural Transformation under Colonialism: The Case of Taiwan," *Journal of Economic History* 28:3 (1968): 313–40; and Yujiro Hayami and Verno W. Ruttan, "Korean Rice, Taiwan Rice, and Japanese Agricultural Stagnation: Economic Consequences of Colonialism," *Quarterly Journal of Economics* 84:4 (1970): 562–89. Contrarily, Mizoguchi Toshiyuki showed a rapid rise in rural and industrial real wages from the 1910s on, with a peak in 1930 and a slow decline thereafter, although wages remained above the level of the 1910s. Based on a similar estimation, Ho Yhimin concluded that rural consumption rose, which implies that the rural sector retained a larger share of the output gains in agriculture than food availability data suggest. See Mizoguchi Toshiyuki, "Consumer Prices and Real Wages in Taiwan and Korea under Japanese Rule," *Hitotsubashi Journal of Economics* 13:1 (1972): 40–56; and Ho Yhimin, "Taiwan's Agricultural Transformation under Colonialism: A Critique," *Journal of Economic History* 31:3 (1971): 678–79.

[152] Ho, "Agricultural Transformation under Colonialism," 336.

[153] Zhang Hanyu, "A Study of the Living Conditions of Farmers in Taiwan, 1931–1950," in Zhang Hanyu, *Economic Development and Income Distribution in Taiwan: The Essays of Dr. Chang Han-Yu* (Taipei: Sun Ming, 1983), 4:65–111.

[154] Samuel Ho published his book in 1971 and revised it in 1978. See Samuel P. S. Ho, *The Developmental Policy of the Japanese Colonial Government in Taiwan, 1895–1945* (New Haven: Yale University Press, 1971); and Ho, *Economic Development of Taiwan.* For the book review and comparison, see Ho Yhimin, "Review of Samuel P. S. Ho, *Economic Development of Taiwan, 1860–1970,*" *Economic Development and Cultural Change* 28:3 (1980): 637–44.

[155] Ho, *Economic Development of Taiwan,* 96–98.

[156] Yeh Shujen. "Economic Growth and the Farm Economy in Colonial Taiwan, 1895–1945," PhD diss., University of Pittsburg, 1991, 202–34.

[157] Lai He, "Asi," in Li Nanheng, ed., *Lai He quanji* (The Collected Works of Lai He) (Taipei: Mintan, 1979), 336.

[158] Just as political decolonization has been studied in Taiwan for over fifty years, postcolonialism became popular in the 1980s with an exclusive focus on cultural studies. See Liao Binghui, *Huiku xiandai: Hoxiandai yu hozhimin lunwenji* (Reviewing Modernity: Articles on Postmodernity and Postcolonization) (Taipei: Maitian, 1994), 18. According to Warwick Anderson, "A postcolonial perspective suggests fresh ways to study the changing political economies of capitalism and science, the mutual reorganisation of the global and the local, the increasing transnational traffic of

people, practices, technologies, and contemporary contests over intellectual property." Warwick Anderson, "Postcolonial Technoscience," *Social Studies of Science* 5–6 (2002): 643. Current studies of colonial medicine in Taiwan have not yet matched the criteria he proposed.

Conclusion

[1] The Rangaku (Dutch studies; for a brief discussion, see chap. 1) in the late Tokugawa period created a framework of support for the Meiji Restoration and provided a stable foundation for westernization. See Harry Harootunian, *Toward Restoration* (Berkeley: University of California Press, 1984), xix, xvi; and *Things Seen and Unseen: Discourse and Ideology in Tokugawa Nativism* (Chicago: University of Chicago Press, 1988).

[2] A Whiggish optimism and confidence in scientific or modern Western medicine was prevalent between the mid–nineteenth and mid–twentieth centuries. Japan after the 1870s was hardly an exception. For a brief but inspiring discussion of the Japanese attitude toward Western science, see Satofuka Fumihiko, "Some Aspects of the Debate on the Scientific Tradition in Japan," *Historia Scientiarum* 2 (1992): 61–69.

[3] Daniel R. *Headrick, The Tools of Empire: Technology and European Imperialism in the Nineteenth Century* (Oxford: Oxford University Press, 1981).

[4] Lenore *Manderson, "Wireless Wars in the Eastern Arena: Epidemiological Surveillance, Disease Prevention, and the Work of the Eastern Bureau of the League of Nations Health Organisation, 1925–1942," in Paul Weindling, ed., International Health Organisations and Movements, 1918–1939 (Cambridge: Cambridge University Press, 1995), 109–33.*

[5] George W. Basalla, "The Spread of Western Science: A Three-Stage Model Describes the Introduction of Modern Science into Any Non-European Nation," *Science* 3775 (1967): 611–22.

[6] "[Postwar] Japanese historians of science have sought to develop Basalla's model for, as Blussé has noted, the historiography of expansion in Japan has tended to justify Japan's 'right' to expand overseas in Asia." Morris Fraser Low, "The Butterfly and the Frigate: Social Studies of Science in Japan," *Social Studies of Science* 19:2 (1989): 320. See also L. Blussé, "Japanese Historiography and European Sources," in P. C. Emmer and W. L. Wesseling, eds., *Reappraisals in Overseas History: Essays on Post-war Historiography about European Expansion* (The Hague: Martinus Nijhoff for Leiden University Press, 1979), 193–221.

[7] For example, see André Gunder Frank, *Capitalism and Underdevelopment in Latin America* (New York: Monthly Review Press, 1969); and Immanuel Wallerstein, *The Modern World System* (New York: Academic Press, 1974). Many critiques, however, contained a similar of center-periphery pattern and diffusionist models of economy. For

the review of these critiques, see Gilbert M. Joseph, "Close Encounters: Toward a New Cultural History of U.S.–Latin American Relations," in Gilbert M. Joseph, Catherine C. LeGrand, and Ricardo Salvatore, eds., *Close Encounters of Empire: Writing the Cultural History of U.S.–Latin American Relations* (Durham and London: Duke University Press, 1998), 3–46.

[8] David Wade Chambers, "Period and Process in Colonial and National Science," in Nathan Reingold and Marc Rothenberg, eds., *Scientific Colonialism: A Cross-Cultural Comparison* (Washington, DC: Smithsonian Institution Press, 1987), 314. See also David Wade Chambers and Richard Gillespie, "Locality in the History of Science: Colonial Science, Technoscience, and Indigenous Knowledge," in Roy MacLeod, ed., *Nature and Empire: Science and the Colonial Enterprise, Osiris* 15 (2000): 231.

[9] Paolo Palladino and Michael Worboys, "Science and Imperialism," *Isis* 84 (1993): 99–100.

[10] Thomas McKeown, *The Role of Medicine: Dream, Mirage, or Nemesis* (London: Nuffield Provincial Hospitals Trust, 1976); *The Rise of Modern Population* (New York: Academic Press, 1976). Unfortunately, while this viewpoint has influenced many contemporary studies of demography, as well as public health, it has not yet been applied to colonial medicine in Taiwan.

[11] Along with Taiwanese historians, some Korean scholars have adopted Western views on colonial medicine. For example, see Park Yunjae, "Medical Policies toward Indigenous *Medicine* in Colonial Korea and India," *Korea Journal* 46:1 (2006): 198–224.

[12] Andrew Cunningham and Bridie Andrews, eds., *Western Medicine as Contested Knowledge* (Manchester: Manchester University Press, 1997), 12.

[13] Warwick Anderson, *Colonial Pathologies: American Tropical Medicine, Race, and Hygiene in the Philippines* (Durham: Duke University Press, 2006). Anderson provides an excellent discussion of the literature on colonial medicine and the contextualization of medical practice in colonial territory.

[14] Basalla, "The Spread of Western Science," 617.

[15] Medical westernization in Japan began in the 1870s, roughly twenty years before the occupation of Taiwan, and medical resources such as manpower and facilities were still insufficient in the 1890s. For the details, see chapter 1.

[16] Naikaku Tôkekyoku, ed., *Meiji go nen ikô wagakoku no jinkô* (The Population of Our Country since Meiji 5 Year) (Tokyo: Naikaku Tôkekyoku, 1930).

[17] See chapter 4.

[18] As discussed in the introduction and chapter 1, Gotô Shinpei's theory of *Biologische Principien* has been portrayed as a guide for Japanese colonial medicine in Taiwan

by many Taiwanese historians. However, close observation might reveal that he had much less influence and accomplished less than Takagi Tomoe did. For a good example of Taiwanese historians on Gotô Shinpei's theory of *Biologische Principien*, see Fan Yanqiu, "Xinyixue zai Taiwan de shijian" (The Practice of New Medicine in Taiwan [1898–1906]), *Xinshixue* (New History) 9:3 (1998): 49–86.

[19] Based on Gotô Shinpei's educational background and the contemporary documents discussed in chapter 2, I hardly agree with Mark Peattie's characterization of Gotô as "superbly trained in the medical profession in Germany, [and] widely read in the contemporary literature of colonialism." Mark Peattie, "Japanese Attitudes toward Colonialism, 1895–1945," in Roman Myers and Mark Peattie, eds., *The Japanese Colonial Empire, 1895–1945* (Princeton: Princeton University Press, 1984), 83.

[20] Takekoshi Yosaburo, *Japanese Rule in Formosa*, trans. George Braithwaite (London: Longmans, 1907), vii.

[21] Although Ôjima Masamitsu admired Takagi's contribution to medical services and his endless efforts to promote clinical medicine in Taiwan, he criticized the whole medical system in Taiwan for being under the control of clinicians, a group of moderate professionals who knew nothing about the virtues of the laboratory medicine taught exclusively in imperial universities. Ôjima Masamitsu, "Ochipo o hiroite" (Picking Spikes), in Du Congming, ed., *Takagi Tomoe sensei tsuiokushi* (Collection in Remembrance of Takagi Tomoe) (Tokyo: Takagi Tomoe kinenji iinkai, 1957), 21–22.

[22] The malariologist Morishita Kaoru hoped the data he collected in Taiwan would benefit ongoing research on malaria treatments in Japan. Morishita Kaoru, *Maraia no bôekigaku to yobô: Taiwan ni okeru Nihon tôji jitai no kiroku to kenkyû* (The Prevention and Precaution of Malaria: Records and Research in Taiwan under Japanese Rule) (Tokyo: Nippon itaikikuya, 1976), 125–29.

[23] The teacher-student model is another concept favored by historians of science to explain the "long-term, one-way traffic in knowledge [that] has occurred from 'West' to 'East.'" See Low, "The Butterfly and the Frigate," 328–29.

[24] I do not mean that the Taiwanese doctor was a tool of the colonial government, as Yao Rendo suggests, but I do believe the Taiwanese doctor was trained to appreciate Japanese teachers and their norms. Yao Rendo, Review of Miriam Ming-cheng Lo, *Doctors within Borders: Professions, Ethnicity, and Modernity in Colonial Taiwan, Taiwanese Sociology* 4 (2002): 252–57. I simply mean that in bringing education in modern medicine to Taiwan the Japanese filled most teaching positions with Japanese nationals.

[25] For her illustration of the argument of Taiwanese doctors' self-identity as the colonized, see Miriam Ming-cheng Lo, *Doctors within Borders: Professions, Ethnicity, and Modernity in Colonial Taiwan* (Berkeley: University of California Press, 2002), 193.

[26] As Morris Fraser Low notes in "The Butterfly and the Frigate," the teacher-student relationship is very traditional and highly valued in many Confucian-influenced cultures, including those of Japan and China.

[27] Ogata Norio, *Saikin heno chôsen: Nihon no saikingakushi* (Challenges to Bacteria: The History of Bacteriology in Japan) (Tokyo: Nippon hôsô shuppan kyôka, 1940), 184.

[28] For cases and general feelings about this attitude, see Guo Wenhua and Yeh Lin, "Yixue yu renwen lishi de jiaohui: Fang Zhuang Yungming tan Taiwan yixueshi" (The Interaction between Medicine and Humanity: An Interview with Zhuang Yunmin on Taiwan's Medical History), *Yiwang* (Hope) 8 (1995): 19–21.

[29] Takagi Tomoe, "Dôkakai ni tsuite (taishô nana nen)" (To the Society of Assimilation. Taishô 4 Year)," in Du Congming, *Takagi Tomoe sensei tsuiokeshi*, 52.

[30] Ibid.

[31] Quoted in Shinobu Seiizaburô, *Gotô Shinpei: Kagakuteki seiijika no syôgai* (Gotô Shinpei: The Career of a Scientific Politician) (Tokyo: Hakubunkan, 1941), 133–34.

[32] Kitaoka Shinichi, *Gotô Shinpei: Gaikô to Pojon* (Gotô Shinpei: Diplomacy and Vision) (Tokyo: Chuokoronsha, 1988), 38–41. Kitaoka's interpretation appears to have influenced many Taiwanese scholars, who understand Gotô's metaphor not as racist but as reflecting his interest in applying biological principles to scientific colonization in Taiwan. See Xu Jidun, *Taiwan jindai fazhanshi* (The Modern History of Development in Taiwan) (Taipei: Qienwei, 1996), 267.

[33] Ernst Klee, *Deutsche Medizin im Dritten Reich: Karrieren vor und nach 1945* (German Medicine during the Third Reich: Its Development before and after 1945) (Frankfurt am Main: Fischer, 2001), 93.

[34] Zheng Zhimin, "Zhimin yangban huo tairen yingxiong: Shirun Du Congmin yu rizhishiqi Taiwan de yixue jiaoyu" (A Colonist's Sample or a Taiwanese Hero: The Studies of Du Congming and Medical Education in the Japanese-Ruled Period), *Taiwan tushuguan guanli jikan* (Taiwanese Journal of Library Management) 1:1 (2005): 104–5.

[35] William McNeill, *Plagues and Peoples* (Oxford: Basil Blackwell, 1977).

[36] Sheldon Watts, *Epidemics and History: Disease, Power, and Imperialism* (New Haven: Yale University Press, 1997), 207.

[37] Ibid., 167–212, 269–79.

[38] Farley stated that "the author does, perhaps, attempt to do too much. The reader is often led away from the central focus of the disease as Watts cuts broad swaths through periods of history and leaves the reader grasping at various -isms with which many will not be familiar." John Farley, Review of Sheldon Watts, *Epidemics and History: Disease, Power, and Imperialism, Canadian Bulletin of Medical History* 16:2 (1999): 388.

[39] Zaheer Baber, "Colonizing Nature: Scientific Knowledge, Colonial Power, and the Incorporation of India into the Modern World-System," *British Journal of Sociology* 52:1 (2001): 48.

[40] The arms of the policeman-bodhisattva on one poster not only caught thieves and assisted those in need but also administered inoculations and performed nursing tasks. Taihokushû keimubu, ed., *Taihoku keisatsu eisei tenrankai shashinchô* (Photo Album of the Taihoku Prefecture Police Hygiene Exhibition) (Taihoku: Taiwan nichinichi simposha, 1926), 44.

[41] "Ping jingcha weisheng zhanlanhui de jiazhi" (On the Value of the Police Hygiene Exhibition), *Taiwan minpo* 82 (1925).

[42] Although she focuses on the education of Native Americans, I found that Cathryn McConaghy's inspiring phrase "the indigenous people" become objects to be "done to, talked about, and lifted up by the efforts of those white people who are capable and who know," can also be applied to colonial Taiwan. Cathryn McConaghy, *Rethinking Indigenous Education: Culturalism, Colonialism, and the Politics of Knowing* (Flaxton, Queensland, Australia: Post Pressed, 2000), 148.

[43] David Arnold, "Medicine and Colonialism," in William F. Bynum and Roy Porter, eds., *Companion Encyclopedia of the History of Medicine* (London: Routledge, 1993), 2:1411.

[44] Hobsbawm used *nations* in the original statement, but it would also be true when we consider his argument in the context of building a modern colony. Eric Hobsbawm, *Nations and Nationalism* (Cambridge: Cambridge University Press, 1991), 10.

[45] Arnold, "Medicine and Colonialism," 2:1406.

[46] Baber, "Colonizing Nature," 46. The author describes the process of building the modern Indian nation-state. However, the statement could also be applied to the Japanese colonial government's attempt to build a modern colony.

[47] Megan Vaughan, *Curing Their Ills* (Oxford: Polity, 1991), 60.

[48] Soma Hewa, *Colonialism, Tropical Disease, and Imperial Medicine: Rockefeller Philanthropy in Sri Lanka* (Washington, DC: University Press of America, 1995), 14, 68.

[49] John Farley, Review of Soma Hewa, *Colonialism, Tropical Disease, and Imperial Medicine, Bulletin of the History of Medicine* 70:4 (1996): 723–24.

[50] Charles Rosenberg and Janet Golden, eds., *Framing Disease: Studies in Cultural History* (New Brunswick, NJ: Rutgers University, 1992), xv.

[51] George Rice and E. Palmer, "Pandemic Influenza in Japan, 1918–19: Mortality Patterns and Official Responses," *Journal of Japanese Studies* 19.2 (1993): 389–420.

[52] Cai Chenghau, "Bingdu, tingke, chucao: Xibanya liukan qinxixia de Taiwan (1918–20)" (Virus, Suspending Class, and Hunting Head: Taiwan under the Invasion of Spanish Flu (1918–1920)," in *Proceedings of the Conference of Medical Humanity* (Taipei: Taipei Medical University, 2004), 28.

[53] Vaughan, *Curing Their Ills*, 25.

[54] Western scholars have contributed much to such studies. See, for example, Robert Fogel et al., eds., "Secular Changes in American and British Stature and Nutrition," *Journal of Interdisciplinary History* 14:2 (1983): 445–81; and John Komlos, ed., *Stature, Living Standards, and Economic Development: Essays in Anthropometric History* (Chicago: University of Chicago Press, 1994).

[55] David Arnold, *Colonizing the Body: State Medicine and Epidemic Disease in Nineteenth-Century India* (Berkeley: University of California Press, 1993), 9–10.

[56] By "biomedicine," I simply mean the application of the principles of the natural sciences, especially biology and bacteriology, to medical therapy.

[57] Shula Marks, "What Is Colonial about Colonial Medicine and What Has Happened to Imperialism and Health?" *Social History of Medicine* 10:2 (1997): 205–19; Warwick Anderson, "Postcolonial Histories of Medicine," in Frank Huisman and John Harley Warner, eds., *Locating Medical History: The Stories and Their Meanings* (Baltimore: Johns Hopkins University Press, 2004), 285–306. Anderson states, "Historians of colonial medicine are now more likely to discern a deeper collusion between medicine and empire: the political economists among them describe more plausibly a colonial production of disease, and the more literary of them analyze medicine and public health as technical discourses of colonialism." Warwick Anderson, "Where Is the Postcolonial History of Medicine?" *Bulletin of the History of Medicine* 72:3 (1998): 523.

[58] My understanding of decolonization is inspired by current cultural studies of postcolonialism. Decolonization could be more a social and conceptual process than a political one, a process that decolonizes the social values and norms that the colonist inserted into the colonial society and neutralizes their interference with postcolonial society. Therefore, decolonization requires "an imaginative creation of a new form of consciousness and way of life." Such a process involves all parties in colonization and reflects "the relationship between power and culture, domination and the imaginary." Jan Nederveen Pieterse and Bhikhu Parekh, "Shifting Imaginaries: Decolonization,

Internal Decolonization, and Postcoloniality," in Jan Nederveen Pieterse and Bhikhu Parekh, eds., *The Decolonialization of Imagination: Culture, Knowledge, and Power* (London: Zed, 1995), 1–15.

Selected Bibliography

Three archival institutes provided major assistance for writing this book. Their holdings include not only important archives but also well-preserved books and journals published before 1945 that were essential to my research. They are (in alphabetical order) the National Archives of Japan, Tokyo; Rockefeller Archive Center, New York; and Taiwan Historica, Nantou, Taiwan.

This selective bibliography of documents related to Japanese colonial medicine in Taiwan includes books and articles by numerous authors, official documents, newspapers, pamphlets, and even pharmaceutical catalogues. Many early articles are not included here because many journals that predate the 1930s were later rebound by different institutions and the volumes renumbered, a situation that caused great difficulty in the early stages of research for this book. Articles from *Taiwan igakukai zasshi*, *Taiwan shinpo*, *Taiwan nichinichi shinpo*, and *Taiwan minpo* were omitted for this reason. Fortunately, the digitizing of archives and older publications in Taiwan has preserved these important articles. It is now possible to search *Taiwan igakukai zasshi* (nos. 1–480, 1902 to 1945) online via the Academia Sinica website—www.sinica.edu.tw. The archive of Taiwan Sôtokufu, which includes *Sôtokufu fupo*, *Taiwan Sôtokufu Archives*, and *Taiwan shiryo kôhon* (Collection of Taiwanese Historical Materials) can be accessed, with permission, from the Taiwan Historica website—www.th.gov.tw.

Despite its selective nature I hope that this bibliography will be useful to readers interested in the field of Japanese colonial medicine.

Government Reports, Journals, and Newspapers

The large number of medical and hygienic journals, newspapers, and government reports published during the colonial period provided essential material with which to gauge the impact of Japanese colonial medicine in Taiwan. I have listed only those periodicals that I reviewed systematically for the research. In all cases, the periodicals were part of the collections of the libraries at either Academia Sinica or the Taiwan Historica, both located in Taiwan. A small number of periodicals were accessed at the General Library of Tokyo University and the National Diet Library, Tokyo.

Government Reports

Chûô Eisei Kyoku (Central Bureau of Sanitation), ed. (*Eisei Kyoku Nenpo*) *Annual Report of the Central Sanitary Bureau.* Tokyo: Central Sanitary Bureau, various issues.

Far Eastern Association of Tropical Medicine, ed. *Transactions of Biennial Congress Held at Hong Kong.* Hong Kong: Far Eastern Association of Tropical Medicine, 1912.

Government-General of Taiwan (Taiwan Sôtokufu), ed. *Statistical Summary of Taiwan.* Tokyo: Japan Times Press, 1912.

Keijo igaku senmon gakkô (Keijo Medical College). *Keijo igaku senmon gakkô ichiran* (Handbook for Keijo Medical College). Keijo: Kiejyo igaku senmon gakkô, 1931.

Koseisho, ed. *Iseihyakunenshi* (The Hundred-Year History of Medical Regulations). Tokyo: Koseishoimukyoku, 1976.

League of Nations, ed. *Health Organisation in Japan* (League of Nations Report). Tokyo: League of Nations, Japan Office, 1925.

Minseibu Keisatsuka, ed. *Minsei taiyô* (Summary of Civil Affairs). Taihoku: Taiwan Sôtokufu, various issues.

Monbusho, ed., *Monbusho Nenpo* (Annual Reports of the Ministry of Education). Tokyo: Monbusho, various years.

Naikaku Tôkekyoku, ed. *Meiji go nen ikô wagakoku no jinkô* (The Population of Our Country since Meiji 5 Year). Tokyo: Naikaku Tôkekyoku, 1930.

Naimusho, ed. *Naimusho Nenpo* (Annual Report of the Ministry of Home Affairs). Tokyo: Naimusho, various years.

Naimusho Eiseikyoku, ed. *Isei gojônen shi* (The Fifty-Year History of the Medical System). Tokyo: Obunkai, 1925.

Nihon gôdôtsû shinsha, ed. *Taiwan taikan* (Overview of Taiwan). Taihoku: Nihon gôdôtsû shinsha, 1932.

Ninoshima rinji rikugun kenekijo, ed. *Ninoshima rinji rikugun kenekijo gyômu houkoku kouhen* (Business Report of the Army Quarantine Institute at Ninoshima). Tokyo: Ninoshima rinji rikugun kenekijo, 1896.

Nippon ijishinôsha, ed. *Nippon ijirenkan* (Annual Account of Registered Doctors in Japan). Tokyo: Nippon ijishinôsha, 1939.

Office of Inspector-General of Customs, ed. *Customs Medical Report (1876–77).* Shanghai: Inspector-General of Customs, 1886.

Sanitary Sector of the Government of Taiwan Governor-General, ed. *The Sanitation Regulation in Taiwan.* Taihoku: Sanitary Sector of the Government of Taiwan Governor-General, 1900.

Taichûchô, ed. *Taichûchô kyoiku eisei tenrankai shashinchô* (Photo Album of the Taichû Education Hygiene Exhibition). Taihoku: Arita shashinkan, 1918.

Taihoku igakkô, ed., *Sôritsu nijugo shyônen shukugakiji* (The Archive Collection of Twenty-five Years of Transformation). Taihoku: Taihoku igakkô, 1930.

Taihokushû keimubu, ed. *Taihoku keisatsu eisei tenrankai kiroku* (Record of the Taihoku Prefecture Police Hygiene Exhibition). Taohoku: Taiwan nichinichi simposha, 1926.

————. *Taihoku keisatsu eisei tenrankai shashinchô* (Photo Album of the Taihoku Prefecture Police Hygiene Exhibition). Taihoku: Taiwan nichinichi simposha, 1926.

Taiwan eipôsha, ed. *Taiwan eisei nenkan* (Taiwanese Annals of Hygiene). Taihoku: Taiwan eipôsha, 1932.

Taiwan igakukai, ed. *Taiwan eisei gaiyô* (Summary of Sanitation in Taiwan). Taihoku: Taiwan igakukai, 1913.

Taiwan Sôtokufu, ed. *Taiwan Sôtokufu minseijibu seiseki taiyô* (Summary of Works of Civil Affairs in Taiwan). Taihoku: Taiwain Sôtokufu, 1897.

————. *Taiwan Pesutoryûkôkj: Meiji 29 nen* (Taiwan's Record of the Pest Epidemic of Meiji 29 Year). Taihoku: Taiwan Sôtokufu, 1898.

————. *Taiwan Pesuto ryûkôkji: Meiji 31 nen* (Taiwan's Record of of the Pest Epidemic of Meiji 31 Year). Taihoku: Taiwan Sôtokufu, 1900.

————. *Eisei kaipo: Tennentô* (Summary Report on Sanitation: Smallpox). Taihoku: Taiwan Sôtokufu, 1926.

————. *Taiwan eisei kaiyô* (Summary of Sanitation in Taiwan). Taihoku: Taiwan Sôtokufu, 1913.

————. *Taishô 9 nen Taiwan tôkei yôran* (Satistical Summary of Taiwan in Taishô 9 Year). Taihoku: Taiwan Sôtokufu, 1916.

————. *Korera) byô ryûkôji: Taishô 8, 9 nen* (Record of the Cholera Epidemic of Taishô 8 and 9 Year). Taihoku: Taiwan Sôtokufu, 1923.

————. *Dai ichi kai eisei chôsa houkoku* (The First Public Health Investigation). Taihoku: Taiwan Sôtokufu, 1931.

Taiwan Sôtokufu Chûô kenkyûsho, ed. *Taiwan Sôtokufu Chûô kenkyûsho eiseibu nenpo* (Annual Report of the Central Research Institute of Taiwan Sôtokufu). Taihoku: Taiwan Sôtokufu Chûô kenkyûsho, 1922.

————. *Taiwan Sôtokufu Chûô kenkyûsho eiseibu gyôseiki* (General Report of the Hygiene Section of the Central Research Institute of Taiwan Sôtokufu). Taihoku: Taiwan Sôtokufu Chûô kenkyûsho eiseibu, 1922.

————. *Chûô kenkyûsho eiseibuji gyôji ikô keikka kusho* (General Report of the Achievements of the Hygiene Section of the Central Research Institute). Taihoku: Chûô kenkyûsho eiseibu, 1930.

————. *Taiwan Sôtokufu Chûô kenkyûsho eiseibu gyôseiki* (General Report of the Hygiene Section of of the Central Research Institute of Taiwan Sôtokufu). Taihoku: Taiwan Sôtokufu Chûô kenkyûsho eiseibu, 1942.

Taiwan Sôtokufu igakkô, ed. *Sôtokufu igakkô ichiran* (Overview of the Sôtokufu Medical School). Tahoku: Sôtokufu igakkô, 1905.

Taiwan Sôtokufu igaku senmon gakkô, ed. *Sôtokufu igaku senmongakkô ichiran* (Overview of the Sôtokufu Medical College). Taihoku: Sôtokufu igaku senmon gakkô, 1922.

————. *Sôtokufu igaku senmon gakkô ichiran* (Overview of the Sôtokufu Medical College). Taihoku: Taiwan Sôtokufu igaku senmon gakkô, 1933.

Taiwan Sôtokufu minsebu, ed. *Minsetsu teiyô* (Summary Report of Civil Affairs). Taihoku: Taiwan Sôtokufu, 1898.

————. *Taiwan eisei gaiiyô* (Summary of Hygiene in Taiwan). Taihoku: Taiwan Sôtokufu, 1913.

Taiwan suidô kenkyûkai, ed. *Taiwan suidôji* (Taiwan's Water System). Taihoku: Taiwan suidô kenkyûkai, 1941.

Journals and Newspapers

Ninhon ishi shinpo (Japan's New Report of MedicalAffairs) (1943–present)
Taiwan igakukai zasshi (Journal of Formosan Medical Association) (1902–45)
Taiwan minpo (Taiwan People's Newspaper) (1923–41)
Taiwan nichinichi shinpo (Taiwan New Daily) (1898–1944)
Taiwan shinpo (Taiwan News) (1896–98, 1944–45)
Taiwan Sôtokufu fupo (Report of the Taiwan Governor-General Government) (1895–1945)

Publications

Ackerknecht, Erwin H. *Rudolf Virchow: Doctor, Statesman, and Anthropologist.* Madison: University of Wisconsin Press, 1953.

Amano Ikuo. *Kyôseii senmon gakkô ron* (On the Special College in the Old Educational System). Tokyo: Tamagawa University Press, 1993.

Anderson, Warwick. "Where Is the Postcolonial History of Medicine?" *Bulletin of the History of Medicine* 72:3 (1998): 522–30.

————. "Postcolonial Technoscience." *Social Studies of Science* 5–6 (2002): 643–58.

Arnold, David. "Medical Priorities and Practice in Nineteenth-Century British India." *South Asia Research* 5 (1985): 167–83.

————. *Colonizing the Body: State Medicine and Epidemic Disease in Nineteenth-Century India.* Berkeley: University of California Press, 1993.

————. *The Problem of Nature: Environment, Culture, and European Expansion*. London: Blackwell, 1996.

Arnold, David, ed. *Imperial Medicine and Indigenous Societies*. Manchester: Manchester University Press, 1988.

————. *Warm Climates and Western Medicine: The Emergence of Tropical Medicine, 1500–1900*. Amsterdam: Rodopi, 1996.

Baber, Zaheer. "Colonizing Nature: Scientific Knowledge, Colonial Power, and the Incorporation of India into the Modern World-System." *British Journal of Sociology* 52:1 (2001): 37–58.

Baelz, Erwin [Dokutoru Berutsu]. "Nippon jinsho kairyôron" (On the Improvement of the Japanese Race). *Dainipon shiritsu eiseikai zasshi* (Journal of the Japanese Private Society of Hygiene) 43 (1886): 3–26.

————. *Awaken Japan: The Diary of a German Doctor Erwin Baelz*. Ed. Toku Baelz, trans. Eden and Cedar Paul. New York: Viking, 1932.

Baldry, Peter E. *The Battle against Bacteria: A History of the Development of Antibacterial Drugs for the General Reader*. Cambridge: Cambridge University Press, 1965.

Balfour, M. C. "Letter No. 109 from M. C. Balfour to Dr. W. A. Sawyer (N.Y.) 5/21/1940," R. G. 1.1, series 609, Japan, box 3, folder 17, Rockefeller Archives.

Barclay, George W. *Colonial Development and Population in Taiwan*. Princeton: Princeton University Press, 1954.

Basalla, George. "The Spread of Western Science: A Three-Stage Model Describes the Introduction of Modern Science into Any Non-European Nation." *Science* 3775 (1967): 611–22.

Bernd, Martin. *Japan and Germany in the Modern World*. Oxford: Berghahn, 1995.

Bideau, Alain, Bertrand Desjardins, and Hector Perez Brignoli, eds. *Infant and Child Mortality in the Past*. Oxford: Clarendon, 1997.

Blacker, Carmen. *The Japanese Enlightenment: A Study of the Writing of Fukuzawa Yukichi*. London: Cambridge University Press, 1964.

Blyden, Nemata. Review of David Eltis, ed., *Coerced and Free Migration: Global Perspectives (the Making of Modern Freedom)*. *American Historical Review* 109:1 (2004): 143–44.

Bowers, John. *When the Twain Meet: The Rise of Western Medicine in Japan*. Baltimore: Johns Hopkins University Press, 1980.

————. "The Odyssey of Smallpox Vaccination." *Bulletin of the History of Medicine* 55 (1981): 17–33.

Bowker, Geoffrey C., and Susan Leigh Star. *Sorting Things Out: Classification and Its Consequences*. Cambridge: MIT Press, 2000.

Broman, Thomas. "Rethinking Professionalization: Theory, Practice, and Professional Ideology in Eighteenth-Century German Medicine." *Journal of Modern History* 67:4 (1995): 835–72.

Burk, Ardath W. *The Modernizers: Overseas Students, Foreign Employees, and Meiji-Japan.* New York: Boulder, 1985.

Butterfield, Herbert. *The Whig Interpretation of History.* Harmondsworth, Middlesex: Pelican, 1973.

Bynum, William, and Roy Porter, eds. *Companion Encyclopedia of the History of Medicine* (2 Volumes). London: Routledge, 1993.

Cai Chenghao. "Bingdu, tingke, chucao: Xibanyaliukan qinxixia de Taiwan (1918–1920)" (Virus, Suspending Class, and Hunting Head: Taiwan under the Invasion of Spanish Flu (1918–1920). In *Proceedings of the Conference of Medical Humanity.* Taipei: Taipei Medical University, 2004.

Cao Yunghe, ed. *Rijuqianqi Taiwan beipu shizhang jishi: Weisheng pian* (Record of Administrative Works in Northern Taiwan during the Early Japanese-Ruled Period: Sanitation). Taipei: Taipeishi wenxian weiyunhui, 1986.

Cao Yunghe, ed. *Cao Yunghe xiansheng pashi shouqing lunwenji* (Collection Celebrating the Eightieth Birthday of Mr. Cao Yunghe). Taipei: Lexue, 2001.

Cartwright, Frederick. *A Social History of Medicine.* London: Longman, 1977.

Cartwright, Hamilton. "Vaccination in Japan." *Lancet,* May 25, 1889, 1051–53.

Chen, C. T., Y. T. Wu, and H. C. Hsieh. "Differences in Detectability of Minor Splenomegaly through Variation in the Recumbent Position of the Patient." *Taiwan yixhuxhui zhachi* 53:9 (1954): 561–67. Formerly *Taiwan igakkukai zasshi.*

Chen Jinsheng. "Rijushiqi Taiwanyapian jianjinzhengce zhiyanjiu (1895–1930)" (The Gradualist Policy of Opium Prohibition in Japanese-Occupied Taiwan). MA thesis, National Taiwan University, 1988.

Chen Kuanzhang. "Rinkozhuanxing de xingshidontai" (The Dynamic Form of Demographic Transition). *Rikoxuekan* (Journal of Population Studies) 8 (1985): 1–23.

Chen Kuanzhang and Yeh Tienfeng. "Rijushidai yilai Taiwan diqu renko nianling zucheng zhi bianqian" (Changes in Age Cohorts of the Taiwanese Population since the Japanese-Occupied Period). *Taiwandaxue renkoxuekan* (National Taiwan University Journal of Demography) 6 (1982): 99–114.

Chen Shaoxin. *Taiwan de renkou bianqian yu shehui bianqian* (Population and Social Change in Taiwan). Taipei: Lianjing, 1985.

Chen Shufen. *Zhanhou zhiyi: Taiwande gonggongweisheng wenti yu jianzhi* (Postwar Epidemics: Problems and Formations of Public Health in Taiwan). Taipei: Daoxiang, 2000.

Chen Yenhong. "Hoten Xinping (Gotô Shinpei) cai taizhimingzhengci zhi yenju" (A Study of Gotô Shinpei's Colonization Policies in Taiwan). MA thesis, Danjiang University, 1987.

Chen Yungxin. "Cong jenwen fangmian tantao gujin yixue liu" (From the Viewpoint of Humanity to Study Medical Ethics in the Past and Present). Comp. Chen Chongquang. *Newsletter of Mackey Memorial Hospital* 1:5 (1991): 29–32.

———. *Taiwan yiliao fazhanshi* (The Development History of Medicine and Therapy in Taiwan). Taipei: Yuedan, 1997.

Chugai maiji shinbunsha, ed. *Yakushin Taiwan taikkan* (Overview of Leap-Forward Taiwan). Tokyo: Chugai maiji shinbunsha, 1941.

Chorover, Stephan L. *From Genesis to Genocide: The Meaning of Human Nature and the Power of Behavior Control.* Cambridge: MIT Press, 1979.

Cortazzi, Hugh. *Dr. Willis in Japan, 1862–1877: British Medical Pioneer.* London: Athlone, 1985.

Craig, Albert M. *Choshu in the Meiji Restoration.* Lanham, MD: Lexington, 2000.

Crosby, Alfred. *Ecological Imperialism: The Biological Expansion of Europe, 900–1900.* Cambridge: Cambridge University Press, 1993.

Cunningham, Andrew, and Bridie Andrews, eds. *Western Medicine as Contested Knowledge.* Manchester: Manchester University Press, 1997.

Curtin, Philip D. *Death by Migration: Europe's Encounter with the Tropical World in the Nineteenth Century.* Cambridge: Cambridge University Press, 1989.

Dahrendorf, Ralf. *Society and Democracy in Germany.* New York: Anchor, 1969.

Dainibon seiyaku kabushikikaisha, comp. *Shiyaku yôran* (Handout of New Medicine). Osaka: Dainibon seiyaku kabushikikaisha, 1932.

Danjian University, ed. *Taiwanshi guoji xueshu yentaohui: Shehui, jingji yu kentuo* (International Conference on Taiwanese History: Society, Economy, and Exploitation). Taipei: Danjian University, 1995.

Dennie, Charles. *A History of Syphilis.* Springfield, IL: Charles C. Thomas, 1962.

Department of Health, ed. *Malaria Eradication in Taiwan.* Taipei: Executive Yuan, 1991.

Desowitz, Robert S. *Who Gave Pinta to the Santa Maria? Torrid Diseases in a Temperate World.* New York: Norton, 1997.

Dieckhofer, Klemens, and Kaspari Christoph. "Die Tatigkeit des Sozialhygienikers und Eugenikers Alfred Grotjahn (1869–1931) als Reichstagsabgeordneter der SPD," (The Works of Social Hygienist and Eugenicist Alfred Grotjahn [1869–1931] as a Parliamentary Delegate of the SPD). *Medizinhistorische Journal* (Journal of Medical History) 21 (1986): 308–31.

Du Congming. *Du Congming yenlunji* (Words of Du Congming). Taipei: Du Congming boshi jinian jiangxuejin quanliweiyuanhui, 1955.

———. *Du Congming huiyilu* (Memoir of Du Congming). Taipei: Du Congming boshi jinian jiangxuejin quanliweiyuanhui, 1973.

———. *Huiyilu* (Memoir). 8 Volumes. Taipei: Longwen, 1989.

———. *Zhongxi yixueshilüe* (A Brief History of Chinese and Western Medicine).(Kaohsiung: Kaohsiung Medical College, 1959),

Du Congming, ed. *Takagi Tomoe sensei tsuiokushi* (Collection in Remembrance of Takagi Tomoe). Tokyo: Takagi Tomoe kinenji iinkai, 1957.

Dube, Saurabh, Ishita Banerjee Dube, and Edgardo Lander, eds. *Critical Conjunctions: Foundations of Colonialism and Formations of Modernity.* Durham: Duke University Press, 2002.

Easterlin, Richard A., ed. *Population and Economic Change in Developing Countries.* Chicago: University of Chicago Press, 1980.

Edmonds, Richard Louis, and Steven M. Goldstein, eds. *Taiwan in the Twentieth Century: A Retrospective View.* China Quarterly Special Issues, new ser., no. 1. Cambridge: Cambridge University Press, 2001.

Emmer, P. C., and W. L. Wesseling, eds. *Reappraisals in Overseas History: Essays on Post-war Historiography about European Expansion.* The Hague: Martinus Nijhoff for Leiden University Press, 1979.

Fan Pingzhen. "A Review of Filariasis Study Focusing on Eradication in Quemoy." *Parasitology of National Yang-min Medical College,* special issue (1982): 134–88.

Fan Tianji. "Jiyaobao: Banshijiqian de jijiu xiang" (Jiyaobao: The First-Aid Box a Half Century Ago). *Mingshengbao* (Mingsheng Daily), October 13, 2001. Fan Yanqiu. "Rijuqianqi Taiwanzhi gonggongweisheng: Yi fangyi weizhongxin zhiyanjiu" (Public Health Policy during the Early Japanese Occupation: A Study Focusing on Epidemic Prevention). MA thesis, National Taiwan Normal University, 1994.

———. "Xinyixue zai Taiwan de shijian" (The Practice of New Medicine in Taiwan). *Xinshixue* (New History) 9:3 (1998): 49–86.

———. "Ribendiguo fazhanxia zhimindi Taiwan de jenzhuangweisheng" (Racial Hygiene in Colonial Taiwan under the Japanese Empire). PhD diss., Zhengzhi University, 2001.

———. "Redai fengtuxunhua, riben diguoyixue yu zhimindi jenzhuanglun" (Tropical Acclimatization, Japanese Imperial Medicine, and Racial Discourses in the Colony). *Taiwan shehui yenjui jikan* (Radical Quarterly of Social Studies) 57 (2005): 87–132.

————. *Yibing, Yixue yu Zhiming Xiandaixing: Rizhi Taiwan yixueshi* (Epidemics, Medicine, and Colonial Modernity: History of Medicine in Japan-ruled Taiwan). Taipei: Daoxiang, 2005.

Fan Zuoxun, ed. *Taiwan yauxue shi* (History of Taiwan Pharmaceuticals) Taipei: Zhenshi yauxue jijinhuei, 1991.

Farley, John. Review of Soma Hewa, *Colonialism, Tropical Disease, and Imperial Medicine. Bulletin of the History of Medicine* 70:4 (1996): 723–24.

————. Review of Sheldon Watts, *Epidemics and History: Disease, Power, and Imperialism. Canadian Bulletin of Medical History* 16:2 (1999): 387–88.

Farris, William W. *Population, Disease, and Land in Early Japan, 645–900.* Cambridge: Harvard University Press, 1985.

Fogel, Robert W., Stanley L. Engerman, Roderick Floud, Gerald Friedman, Robert A. Margo, Kenneth Sokoloff, Richard H. Steckel, T. James Trussell, Georgia Villaflor, and Kenneth W. Wachter. "Secular Changes in American and British Stature and Nutrition." *Journal of Interdisciplinary History* 14:2 (1983): 445–81.

Forest, Robert, and Orest Ranun, eds. *Biology of Man in History: Selections from the Annals, Economics, Societies, Civilisation.* Trans. Elborg Forster and Patricia Ranun. Baltimore: Johns Hopkins University Press, 1975.

Fredrickson, George. *Racism: A Short History.* Princeton: Princeton University Press, 2002.

Fruhstuck, Sabine. *Colonizing Sex: Sexology and Sex Control in Modern Japan.* Berkeley: University of California Press, 2003.

Fu Dawei. *Yaxiya de xinshengti* (The Asian New Body). Taipei: Socio, 2005.

Fujii Namiku, ed. *Nihon igaku bunka nenbyô* (The Cultural Annals of Japanese Medicine). Tokyo: Nishin shôin, 1928.

Fujikawa Yû. "Eiseigaku ni ukeru jinruigakuno hidobi sakainoshiso" (Social Thoughts about the Evolution of Hygienic Studies). *Dai Nippon eisei shiryo zasshi* (Great Japan Journal of Hygienic Materials) 309 (1909): 6–9.

Fujimoto Hajime, ed. *Yakkyoku kampo: Sono reimei kara* (Chinese Medicine in Pharmacies: From the Beginning). Tokyo: Nippon yakkyoku kyoreikai, 1997.

Furuno Naoya. *Taiwan jindaihui mishi* (The Myth of Taiwan's Modernization). Kaohsiung: Diyi, 1994.

Garrison, Fielding. *History of Medicine.* Philadelphia: Saunders, 1960.

Gellately, Robert. "Medicine and Collaboration under Hitler." *Canadian Journal of History* 26:3 (1991): 479–85.

Gotô Shinpei. *Eisei seidôron* (On the Sanitation Administration). Tokyo: Daiusha, 1890.

————. *Nippon shokumin seisaku iiban* (A Case of Japanese Colonization Policy). Tokyo: Tokushoku shinpo, 1921.

————. *Kokka eisei genri* (The Principles of State Hygiene). Reprint. Tokyo: Chikuma shobô, 1964.

Guo Wenhua. "Taiwan yiliaoshi yanjiu de huigu: Yi xueshu mailuo weizhungxin de tantao" (A Review of Studies on Taiwan's Medical History: A Discussion Centered on the Thread of Academic Thought). *Taiwan shiliao yanjiu* (Studies of Taiwanese Historical Materials) 8 (1996): 60–57.

Guo Wenhua and Ye Lin. "Yixue yu jenwen lishi de jiaohui: Fang Zhuang Yunmin tan Taiwan yixueshi" (The Interaction between Medicine and Humanity: An Interview with Zhuang Yunmin on Taiwan's Medical History). *Yiwang* (Hope) 8 (1995): 19–23.

Hackett, Roger F. *Yamagata Aritomo in the Rise of Modern Japan, 1838–1922.* Cambridge: Harvard University Press, 1972.

Han Min. *Gendai Nihon no senmon gakkô: Kôto shokugyô kyôiku no igi to kadai* (The Special College in Modern Japan: The Beginning of Vocational Education). Tokyo: Tamagawa daigaku shuppanbu, 1996.

Hara shobô, comp. *Meiji hyakunenshi* (The Hundred-Year History of the Meiji Era). Tokyo: Hara shobô, 1973.

Harootunian, Harry. *Toward Restoration.* Berkeley: University of California Press, 1984.

————. *Things Seen and Unseen: Discourse and Ideology in Tokugawa Nativism.* Chicago: University of Chicago Press, 1988.

Harrington, Anne. *Reenchanted Science: Holism in German Culture from Wilhelm II to Hitler.* Princeton: Princeton University Press, 1996.

Harrison, Mark. *Public Health in British India: Anglo-Indian Preventive Medicine, 1859–1914.* Cambridge: Cambridge University Press, 1994.

————. *Climates and Constitutions: Health, Race, Environment, and British Imperialism in India, 1600–1850.* New Delhi: Oxford University Press, 1999.

Hata Chôsan, Kuriyagawa shô, and Takeishi Hirodan. *Gentai iyakuhin no jisai* (Progress in Modern Medical Treatment). Tokyo: Nansandô, 1950.

Hayase Yukitoshi. "Problems of the Separation of Prescription and Dispensing." *Yakugaku zasshi* (Journal of Pharmaceutical Studies) 123:3 (2003): 121–32.

Hays, Jo. *The Burdens of Disease: Epidemics and Human Response in Western History.* New Brunswick, NJ: Rutgers University Press, 1988.

Headrick, Daniel R. *The Tools of Empire: Technology and European Imperialism in the Nineteenth Century.* Oxford: Oxford University Press, 1981.

Hewa, Soma. *Colonialism, Tropical Disease, and Imperial Medicine: Rockefeller Philanthropy in Sri Lanka.* Washington, DC: University Press of America, 1995.

Hino Shuitsu. "Gotô Shinpei 'kokka eisei genri' shiriron no sengen" (Gotô Shinpei's kokka eisei genri: A Declaration of Self-Interest Thought). *Nihon isigakushi zasshi* (Journal of the Japan Society of Medical History) 34:1 (1988): 79–81.

———. "Gotô Shinpei no eisei gyôseiron no itchisei ni tsuite" (The Concepts of Gotô Shinpei's *On the Sanitation Administration*). *Nihon ishigaku zasshi* 34:3 (1988): 1–29.

Hirakawa Sukehirô. "Changing Japanese Attitudes toward Western Learning: Dr. Erwin Baelz and Mori Ogai." *Contemporary Japan* 29 (1968): 138–57.

Hiroshi Nishiura. "Epidemiology of a Primary Pneumonic Plague in Kantoshu, Manchuria, from 1910 to 1911: Statistical Analysis of Individual Records Collected by the Japanese Empire." *International Journal of Epidemiology* 35:4 (2006): 1059–65.

Hiroshige Tôru. *Kagaku no shakaishi* (The Social History of Science). Tokyo: Chûô koronsha, 1973.

Ho, Samuel P. S. "Agricultural Transformation under Colonialism: The Case of Taiwan." *Journal of Economic History* 28:3 (1968): 313–40.

———. *The Developmental Policy of the Japanese Colonial Government in Taiwan, 1895–1945.* New Haven: Yale University Press, 1971.

———. *Economic Development of Taiwan, 1860–1970.* New Haven: Yale University Press, 1978.

Ho Yhimin. "Taiwan's Agricultural Transformation under Colonialism: A Critique." *Journal of Economic History* 31:3 (1971): 672–81.

———. Review of Samuel P. S. Ho, *Economic Development of Taiwan, 1860–1970. Economic Development and Cultural Change* 28:3 (1980): 637–44.

Hobsbawm, Eric. *Nations and Nationalism.* Cambridge: Cambridge University Press, 1991.

Hong Minling, ed. *Riju chuqi zhi yapian zhengce* (Opium Policy in the Early Japanese-Occupied Period). Taichung: Historical Research Commission of Taiwan Province, 2 Volumes, 1978.

Honigsbaum, Frank. *The Division in British Medicine: A History of the Separation of General Practice from Hospital Care, 1911–1968.* London: Kegan Paul, 1979.

Horiuchi Takao. "Haiso ekikô" (Epidemics from Black Rats). *Taiwan ishi zasshi* (Taiwan Medical Affairs) 1:3 (1899): 14–22.

———. "Sôki shindan no konnan oyobi ni byoroi" (The Pathology and Diagnosis of Plague). *Taiwan ishi zasshi* 2:2 (1900): 1–15. Later *Taiwan igakukai zasshi.*

————. "Bankin Taiwan ni okeru eiseijôtai gakuten no genin to sono kyûkyûsaku" (The Latest Developments and Research on Hygiene in Taiwan). *Taiwan jipo* (March 1921): 53–61.

————. "Taiwan jôgunki" (Army Service in Taiwan). *Minsoku Taiwan* (Taiwanese Folklore) 10 (1942): 2–6.

Hoshino Tetsuo. *Kenkozoshin no tame no chishiki* (Knowledge to Improve Health). Tokyo: Eiseibunka shisôkai, 1929.

House, Edward. *Japanese Expedition to Formosa.* Tokyo: [s.n.], 1875.

Huang Dengyun. "Taiwan Peingtong te wandanshô to ryukrusyo ni okeru bankerofuto shisoshô no ikigaku no chôsa" (The Epidemiological Investigation of *Bancrofti* at Wendan and Liuqiu of Peington, Taiwan). *Acta Japonia Medicina Tropicalis* 1:2–3 (1939): 411–35.

Huang Wu-Dar, Ja-Haur Tsay, and Naito Akira. "The Evolution of Building Legislation in Colonial Taiwan: Case Studies in Taipei City." *Jianzhu xuebao* (Journal of Architecture) 23 (1997): 99–127.

Huang Wudong. *Huang Wudong huiyilu: Taiwan zhanglaojiaohui fazhanshi* (Memoir of Huang Wudong: The Development History of the Taiwan Presbyterian Church). Taipei: Qianwei, 1990.

Huang Zhaotong. *Taiwan zongdufu* (The Taiwanese Government of the Governor-General). Trans. Huang Yinzhe. Taipei: Qinwei, 2002.

Huerkamp, Claudia. "The History of Smallpox Vaccination in Germany: A First Step in the Medicalization of the General Public." *Journal of Contemporary History* 20 (1985): 617–35.

Huisman, Frank, and John Harley Warner, eds. *Locating Medical History: The Stories and Their Meanings.* Baltimore: Johns Hopkins University Press, 2004.

Hume, John. "Colonialism and Sanitary Medicine: The Development of Preventive Health Policy in the Punjab, 1860 to 1900." *Modern Asian Studies* 20:4 (1986): 703–24.

Iijima, Wataru. *Pesuto to kindai chugoku* (Plague and Modern China). Tokyo: Kemmbun shuppan, 2000.

————. *Mararia to teikoku* (Malaria and Empire). Tokyo: University of Tokyo Press, 2005.

Ikeda Takuichi, ed. *Sinjidai no Taiwan kenchiku* (Taiwan's Architecture in the New Age). Taihoku: Daiiminsha, 1937.

Isei hyakunenshi furo: Eisei tô kei karamita isei hykunen no ayomi (The Hundred-Year History of Isei, Appendix: Reviewing the Hundred-Year History of Sanitation Statistics). Tokyo: Kôseishô, 1976.

Iseki Kurô. *Hihan enkyû hakushi jinbutu igakuhen* (Comments on and Studies of People with Doctoral Titles: The Medical Professionals). Tokyo: Hattensha, 1925.

Ishii Takeo. "Maruyama Yosito bokushi no jinyô de Taiwan no iryoshi hakase ate no shokan o note" (Reading after Dr. Maruyama Yoshito's Recent Works of Taiwan's Medical and Hygienic History). *Tokyo ishi shinji* (Tokyo New Medical Magazine) 74:11 (1957): 44.

Ishikawa Nobuo. *Kameikangogaku* (The Simplified Textbook of Nursing). Tokyo: Nanzandô, 1939.

Itazawa Syôgokô. *Tenrento ni kansuru kenkyu* (Studies Related to Smallpox). Tokyo: Tobôdô, 1925.

Itô Ginchirô. *Kike Gotô Shinpei* (An Excellent Figure: Gotô Shinpei). Taihoku: Kiyomizu Shoten, 1944.

Izumi Hyonosuke. "Eiseigakusha Tsuboi Jirô no keireki to gyuseki" (The Career and Studies of the Hygienist Tsuboi Jirô). *Nihon ishigaku zasshi* 36:3 (1993): 3–33.

Jannetta, Ann. *Epidemics and Early Modern Japan.* Princeton: Princeton University Press, 1987.

Jannetta, Ann, and Samuel H. Preston. "Two Centuries of Mortality Change in Central Japan: The Evidence from a Temple Death Register." *Population Studies*, Vol. 45, No. 3 (1991): 417–36.

Jansen, Marius, ed. *The Cambridge History of Japan*, Vol. 5. Cambridge: Cambridge University Press, 1989.

Jiang Tingfu. *Zuijinsanbainian dongbeiwaihuanshi* (The History of Foreign Invasions of Manchuria in the Last Three Hundred Years). Taipei: Zhongyangri baoshe, 1953.

Jiaotong bu (Transportation Bureau), ed. *Taiwansheng jiaotong jianshe* (The Development of Transportation in Taiwan). Taizhung: Taiwanshengzhegfu, 1987.

Jingdian zhazhi, ed. *Cirri yenyen: Taiwan* (The Sun Was Burning: Taiwan). Taipei: Jingdian zhazhi, 2005.

Johnston, William. "Disease, Medicine, and the State: A Social History of Tuberculosis in Japan, 1850–1950." PhD diss., Harvard University, 1987.

———. *The Modern Epidemic: A History of Tuberculosis in Japan.* Cambridge: Council on East Asian Studies, Harvard University, 1995.

Katô Naoshi. "Taiwan no eisei" (Taiwan's Sanitation). *Taiwan kyôkaii kaipo* 46 (1910): 25.

Kato Shigeo. "Shanhai shizen kagaku kenkyujyo no setsuritsu kouso" (The Establishment Plan for the Shanghai Institute for Natural Science). *Nenpo kagaku gijutsu, shakai* (Japanese Journal of Science, Technology, and Society) 6 (1997): 1–34.

Kawakami On and Nakagawa Yurezô, eds. *Iryô seido* (The Medical Service System). Tokyo: Nihon hyôlon sha, 1974.

Kawakami Take and Agarihayashi Shigerû. *Kunisaki Teido.* Tokyo: Kubisoshobo, 1970.

Kawakami Take and S. Kanbayashi, eds. *Kunisaki Teido, teiko no igakusha* (Kunisaki Teido as a Medical Scientist of Resistance). Tokyo: Kieso Shobo, 1970.

Kawakami Take and Y. Komiya, eds. *Iryo shakai ka no dohyo* (The Process of Socializing Medicine). Tokyo: Keiso Shobo, 1969.

Keene, Donald. *The Japanese Discovery of Europe.* Stanford: Stanford University Press, 1969.

Kenji Maki. *Nihon hôken seido seritsu shi* (The History of the Establishment of the Japanese Feudal System). Tokyo: Shimizu Kôbundô shobô, 1969.

Keishicho (The Police Force), ed. *Keishichoshi* (History of the Police Force). Tokyo: Keishichoshi hensan iinkai, 1949.

Kinebuchi Yoshifusa. *Taiwan shakai jigyôshi* (History of the Social Welfare Business in Taiwan). Taihoku: Tokuyûkai, 1940.

Kiple, Kenneth F., ed. *The Cambridge World History of Human Disease.* Cambridge: Cambridge University Press, 1993.

Kitaoka Shinichi. *Gotô Shinpei: Gaikô to Pojon* (Gotô Shinpei: Diplomacy and Vision). Tokyo: Chuokoronsha, 1988.

Kitasato Kenkyujo (Kitasato Institute), ed. *Kitasato kenkyujo gojunenshi* (The Fifty-Year History of the Kitasato Institute). Tokyo: Kitasato Kenkyujo, 1966.

———. *Kitasato Shibasaburo den* (The Biography of Kitasato Shibasaburo). Tokyo: Kitasato Kenkyujo, 1932.

Klee, Ernst. *Deutsche Medizin im Dritten Reich: Karrieren vor und nach 1945* (German Medicine during the Third Reich: Its Development before and after 1945). Frankfurt am Main: Fischer, 2001.

Kobayashi Hiroshi, ed. *Hikone shi no mararia taisaku* (The Elimination of Malaria in Hikone City). Hikone City: Hikone shi eiseika, 1951.

Komiya Yoshitaka. "Mararia boatsu no ichijuyo shudan toshiteno anoferesu bokumetsu ni tsuite" (On the Anti-anopheles Method of Malaria Control). *Toa igaku* (East Asian Medicine) 1 (1940): 167–88.

Komlos, John, ed. *Stature, Living Standards, and Economic Development: Essays in Anthropometric History.* Chicago: University of Chicago Press, 1994.

Kono eshidan gunibu, ed. *Seitai eiseihô* (Modern Hygienic Laws). Tokyo: Rikugunsho, 1896.

Kraas, E., and Y. Hiki, eds. *300 Jahre deutsch-japanische Beziehungen in der Medizin* (Three Hundred Years of German-Japanese Relations in Medicine). Tokyo: Springer-Verlag, 1992.

Kuraoka Hikosuke. *Taiwan ni okeru pesuto no ryûkôbyôgaku kenkyû* (An Epidemiological Study of Pests in Taiwan). Taihoku: Taiwan igakukai, 1920.

Kure Shosan. *Kure Shosan zanshô* (Bibliography of Kure Shosan). Kyoto: Shibunkaku, 1982.

League of Nations, Japan Office, ed. "Public Health Organisation and Administration in Kwantung Province and the Territory Attached Thereto." In *Health Organisation in Japan.* League of Nations Report C.H.332, 1925, 270–80.

Li Chongsi. "Ribanshidai Taiwan jingcha zhidu zhi yenchiu" (The Police System in Taiwan during the Japanese Period). MA thesis, National Taiwan University, 1996.

Li Denghui. *Taiwan nongye fazhan de jingji fenxi* (Economic Analysis of Agricultural Development in Taiwan). Taipei: Lianjin, 1980.

Li Nanheng, ed. *Lai He quanji* (The Collected Works of Lai He). Taipei: Mintan, 1979.

Li Shang-jen. Review of David Arnold, *Colonizing the Body: State Medicine and Epidemic Disease in Nineteenth-Century India. Xinshixue* (New History) 10:4 (1999): 159–67.

——. "Yixue, diguozhuyi yu xiandaixing daodu" (Medicine, Imperialism, and Modernity: An Introduction). *Taiwan shehui yenjiu jikan* 54 (2004): 1–16.

Li Xinfang. "Jidujiao yu Taiwan yiliao weisheng de xiandaihua: Yi Zhanghua jidujiao yiyuan weizhongxin zhi tantao" (Christianity and the Modernization of Taiwanese Medicine and Public Health: A Study of the Zhanghua Christian Hospital). MA thesis, National Taiwan Normal University, 1989.

Liao Binghui. *Huiku xiandai: Hoxiandai yu hozhimin lunwenji* (Reviewing Modernity: Articles on Postmodernity and Postcolonization). Taipei: Maitian, 1994.

Lin Jichong, ed. *Taida yiyun bainianshi (I) Rizhishiqi (1897–1945)* (The Hundred-Year History of the Medical School of National Taiwan University: The Japanese-Occupied Period [1897–1945]). Taipei: National Taiwan University Medical College, 1997.

Lin Ruiming, ed. *Lai Ho quanji: Xiaoshuojuan* (The Collected Works of Lai Ho: The Novels). Taipei: Qianwei, 2000.

Liu Jianhan, ed. *Rijuqianqi Taiwan beibushicheng jishi* (Record of Administrative Works in Northern Taiwan during the Early Japanese-Ruled Period). Taipei: Taipeishi wenxian weiyuanhui, 1986.

Liu Shiyung. "Zhanqian riwen yixue quanxi shumu" (Medical Books in the Prewar Period). Research report submitted to the Japan-Taiwan Exchange Center, Taipei, 1998.

————. "1930 niendai rizhishiqi Taiwan yixue de tezhe" (The Characteristics of Taiwanese Medicine in the 1930s Japanese-Ruled Period). *Taiwanshi yenjiu* (Taiwanese Historical Research) 4:1 (1999): 97–147.

————. "Public Health Investigation and Statistics in Colonial Taiwan." In *Introduction: The Archives of Social Affairs in Colonies—Taiwan*, 1–21. Tokyo: Modern Information Publishers, 2001.

————. "'Qingjie,' 'weisheng' yu 'paojian': Rizhishiqi Taiwanshehui gonggong weisheng guannia zhi zhuanbian" (Sanitation, Hygiene, and Public Health: Changing Thoughts on Public Health in Colonial Taiwan). *Taiwanshi yenju* 8:1 (2001): 41–88.

————. "Rizhishiqi Taiwandiqu de jibienjiego yenbian" (Changing Disease Patterns in Colonial Taiwan). *Xinshixue* (New History) 13:4 (2002): 165–208.

————. "Building a Strong and Healthy Empire: The Critical Period of Building Colonial Medicine in Taiwan." *Japanese Studies* 23:4 (2004): 301–13.

————. "Differential Mortality in Colonial Taiwan (1895–1945)." *Annales Démographie Historique* 1 (2004): 229–47.

Liu Ts'ui-jung and Liu Shiyung. "Disease and Mortality in the History of Taiwan." *Taiwanshi yenjiu* 4:2 (1998): 90–132.

Liu Ts'ui-jung, James Lee, David Sven Reher, Saito Osamu, and Wang Fang, eds., *Asian Population History.* Oxford: Oxford University Press, 2001.

Lo, K. K., L. Y. Chong, and Y. M. Tang, eds. *Social Hygiene Handbook.* Hong Kong: Social Hygiene Service, Department of Health, 1994.

Lo, Miriam Ming-cheng. "Between Ethnicity and Modernity: Taiwanese Medical Students and Doctors under Japan's Kominka Campaign, 1937–1945." *positions* 10:2 (2002): 285–332.

————. *Doctors within Borders: Profession, Ethnicity, and Modernity in Colonial Taiwan.* Berkeley: University of California Press, 2002.

Low, Morris Fraser. "The Butterfly and the Frigate: Social Studies of Science in Japan." *Social Studies of Science* 19:2 (1989): 313–42.

Lowood, Henry. Review of Geoffrey C. Bowker and Susan Leigh Star, *Sorting Things Out: Classification and Its Consequences. Technology and Culture* 42:2 (2001): 392–93.

Mackay, George. *From Far Formosa: The Island, Its People, and Missions.* New York: F. H. Revell, 1896.

Macleod, Roy, and Milton Lewis, eds. *Disease, Medicine, and Empire*. London: Routledge, 1988.

Maki Kenji. *Nihon hôken seido seritsu shi* (History of the Establishment of the Japanese Feudal System). Tokyo: Shimizu Kôbundô shobô, 1969.

Marks, Shula. "What Is Colonial about Colonial Medicine and What Has Happened to Imperialism and Health?" *Social History of Medicine* 10:2 (1997): 205–19.

McConaghy, Cathryn. *Rethinking Indigenous Education: Culturalism, Colonialism, and the Politics of Knowing*. Flaxton, Queensland, Australia: Post Pressed, 2000.

McKeown, Thomas. *The Rise of Modern Population*. New York: Academic Press, 1976.

———. *The Role of Medicine: Dream, Mirage, or Nemesis*. London: Nuffield Provincial Hospitals Trust, 1976.

McNeill, William. *Plagues and Peoples*. Oxford: Basil Blackwell, 1977.

Minasaki Takena. *Igaku to eisei: Nanhô seikatsu hitsuju* (Medicine and Hygiene: The Way to Live in the South). Tokyo: Kyoizai sha, 1937.

Ming-cheng Lo, "From National Physicians to Medical Modernists: Taiwanese Doctors under Japanese Rule," (Ph.D. Diss., University of Michigan, 1996).

Miora Seikô. "Gotô Shinpei shoron: Nagoya ikanjidai kara eiseikyoku made no sokubakukento" (A Brief Bibliography of Gotô Shinpei: From a Medical Officer in Nagoya to the Chief Deputy of the Central Sanitation Bureau). *Ritsumeikanhôgakû* (Studies in the Law of Ritsumeikan) 3 (1980): 723–51.

Mirzaee, Mohammad. "Trends and Determinants of Mortality in Taiwan, 1895–1975." PhD diss., University of Pennsylvania, 1979.

Miyahara Daisuke. *Mararia no chiryô* (Malaria Treatment). Taihoku: Taiwan Sôtokufu, 1939.

Miyahara Hatsuo. "Mararia no chiryo" (A Treatment for Malaria). *Kyudai iho* (Kyushu University Medical Journal) 12:6 (1938): 1–8.

———. "Taikoku no mararia chyôsa owarite" (About the Empire and the Malaria Survey). *Taiwan no ikai* (Taiwan's Medical Circle) 2:6 (1943): 330–33. Miyamoto Shinobu. *Mori Ôgai no igaku shisô* (The Medical Thought of Mori Ôgai). Tokyo: Keisô shobô, 1979.

Mizoguchi Toshiyuki. "Consumer Prices and Real Wages in Taiwan and Korea under Japanese Rule." *Hitotsubashi Journal of Economics* 13:1 (1972): 40–56.

Moolton, S. E. "Measures Taken for Reform of Medical Education in Japan." *Nippon ishi shinpo*, February 27, 1946.

Mori Ôgai. *Ôgai zensyu* (The Collected Works of Ôgai) 38 volumes. Tokyo: Iwanami shoten, 1952.

Morishita Kaoru. *Maraia no bôekigaku to yobô: Taiwan ni okeru Nihon tôji jitai no kiroku to kenkyû* (The Prevention and Precaution of Malaria: Records and Research in Taiwan under Japanese Rule). Tokyo: Nippon itaikikuya, 1976.

Morishita Kaoru, and T. Katagai. "Examination of the Blood Meals of Formosan Anophelines by Precipitin Tests." *Journal of Zoology* 45 (1933): 122–41.

Morishita Kaoru, Y. Komiya, and H. Matsubayashi, eds. *Nihon niokeru kiseichugaku no hattastu* (The Study of Parasites in Japan) 2 volumes. Tokyo: Meguro Kiseichukan (Meguro Parasite Museum), 1961.

Morôka Son and Shimakage Chikai. *Idôgakushinron* (The New argument of Medical Ethnicity). Tokyo: Taito, 1937.

Müller-Hill, Benno. *Murderous Science: Elimination by Scientific Selection of Jews, Gypsies, and Others, Germany, 1933–1945.* Oxford: Oxford University Press, 1988.

Myers, Roman, and Mark Peattie, eds. *The Japanese Colonial Empire, 1895–1945.* Princeton: Princeton University Press, 1984.

Nagaki Daiizô. *Kitasato Shibasaburu to sono ichimon* (Kitasato Shibasaburu and His Pupils). Tokyo: Keio University Press, 1992.

Nagaoka Masami, ed. *Syokuminchi shakaijigu kankei shiryoshu* (A Collection of Colonization Materials). Tokyo: Kinkendai shiryokankokai, 2000.

Nakamura Humio. *Mori Ôgai to Meiji kokka* (Mori Ôgai and the Meiji State). Tokyo: Sanichi shubô, 1992.

Nakano Misao. *Kôkoku ishi dainenbyô* (Great Japan's Annals of Medical Affairs). Tokyo: Nankôdô, 1942.

———. "Meiji shoki no eiseigaku" (Hygienic Studies in the Early Meiji Period). *Nihon Ishigaku zasshi* 5:1 (1954): 31–32.

Nathan, Carl F. *Plague Prevention and Politics in Manchuria, 1910–31.* Cambridge: Harvard University Press, 1967.

Ninomi Fujiaki. "Eiji zenhanki oshui rugakusei ni tsuite" (On Overseas Students in the First Half of the Meiji Period). *Nihon ishigaku zasshi* 33:4 (1987): 54–60.

Nippon minzogu eiseikai (Japanese Society of Racial Hygiene), ed. "Kantogo" (Words on Cover Page). *Nihon minzoku eisei gakkaishi* (Journal of the Japanese Society of Racial Hygiene) 1:1 (1930): 1–3.

Nippon yakgaku kyokai, (Japan Society of Pharmacology) ed. *Rinjyo iyaku soho zenron* (A Collection on Clinical Prescriptions). Tokyo: Meishinto, 1938.

Nishida shôki, ed. *Nihon saikingakkai no 50 nen* (Fifty Years of the Japanese Society of Bacteriology). Tokyo: Nihon saikin gakkai, 1978.

Ôda Toshiro. "Takagi Tomoe hakase ate no shokan wo mite senjin wo shinobu" (Reading a Letter by Takagi Tomoe and Thinking about the Pioneers). *Nippon ishi shinpo* No. 2782, (1977).

————. *Taiwan igaku gojûnen* (The Fifty-Year History of Taiwanese Medicine). Trans. Hong Youshi. Taipei: Qianwei, 1995.

Ôda Toshiro and Morishita Kaoru. *Mararia no bôatsu* (The Prevention and Eradication of Malaria). Taihoku: Taiwan Sôtokofu, 1939.

Odaka Takeshi. "Naimusho shokan densenbyô kenkyûsho" (The Institute of Infectious Disease under the Ministry of Home Affairs). *Nihon ishigaku zasshi* 35:4 (1989): 1–35.

Odaka Takeshi. *Densenbyô kenkyûjyo* (The Institute of Infectious Disease). Tokyo: Gakkai shuppan senta, 1992.

Ogata Norio. *Saikin heno chôsen: Nihon no saikingakushi* (Challenges to Bacteria: The History of Bacteriology in Japan). Tokyo: Nippon hôsô shuppan kyôka, 1940.

Olds, Kelly. "The Biological Standard of Living in Taiwan under Japanese Occupation." *Economics and Human Biology* 1:2 (2003): 187–206.

Omori, N., and H. Noda. "On an Anopheline Mosquito, *Anopheles arbumbrosus*, Newly Found in Taiwan." *Studia medica Tropicalis* (Formosa) 1 (1943): 83–89.

Onda Shigenobu. *Obeiyakuseichushaku* (Notes on the Pharmaceutical System in Europe and America). Tokyo: Tokyo Insatsukabushikigaisha, 1922.

Ono Yoshirô. *Seiketsu no kindai: Eiseishôka kara kô kinguzzu he* (Sanitation in Modern Times: From Songs of Cleanliness to the Battle against Germs). Tokyo: Kôdansha, 1997.

Ozeki Tsuneo. *Meiji-shoki Tokyodaigaku igakubu sugyosei dosei ichiran* (A Statistical Summary of the Graduates of Tokyo University in the Early Meiji Period). Tokyo: Tokyo University Press, 1991.

Palladino, Paolo, and Michael Worboys. "Science and Imperialism." *Isis* 84 (1993): 91–102.

Park Yunjae. "Medical Policies toward Indigenous Medicine in Colonial Korea and India." *Korea Journal* 16:1 (2006): 198–224.

Passin, Herbert. *Society and Education in Japan.* Tokyo: Teachers College Press, 1965.

Pieterse, Jan Nederveen, and Bhikhu Parekh, eds. *The Decolonialization of Imagination: Culture, Knowledge, and Power.* London: Zed, 1995.

Porter, Dorothy, ed. *The History of Public Health and the Modern State.* Amsterdam: Rodopi, 1996.

Porter, Dorothy, and Roy Porter. "What Was Social Medicine? An Historiographical Essay." *Journal of Historical Sociology* 1:1 (1988): 90–106.

Porter, Roy. "The Doctor and the World." *Medical Sociology News* 9 (1978): 21–28.

———. *The Greatest Benefit to Mankind: A Medical History of Humanity from Antiquity to the Present.* London: Fontana, 1997.

Prakash, Gyan. *Another Reason: Science and the Imagination of Modern India.* Princeton: Princeton University Press, 1999.

Presseisen, Ernest L. *Before Aggression: Europeans Prepare the Japanese Army.* Tucson: University of Arizona Press, 1965.

Proctor, Robert. *Racial Hygiene: Medicine under Nazis.* Cambridge: Harvard University Press, 1988.

Pyle, Kenneth B. "Advantages of Fellowship: German Economics and Japanese Bureaucrats, 1890–1925." *Journal of Japanese Studies* 1:1 (1974): 127–64.

Qin Xienyu [Chin Hsien-yu]. 1998. "Colonial Medical Police and the Postcolonial Medical Surveillance System in Taiwan, 1895–1950s." *Osiris* 13 (1998): 326–38.

Qu Haiyuan and Zhang Yinghua, eds. *Taiwan shehui yu wenhua bianqian* (Changes in Society and Culture in Taiwan). Taipei: Lianjin, 1986.

Rakugatsu Taisô. *Meiji nana nen seban ishi* (The Record of the Conquering Barbarian in Meiji 7 Year). Tokyo: Nihokunibo, 1887.

Ramasubban, Radhika. *Public Health and Medical Research in India: Their Origins and Development under the Impact of British Colonial Policy.* Stockholm: SAREC, 1982.

Reidai igaku kenkyujyo (Institute of Tropical Medicine). *Nekken gojunen no ayumi* (The Fifty-Year History of the Institute of Tropical Medicine). Nagasaki: Reidai igaku kenkyujyo, 1993.

Rice, George, and E. Palmer. "Pandemic Influenza in Japan, 1918–19: Mortality Patterns and Official Responses." *Journal of Japanese Studies* 19:2 (1993): 389–420.

Riedel, Stefan. "Plague: From Natural Disease to Bioterrorism." *Baylor University Medical Center Proceedings* 12:8 (2005): 116–24.

Rosen, George. "What Is Social Medicine? A Genetic Analysis of the Concept." *Bulletin of the History of Medicine* 21 (1947): 674–733.

———. *A History of Public Health.* Baltimore: Johns Hopkins University Press, 1993.

Rosen, George, ed. *From Medical Police to Social Medicine: Essays on the History of Health Care.* New York: Science History Publications, 1974.

Rosenberg, Charles, and Janet Golden, eds. *Framing Disease: Studies in Cultural History.* New Brunswick, NJ: Rutgers University Press, 1992.

Ryo Meishu. *Taiwan tôji to ahen mondaii* (The Rule of Taiwan and Opium Problems). Tokyo: Yamakawasha, 1983.

Sand, René. *Vers la médecine* (Toward Medicine). Paris: Bailliere, 1948.

Satô Shuwasuke. *Takano Chôei.* Tokyo: Iwanami shoten, 1997.

Satofuka Fumihiko. "Some Aspects of the Debate on the Scientific Tradition in Japan." *Historia Scientiarum* 2 (1992): 61–69.

Sawada Ken. *Gotô Shinpei deh* (Biography of Gotô Shinpei). Tokyo: Kôdansha, 1943.

Schirokauer, Conrad. *A Brief History of Japanese Civilization.* New York: Harcourt, Brace, Javanovich, 1993.

Schlumberger, Han G. "Rudolph Virchow, Revolutionist." *Annals of Medical History*, 3rd ser., 4 (1942): 147–53.

Seiji Hishida, "Formosa: Japan's First Colony," *Political Science Quarterly*, Vol. 22, No. 2, 267–81

Setoguchi Akihisa. "Igaku, kiseichôgaku, konchôgaku: Nippon niokeru retaibyôkenkyu no tenkai" (Medicine, Epidemiology, and Public Health: The Beginning of Tropical Medicine in Japan). *Kagakutetsugaku kagakushi kenkyu* 1 (2006): 125–38.

Shimada Akiseki. *Shindan shorei fuiji horei* (Cases of Diagnosis with Related Regulations). Tokyo: Nankodo, 1916.

Shimizu Hideo. *Jiyô eiseikowa* (Stories of Hygiene and Pharmacy). Tokyo: Tomikura shoten, 1925.

Shimizu Tôtarô. *Nippon yakugakushi* (History of Japanese Pharmaceuticals). Tokyo: Nanzandô, 1971.

Shimojyo Kumaichi. "Nanshi kanton chihou ni okeru mararia chosa hokoku" (Report on Malaria in Guangdong, South China). *Tokyo iji shinshi* (Tokyo Medical Journal) 3177 (1940): 116–38.

———. "Nanhôseikatsuken to wa ga retaiigaku kenkyusho" (The Southern Life Cycle and the Study of Tropical Medicine). *Taiwan jipo* 24:1 (1942): 66–70.

Shinobu Seiizaburô. *Gotô Shinpei: Kagakuteki seiijika no syôgai* (Gotô Shinpei: The Career of a Scientific Politician). Tokyo: Hakubunkan, 1941.

Sigerist, Ernest Henry, and Milton Roemer eds., *On the History of Medicine.* New York: MD Publications, 1960.

Siler, William. "A Competing-Risk Model for Animal Mortality." *Ecology* 60 (1979): 750–57.

Small, Albion W. "Some Contributions to the History of Sociology, Section 8: Approaches to Objective Economic and Political Science in Germany— Cameralism." *American Journal of Sociology* 29:2 (1923): 158–65.

Steckel, Richard H. "Stature and the Standard of Living." *Journal of Economic Literature* 33 (1995): 1903–40.

Steel, Robert W., ed. *Geographers and the Tropics: Liverpool Essays.* London: Longmans, 1964.

Sugimoto Mahito. *Mandan: Taiwan no zaisei* (Fullness: the Finance of Taiwan). Taihoku: Matsuda sha, 1929.

Suzuki Tôen. *Taiwan no ho-kô seido* (Taiwan's Ho-Kô System). Taihoku: Taiwan Sôtokufu, 1940.

Suzuki Zenji. *Nihon no yûseigaku: Sono shisô to undôno kiseki* (Eugenics in Japan: Paths of Thought and Activities). Tokyo: Sankyô shuppan, 1983.

Taeuber, Irene. *The Population of Japan.* Princeton: Princeton University Press, 1958.

Taguchi Tsuitatsu. "Ôkokumin no dôryô" (The Poisonous Tumor of Our Nationals). *Tokyo keisai zasshi* (Tokyo Journal of Economy) 790 (1895): 371–72.

Taiwan kyôikukai, ed. (Taiwan Society of Education). *Taiwan kyôiku engakuji* (The Development of Education in Taiwan). Taihoku: Taiwan kyôikukai, 1939.

Taiwan sheng wenxianweiyuanhui, ed. (Taiwan Province Archives Committee). *Taiwansheng tongzhigao* (The unfinished script of the Taiwan Gazette). Nantao: Taiwansheng wenxianweiyuanhui, 1953.

Taiwansheng xingzheng zhang quang gongshu, ed. (The Office of the Chief Executive in Taiwan Province), *Taiwansheng wushiyinianlai tongjitiyao* (A Statistical Summary of Taiwan over the Past Fifty-one Years). Taipei: Taiwansheng xingzheng zhangquang gongshu, 1947.

Taiwan Sôtokufu eiseika, ed. (The Sanitation Section of Taiwanese Governor-General Government). *Taiwan yobôeisei gaikan* (The General Situation of Preventive Hygiene in Taiwan). Taihoku: Taiwan Sôtokufu, 1922.

———. *Nanshi Nanyo no Iryoshisetsu* (The Medical Institutions of South China and Southeast Asia). Taihoku: Taiwan Sôtokufu, 1936.

Taiwan Sôtokufu eiseika, ed. *Mararia bôatsuj* (Preventing Malaria). Taihoku: Taiwan Sôtokufu, 1931.

———. *Taiwan ni okeru ahenseido no kenkyû* (Studies of Taiwan's Opium System). Taihoku: Sôtokufu, 1932.

———. *Taiwan mararia gaikyô* (Summary of Taiwanese Malaria). Taihoku: Taiwan Sôtokufu, 1935.

Taiwan Sôtokufu keimukyoku (The Police Force of Taiwan Government of Governor-General), ed. *Taiwan Sôtokufu keisatsu enkakushi* (History of the Taiwan Sôtokufu Police Force). Taihoku: Morikomu shoji, 1938, Vol. 1 5.

Taiwan Sôtokufu minseibu (The Civil Affairs Section of Taiwan Governor-General Government), ed. *Taiwan ahen seido yôshi* (The Materials of Taiwan's Opium System). Taihoku: Taiwan nichnichshinpo sha, 1898.

Taiwan Sôtokufu senbaigyoku (The Monopoly Bureau of Taiwan Governor-General Government), ed. *Taiwan ahenji* (Opium in Taiwan). Taihoku: Taiwan nichnichshinp sha, 1927.

Takagi Tomoe (Takagi Tomoeda in German). *Die hygienischen Verhaltnisse der Insel Formosa* (Hygienic Conditions on the Island of Formosa). Dresden: Druck von C. C. Meinhold and Sohne, Kgl. Hofbuchdruckerei, 1911.

Takekoshi Yosaburo. *Taiwan tôchishi* (The History of Ruling Taiwan). Taihoku: Minsokoron sha, 1905.

———. *Japanese Rule in Formosa.* Trans. George Braithwaite. London: Longmans, 1907.

Takenaka Masao. *The Development of Social, Educational, and Medical Work in Japan since Meiji.* Brussels: Uitgeverij Van Keulen, 1958.

Takeshi Odaka. "Naimusho shokan densenbyô kenkyûsho" (The Institute of Infectious Disease under the Ministry of Home Affairs). *Nihon ishigaku zasshi* 35:4 (1989): 1–35.

———. *Densenbyô kenkyûsho* (The Institute of Infectious Disease). Tokyo: Sakai shuban senta, 1992.

Takizawa Toshiyuki. "Meiji shoki ishiyosei kyôiku to eisekan" (Related Medical Affairs and Medical Officers in the Early Meiji Period). *Nihon ishigaku zasshi* 38:4 (1991): 45–64.

———. "Kindai Nihon ni okeru shakaieiseigaku riron" (A Brief Discussion of Social Hygiene in Modern Japan). *Nihon ishigaku zasshi* 39:1 (1994): 98–111.

———. "Kindai Nihon ni okeru shakaieiseigaku no tankai to sonotokushitsu" (Concepts behind Social Hygiene in Modern Japan). *Nihon ishigaku zasshi* 40:2 (1995): 7–9.

Tanaka Satoshi. *Eisei tenrankai no yokubô* (The Meaning of Hygiene Exhibitions). Tokyo: Seikyûsha, 1994.

Tanaka Zenritsu. *Taiwan to nanhô shina* (Taiwan and Southern China). Tokyo: Shin shôyôsha, 1927.

Teruoka Gitô ed. *Shakai eiseigaku* (The Study of Social Hygiene) (Tokyo: Iwanami Shoten, 1935).

Tôgô Shi and Saitô Shinro. *Taiwan shokumin hatatsushi* (The Victorious History of Colonization in Taiwan). Taihoku: Kôbunkan, 1916.

Tôkeikyoku (Statistics Bureau), ed. *Nippon jinkôtôkeishôsei* (A Collection of Japan's Demographic Statistics) 10 volumes. Tokyo: Harashobô, 1994.

Tokyo daigaku ikagaku kenkyûjyo (Institute of Medical Science), ed. *Densenbyô kenkyûsho ikagaku kenkyûsho byakunen no ayumi* (The One Hundred Years from the Institute of Infectious Disease to the Institute of Medical Science). Tokyo: University of Tokyo Press, 1992.

Tong Huiwen. "Xingzhang jiankong yu yiliao quixun" (Administrative Structure and Medical Disciplines). MA thesis, Nanhua University, 2004.

Toshiyuki Mizoguchi. "Revising Long-Term National Accounts Statistics of Taiwan, 1912–1990: A Comparison of Estimates of Production Accounts to Expenditure Accounts." In Hitotsubashi University, ed., *The Long-Term Economic Statistics of Taiwan, 1905–1995: An International Workshop*, 1–41. Tokyo: Hitotsubashi University, 1999.

Tsuboi Jirô. "Taiwan no eisei" (Taiwan's Hygiene). *Taiwan ishi zasshi* 1:2 (1899): 1–8.

Tsukahara Togô, ed. *Toajia no kagaku to teikokushogi* (Articles on Science and Technology in East Asia). Tokyo: Kôseisha, 2006.

Tsurumi Tasukuho *Gotô Shinpei*, Vol. 1–4. Tokyo: Kubisôshoten, 1985.

Umakoshi, T. *Kankoku kindai daigaku no seiritsu to tenkai* (The Formation and Development of the Modern University System in Korea). Nagoya: University of Nagoya Press, 1995.

Vaughan, Megan. *Curing Their Ills*. Oxford: Polity, 1991.

Wakabayashi Masahiro and Wu Mizha, eds., *Kuajie de Taiwanshi yenjiu: Yu dongyashi de jiacuo* (The Taiwan Study on the Crossing Zone: Interacting with the History of East Asia). Taipei: Bozhongzhe, 2004.

Wakimura Kohei. "Malaria Control under the Colonial Rule: India and Taiwan." In *Proceedings of the Workshop on Medicine, Colonialism, and Social Changes*. Taipei: Academia Sinica, 1998.

Wang Demu and Chen Wenling. "Rizhishidai yilai Taiwandiqu zhi siwanglu bianqian" (Changes in Mortality Rates in Taiwan since the Japanese-Ruled Period). In *Ershi shiji de Taiwan renko bianqian yentaohui lunwenji* (Proceedings of the Symposium on Demographic Transition in Twentieth-Century Taiwan), 57–78. Taizhong: Zhonggong renko xuehui, 1986.

Wang Junqi. "Rizhishiqi Taiwan yiliao zhi diliyenchiu" (The Geographic Study of Medical Therapy in Japanese-Ruled Taiwan). MA thesis, Chinese Culture University, 1999.

Wang Shiqing. "Rijuchuqi Taiwan zhi jiangbihui yu jieyan yundong" (The Jiangbi Society and the Quit Opium Movement in Early Japanese-

Occupied Taiwan). *Taiwan wenxian* (Taiwanese Historical Materials) 37:4 (1986): 111–52.

Wang Zhiting. *Taiwan jiaoyushihliao shinbian* (The New Edition of Historical Materials on Education in Taiwan). Taipei: Shangwu, 1978.

Washizu Atsuya. *Taiwan keisatsu yonjûnen shiwa* (Historical Account of the Police Force in Taiwan). Taihoku: Washizu Atsuya, 1938.

Wassermann, A., and T. Takaki. "Über tetanusantitoxische Eigenschaften des normalen Centralnervensystems" (Characteristics of the Central Nervous System under the Tetanus Toxicity). *Berliner Klinische. Wochenschrift* 35 (1898): 5–6. Watanabe Seikai. "Asayama Jirô no seibutsugaku to fujôshiso" (Asayama Jirô's Biology and His Views on Survival). *Kagakushi kenkyû* (The Historical Study of Science) 107 (1973): 114–21.

————. *Nihonjin to kindai kagaku: Seiyô heno taiô to kadai* (The Japanese and Modern Science: The Impact on the West and Its Topics). Tokyo: Iwanami shoten, 1976.

Watts, Shelton. *Epidemics and History: Disease, Power, and Imperialism.* New Haven: Yale University Press, 1997.

Wear, Andrew, ed. *Medicine in Society: Historical Essays.* Cambridge: Cambridge University Press, 1992.

Weindling, Paul. "Soziale hygiene und eugenik: Der fall Alfred Grotjahn" (Social Hygiene and Eugenics: The Case of Alfred Grotjahn). *Das Argument: Jahrbuch fur kritische Medizin* (Argument: The Annual of Critical Medicine) (1984): 6–20.

————. "Medicine and Modernisation: The Social History of German Health and Medicine." *History of Science* 24 (1986): 277–301.

————. *Health, Race, and German Politics between National Unification and Nazism, 1870–1945.* Cambridge: Cambridge University Press, 1989.

Weindling, Paul, ed. *International Health Organisations and Movements, 1918–1939.* Cambridge: Cambridge University Press, 1995.

Weishengshu (Department of Health), ed. *Malaria Eradication in Taiwan*, 2 volumes. Taipei: Executive Yuan, 1991.

————. *Taiwan diqu gonggong weisheng fazhanshi* (The History of Public Health in Taiwan). Taipei: Weishengshu, 1995.

Weiss, Sheila Faith. *Race Hygiene, and National Efficiency.* Berkeley: University of California Press, 1987.

Wu Jieru. "Feilao yu feijiehe: Rizhisiqi consumption yu tuberculosis zha Taiwan de jiaohui" (Consumption and Pulmonary Tuberculosis: The Interaction between Consumption and Tuberculosis in Japanese-Occupied Taiwan). MA thesis, Taipei Medical University, 2006.

Wu Jiezun. "Rizhishidai yilai Taiwandiqu jibing zhuanxing mushi zhi tantao" (The Transition Model of Disease Patterns since Japanese Rule in Taiwan). In *Proceedings of the Annual Meeting of the Taiwan Association of Demography*. Taipei: Taiwan Association of Demography, 2006.

Wu Mincha. *Taiwan jindaishi yenchiu* (The Study of Modern Taiwanese History). Taipei: Daoxiang, 1991.

Wu Wenxing. *Rijushihqi Taiwan shihfanjiaoyu zhi yanjiu* (Kaoru Normal Education in the Japanese-Occupied Period). Taipei: National Taiwan University, 1983.

————. "Rijushiqi Taiwan de gaodengjiaoyu" (Higher Education in Japanese-Occupied Taiwan). *Zhungguo lishi xuehui shixue huigan* (Journal of the Chinese Association of History) 25 (1991): 166–69.

Wu, Y. T., and C. T. Chen. "Filariasis Endemic Areas in Taiwan Proper, Part 1: Incidence of Bancroftian Microfilarial Infection among the Native People of Southern Taiwan." *Taiwan yixuehui zhazhi*, vol. 8–9, (1960): 262–72 and 1163–71. Formerly *Taiwan igakkukai zasshi*.

Wu, Y. T., P. T. Tseng, and, C. T. Chen. "Recent Advances in the Study of Filariasis and Its Control in Taiwan." *Gonggongweiseng* (Public Health) 1 (1963): 1–4.

Wu Yulin. *Memories of Wu Lienteh: The Plague Fighter.* Singapore: World Scientific Publishing, 1995.

Wu Zhuoliu. "Taiwanlianqiao" (Taiwanese Forsythia). *Taiwan xinwenxue* (Taiwan New Literature) 1 (1986): 56–63.

Xie Zhenrong. "Ribenzhiminzhuyixia Taiwanweishengzhengce zhiyanjiu" (The Study of Public Health Policy in Taiwan under Japanese Colonialism). MA thesis, Chinese Culture University, 1989.

Xu Jidun. *Taiwan jindai fazhanshi* (The Modern History of Development in Taiwan). Taipei: Qienwei, 1996.

Xu Jienlin. *Taiwan Shiji* (The Great History of Taiwan), 4 volumes. Taipei: Wenyintong, 2001.

Xu Shiju, ed. *Taiwan yiyao weisheng zonglan* (A General Overview of Hygiene in Taiwan). Taipei: Yiyaoxinwenshe, 1972.

Xu Xiqing, ed. and trans. *Taiwan zhongdufu gongwen leizhuan weisheng shiliao huibian* (Sanitation-related Materials of Taiwan Sôtokufu Archives). Nantou: Taiwansheng wenxian weiyunhui, 2000. Xu Xueji, ed. *Taiwan lishi cidian* (Dictionary of Taiwanese History). Taipei: Yuanliu, 2004.

Yamada, H. "The Development of Modern Japanese Pharmaceutical Industry, Part 3: From 1886 to 1906, Coinciding with the Era between the Institution and Issue of *Japanese Pharmacopoeia*, First Edition with Third

Edition (JP I–JP III)." *Yakushigaku zasshi* (Japanese Journal of the History of Pharmacy) 27:2 (1992): 83–95.

Yamaguchi Hidetaka. "The Founding of Taiwan Governor-General Medical College and Its Hope in the Future." Trans. T. C. Han. *Taiwan Historical Materials Studies* 8 (1996): 49–55.

Yamakawa, K. "A History of a Hundred Years of Pharmaceutical Education in Japan." *Yakushigaku zasshi* 29:3 (1994): 446–62.

———. "Historical Sketch of Modern Pharmaceutical Science and Technology, Part 3: From the Second Half of the Nineteenth Century to World War I." *Yakushigaku zasshi* 30:1 (1995): 75–90.

Yanaihara Tadao. *Shokuminchi oyobi shokuminseisaku* (The Colony and the Colonial Administration). Tokyo: Iwanami shoten, 1933.

———. *Teikoku shokika no Taiwan* (Taiwan under Imperialism). Trans. Zhou Xienwei. Taipei: Haixia xueshu, [1988] 1999.

Yang Wenshan. "Trends in Life Expectancy and Cause-Specific Death in Colonial Taiwan, 1906–1935," In *Proceedings of the Conference on Asian Population History*. Taipei: Academia Sinica, 1996.

Yang Yuling. *Yidai yijen Du Congming* (A Doctor Represents a Whole Generation: Du Congming). Taipei: Tienxia, 2002.

Yao Rendo. "Governing the Colonised: Governmentality in the Japanese Colonisation of Taiwan, 1895–1945." PhD diss., University of Essex, 2002.

———. Review of Miriam Lo Ming-cheng, *Doctors within Borders: Professions, Ethnicity, and Modernity in Colonial Taiwan. Taiwanese Sociology* 4 (2002): 252–57.

Yeh Shujen. "Economic Growth and the Farm Economy in Colonial Taiwan, 1895–1945." PhD diss., University of Pittsburg, 1991.

Yiyaoixinwenshe (Publisher of Medical and Pharmaceutical News), ed. *Taiwan yiyao weisheng zonglan* (General Overview of Hygiene in Taiwan). Taipei: Yiyaoixinwenshe, 1972.

Yoshino Shigeru and Aida Toshirô. "Taiwan kaikyô e ken'etsu no kishi" (The Inspected Seashore on the Taiwan Strait). *Kôshû bôeki zasshi* (Journal of Public Epidemic Prevention) 23 (1936): 3–15.

Yujiro Hayami, and Verno W. Ruttan. "Korean Rice, Taiwan Rice, and Japanese Agricultural Stagnation: Economic Consequences of Colonialism." *Quarterly Journal of Economics* 84:4 (1970): 562–89.

Zeigler, J. L. "Editorial: Tropical Splenomegaly Syndrome." *Lancet* 15:1 (1976): 1058–59.

Zhang Hanyu, ed., *Economic Development and Income Distribution in Taiwan: The Essays of Dr. Chang Han-Yu.* Vol. 4. Taipei: Sun Ming, 1983.

Zhang Henghao, ed. 1991. *Yangkui ji* (The Collected Works of Yangkui). Taipei: Qianwei, 1991.

Zhang Jiafang. "Kangxi huangdi jieso jendoshu zhi shijin yu yunyin" (The Time Frame of and Reasons Why the Kangxi Emperor Adopted Variolation). *Zhonghua yishizazhi* (Chinese Journal of Medical History) 26:1 (1996): 30–32.

Zhang Shubing. "Taiwan zai rijushiqi jingcha faling yu fanzui kongzhi" (Regulation of the Police Force and Criminal Control in Japanese-Ruled Taiwan). MA thesis, Fu-jen University, 1986.

————. *Taiwan de riban nongye yimin* (Japanese Agricultural Immigrants in Taiwan). Taipei: Goushiguang, 2001.

Zhang Zhonghan. *Guangfuqian Taiwan zhi gongyehua* (Industrialization in Taiwan prior to World War II). Taipei: Lianjin, 1980.

Zheng Zhimin. "Zhimin yangban huo tairen yingxiong: Shirun Du Congmin yu rizhishiqi Taiwan de yixue jiaoyu" (A Colonist's Sample or a Taiwanese Hero: The Studies of Du Congming and Medical Education in the Japanese-Ruled Period). *Taiwan tushuguan guanli jikan* (Taiwanese Journal of Library Management) 1:1 (2005): 99–123.

Zhou Dingjin. *Jianzhu wuli* (Architectural Physics). Taipei: Xuying wenhua, 1999.

Zhu Zhimou. "Guojia yu gerenguanxi decongzhu" (Reconstructing the Relationship between State and Individual). MA thesis, National Taiwan Normal University, 1998

————. "Zhengfu yu geren guanxi de zaizu: Riling shiqi de Taiwan zilaishui shiye yu caizheng buzhu" (Reconstructing the Relationship between Government and the Individual: The Business of Supplying Water in Japanese-Ruled Taiwan)." In Lin Manhong, ed., *Caizheng yu Jindai Lishi Lunwenji* (The Collection of Finance and Modern History), 551–601. Taipei: Institute of Modern History, Academia Sinica, 1999.

Zhuang Yungming. *Taiwan yiliaoshi: Yi Taida yiyun wei zhuzhou* (The History of Medicine and Therapy in Taiwan). Taipei: Yunliu, 1998.

————. *Han Shiquan yishi de shengming gushi* (The Life of Dr. Han Shiquan). Taipei: Yunliu, 2005.

Index